Zirconia: Material Properties and Surgical Principles for Dental Implants and Restorations

One book, one tree: In support of reforestation worldwide and to address the climate crisis, for every book sold Quintessence Publishing will plant a tree (https://onetreeplanted.org/).

Library of Congress Cataloging-in-Publication Data

Names: Piconi, Corrado, editor. | Özcan, Mutlu, editor.
Title: Zirconia : material properties and surgical principles for dental implants and restorations / edited by Corrado Piconi and Mutlu Özcan.
Other titles: Zirconia (Piconi)
Description: Batavia, IL : Quintessence Publishing Co Inc, [2025] | Includes bibliographical references and index. | Summary: "This text covers the biomechanical and biologic properties of ceramic dental materials, the challenges that remain in the field, and practical considerations such as material selection and surgical implementation so clinicians can confidently meet the diverse needs and wants of every patient who walks through the door"-- Provided by publisher.
Identifiers: LCCN 2024058049 | ISBN 9781647242008 (hardcover)
Subjects: MESH: Zirconium | Dental Implants
Classification: LCC RK667.I45 | NLM QU 180 | DDC 617.6/93--dc23/eng/20250404
LC record available at https://lccn.loc.gov/2024058049

QUINTESSENCE PUBLISHING USA

Quintessence Publishing Co, Inc
411 N Raddant Road
Batavia, IL 60510
www.quintessence-publishing.com

5 4 3 2 1

Editor: Kristen Clark
Production: Angelina Schmelter
Design: Sue Zubek

Printed in Croatia

ZIRCONIA

Material Properties and Surgical Principles for Dental Implants and Restorations

Corrado Piconi
Catholic University Sacro Cuore
Graduate School in Orthopedics and Traumatology
Rome, Italy

Mutlu Özcan, DDS, DMD, PhD
University of Zurich
Center for Dental Medicine
Clinic of Masticatory Disorders and Dental Biomaterials
Zurich, Switzerland

QUINTESSENCE PUBLISHING

Berlin | Chicago | Tokyo
Barcelona | London | Milan | Paris | Prague | Seoul | Warsaw
Beijing | Istanbul | Sao Paulo | Sydney | Zagreb

CONTENTS

FOREWORD

In recent years, dentistry has increasingly moved toward metal-free solutions, and ceramic implants have already established themselves as promising alternatives and supplements to titanium implants. The market for ceramic implants is also undergoing a dynamic change. Although titanium implants still hold the largest market share for dental implants, the demand for metal-free solutions is continuously increasing. Patients are not the only ones who appreciate the excellent biocompatibility and esthetic advantages of ceramic implants. An increasing number of dentists also recognize their potential as a long-term treatment option.

Despite growing scientific evidence to support ceramic implants and the expanding clinical experience with them, numerous questions remain regarding the material properties of ceramics, surgical protocols, standardized treatment concepts, and long-term success rates. This book is intended to help clinicians reach a new level of knowledge about ceramic implantology and to provide them with a sound understanding of this still quite new field. It makes a decisive contribution to the further establishment of ceramic implantology and offers valuable orientation for researchers and practitioners alike.

This work comprises 13 chapters that provide a comprehensive view of ceramic implantology. Starting with materials science, a detailed description of the biomechanical properties of ceramic implants is provided. Subsequently, modern implant designs, surface modifications, and current clinical studies are presented. The extensive clinical section, which describes surgical techniques, prosthetic treatment options, and proven treatment concepts, is particularly valuable. In addition, the book contains case reports that illustrate the application of various ceramic implant systems in practice. It is a reliable reference work to help clinicians integrate ceramic implants safely and successfully into daily practice.

This project was conceived by the members of the Scientific Advisory Board of the European Society for Ceramic Implantology (ESCI) to contribute to the society's goal to disseminate knowledge about ceramic implantology. Nearly all of the authors and contributors are members of the ESCI's scientific advisory board or board of directors, ensuring that the content is at the cutting edge of research and clinical practice. The case studies found in the final chapter were also contributed by ESCI company partners to provide a practical and cross-industry perspective. We would like to thank the authors, contributors, and everyone who has contributed to the creation of this work with their expertise and commitment.

Ceramic implantology has the potential to shape the future of dentistry—and this book is a guide for that exciting journey.

—Dr Jens Tartsch, ESCI President

FOREWORD

As a clinician-scientist, I am honored to be invited by the authors to write a foreword to their new textbook on zirconia. Certainly the current generation of clinician-scientists have been challenged by the rapid changes in dental therapeutics with the digital age. Technologies that existed in dreams have quickly become reality. The printing and milling of materials for the fabrication of complex advanced dental prostheses has become almost routine. Of course there have been bumps in the road with the introduction of new materials and technologies, and the task of Prof Corrado Piconi and Prof Mutlu Özcan and their research colleagues has been to correct and remediate these discovered flaws.

This textbook reviews the factors that make zirconia a reliable dental biomaterial in its first three chapters. It goes on to detail the biologic and biomechanical aspects of zirconia dental implants in chapters 3 to 6. The following three chapters elucidate the hard and soft tissue responses for one- and two-piece zirconia dental implants as well as provide the rationale for using zirconia dental implants. The final three chapters conclude with guided surgical techniques and the ceramic restorative options for zirconia dental implants, with the last chapter detailing case reports from members of the European Society for Ceramic Implantology.

This textbook is a wonderful source of current information regarding zirconia as a restorative and dental implant material, and the dental profession owes a debt of gratitude to the authors for curating the information in an informative and detailed manner.

—Dr Kenneth S. Kurtz, DDS, FACP, FDS, RCPSS (Glasgow), FRCI

Director-Prosthodontic Research,
Graduate Prosthodontics
Montefiore Medical Center/Albert Einstein
College of Medicine
Bronx, New York

Clinical Professor and Director, Division of
Maxillofacial Prosthetics
Stony Brook University School of Dental Medicine
Stony Brook, New York

Clinical Professor and Attending Maxillofacial
Prosthodontist
Zucker School of Medicine at Hofstra/Northwell
Uniondale, New York

CONTRIBUTORS

André Luiz Berbel, DDS, MSc
Private practice
São Paulo, Brazil

Juan Blanco Carrión
Department of Surgery and Medical-Surgical Specialties
University of Santiago de Compostela
Santiago de Compostela, Spain

Loredana Cerroni, DDS, PhD, MS
Chair in Periodontology and Dental Materials
Department of Clinical Science and Translational Medicine
Tor Vergata University of Rome
Rome, Italy

Andre Chen, DDS, PhD, MS
New York University College of Dentistry
New York, New York

Oral Surgery Specialist
Lisbon, Portugal

Jérôme Chevalier, MSc, PhD
National Institute of Applied Sciences of Lyon (INSA-Lyon)
Villeurbanne, France

Luis Gustavo D'Altoé Garbelotto, DDS
Private practice
Zenith Specialized Teaching
Florianópolis, Brazil

Bruno Freitas Mello, DDS, MSc, PhD
Graduate Program in Implant Dentistry
University of South Santa Catarina
Florianópolis, Brazil

Michael Gahlert, DDS, PhD
Hightech Research Center of Cranio-Maxillofacial Surgery
Basel University Hospital
University of Basel
Basel, Switzerland

Sigmund Freud Private University
Vienna, Austria

Franco Giancola, MD, DDS
Private practice
Barcelona, Spain

Sebastian Horvath, DDS, PhD
Department of Preventive and Restorative Sciences
University of Pennsylvania
Philadelphia, Pennsylvania

Department of Prosthodontics
Albert-Ludwigs University
Freiburg, Germany

Claudia Angela Maziero Volpato, DDS, MSc, PhD
Department of Dentistry
Federal University of Santa Catarina
Florianópolis, Brazil

Jochen Mellinghoff, DDS, PhD, MSc
Private practice
Ulm, Germany

Thomas Mehnert, DDS, PhD
Private practice
Cologne, Germany

Mutlu Özcan, DMD, PhD
University of Zurich
Center for Dental Medicine
Clinic of Masticatory Disorders and Dental Biomaterials
Zurich, Switzerland

Michael Payer, MD, DDS, PhD
Clinical Department for Oral Surgery and Orthodontics
Medical University of Graz
Graz, Austria

Andrea Perna, MD, PhD
Department of Orthopedics and Trauma Surgery
Casa Sollievo della Sofferenza Foundation
San Giovanni Rotondo, Italy

Corrado Piconi
Catholic University Sacro Cuore
Graduate School in Orthopedics and Traumatology
Rome, Italy

Alessandro Alan Porporati, PhD
Medical Products Division
CeramTec
Plochingen, Germany

Department of Engineering and Architecture
University of Trieste
Trieste, Italy

Levy Rau, DDS, MSc
Graduate Program in Oral and Maxillofacial Surgery
University of South Santa Catarina

Director
Joana de Gusmão Children's Hospital
Florianópolis, Brazil

Stefan Roehling, DMD
Hightech Research Center of Cranio-Maxillofacial Surgery
Basel University Hospital
University of Basel
Basel, Switzerland

Clinic for Oral and Cranio-Maxillofacial Surgery
Kantonsspital Aarau
Aarau, Switzerland

Jens Tartsch, DMD
President
European Society for Ceramic Implantology

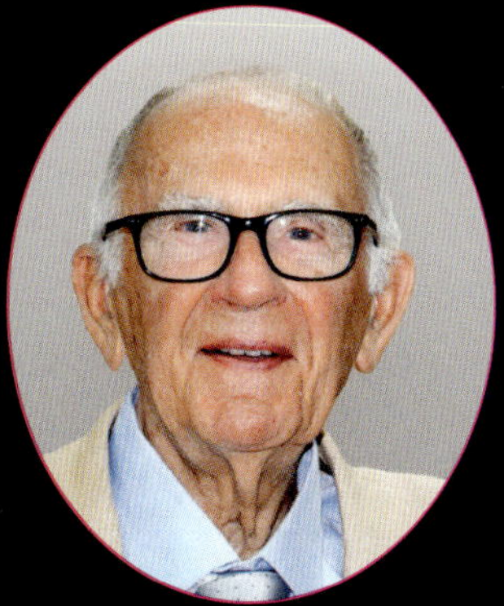

Professor Sami Sandhaus

This book is dedicated to the memory of Professor Sami Sandhaus, who created ceramic implantology.

01

CERAMICS AS DENTAL BIOMATERIALS

Corrado Piconi

This chapter reviews the behavior of the many ceramics used in dentistry. The general behaviors of ceramics are outlined and compared to those of metals. The materials used today in clinical settings are described from a historical perspective, with summaries of their main characteristics and some information on their development.

Introduction to Ceramics

Ceramics are "solid articles which have as their essential component, and are composed in large part of, inorganic nonmetallic materials."[1] In comparison with metals, ceramics exhibit low thermal and electrical conductivity, higher melting temperatures, and no plastic deformation before rupture (Box 1-1). They have been used for centuries to produce bricks and tableware. Only in the last century, however, has their use been extended to other applications. One of the main advances in ceramic technology that made this change possible was the switch from using natural materials to using synthetic raw materials. This expanded the applications of ceramics in many aspects of modern life, ranging from electronics to medicine.

The properties of ceramic oxides are derived from the oxygen atoms present in their molecules. These oxides include magnesia (MgO), titania (TiO_2), zirconia (ZrO_2), and alumina (Al_2O_3), among others. In metals, atoms are bonded together in a cloud of free electrons within the space of the crystal lattice. Ceramic molecules, on the other hand, are directly linked with directional ionic or covalent chemical bonds.

Ceramics can be crystalline solids or amorphous solids. Crystalline solids are characterized by a long-range ordered microstructure formed by atoms arranged in a regular 3D lattice, with the angles and distances between atoms varying according to the specific material. This long-range order is absent in the microstructure of amorphous solids, which exhibit only short-range order. The amorphous microstructure is sometimes termed *glassy microstructure* because it is characteristic of glasses. Crystalline structures are more compact than amorphous ones, and crystalline solids are usually stronger than glassy ones because it is more difficult to break the ordered network of atomic bonds. Figure 1-1 shows the typical microstructure of various ceramic materials.

BOX 1-1 › General behaviors of metals and ceramics

Metals	Ceramics
High number of free electrons	Absence of free electrons
Metallic chemical bonds	Ionic/covalent chemical bonds
Good electrical conductivity	Electrical insulators
Good thermal conductivity	Thermal insulators
Opaque to visible light	Can be transparent or translucent
Plastic strain before fracture	No plastic strain before fracture

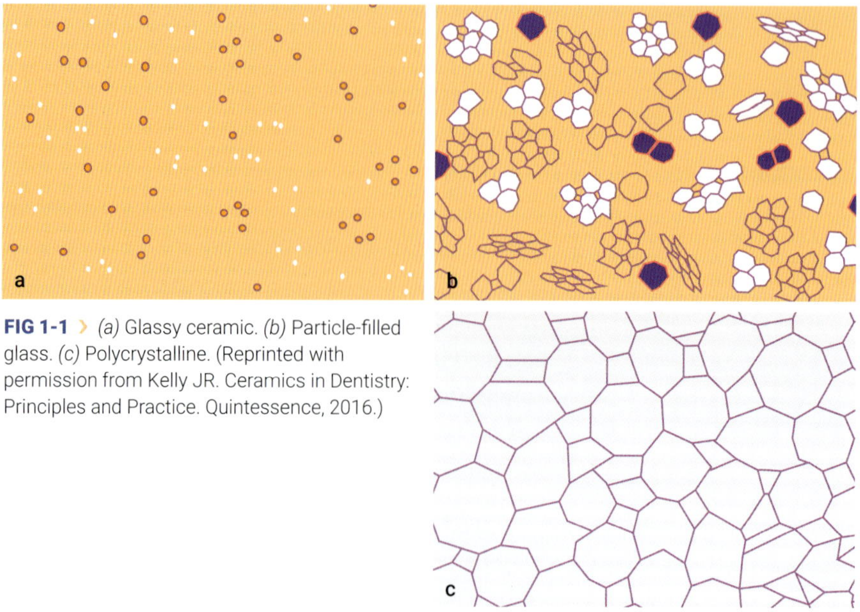

FIG 1-1 › *(a)* Glassy ceramic. *(b)* Particle-filled glass. *(c)* Polycrystalline. (Reprinted with permission from Kelly JR. Ceramics in Dentistry: Principles and Practice. Quintessence, 2016.)

Whatever their structure, ceramics generally have low tensile and bending strength (much lower than those of metallic alloys), although their compressive strength is generally high. Ceramics are also more brittle (less tough) than metals. Material toughness describes how difficult it is for fractures to propagate in a material and eventually lead to rupture. Material toughness is especially relevant in ceramics because linear elastic fracture mechanics tell us that the strength of a material *(σ_R)* is dependent on the ratio between the toughness *(K_{IC})* and the size of the principal critical flaw in the material *(c)*, following Griffith's law[2]:

$$\sigma_R = \frac{K_{IC}}{\sqrt{\pi c}}$$

In addition, ceramics are sensitive to intrinsic flaws in their microstructure—grain boundaries, pores, and inclusions—and to internal stresses and surface defects that may occur during the production process of ceramic devices. This explains why efforts to enhance the strength of ceramics for structural applications are focused on two main areas: *(1)* improving the production process to reduce the number and size of intrinsic flaws and *(2)* developing materials with higher intrinsic toughness.

Although ceramics have low strength and toughness in comparison with metals, ceramics have clear advantages over metals in the oral environment in terms of esthetics and corrosion resistance. From an esthetic viewpoint, metal substructures are limited by their lack of translucency, the metallic ring they exhibit at tooth margins, and the grayish hue they lend to gingival tissues.

Metals are also vulnerable to general and localized corrosion. Local and systemic reactions to the release of metallic ions due to dental device corrosion have been reported in the literature.[3–8] Another benefit of ceramic devices is reduced bacterial surface adhesion.[9,10]

The ceramics currently used in dentistry are essentially composite materials, with some having a glassy phase in their structure. We define a *composite material* (or simply a *composite*) as the combination of two or more materials with different physical and chemical properties into one new material with properties different from those of its components. Two basic types of ceramics are used: those with glass as a component and those without glassy phases in their microstructure. In this book, we devote special attention to zirconia-containing ceramics. Although glass-containing ceramics with metallic structures for added strength are still popular for dental restorations, zirconia ceramics are preferred because of their excellent strength and toughness (important for one- and two-piece dental implants) and their good esthetics (important for metal-free crowns, partial dentures, and complete dentures). Other ceramics, including hydroxyapatite, tricalcium phosphate, calcium sulfate, and bioreactive glasses, are also used in dentistry as scaffolds for the regeneration of bone and to fill bone defects, but these topics are outside the scope of this book.

Glass-Containing Ceramics in Dentistry

A BIT OF HISTORY

The eve of ceramic use in dentistry came during the second half of the 18th century as a consequence of Böttger's discovery of the process to obtain porcelain, which took place in Saxony in 1709.[11] Porcelain was the most sophisticated material available at that time. White, hard, and heat resistant, porcelain seemed to be the ideal denture material to Alexis Duchateau, a Parisian pharmacist who is rightly regarded as the inventor of dental ceramics.[12] After several attempts, Duchateau succeeded in developing a ceramic paste in 1744, from which he manufactured a number of dental appliances, but he was not fully satisfied. He turned to a dentist in Paris, Nicholas Dubois de Chemant, to improve his products from a functional point of view.

De Chemant immediately understood the importance of the discovery and performed extensive experiments in the laboratories of the Manufacture Royale de Porcelaines in Sevés, France, to improve Duchateau's basic mixture. De Chemant published the results of this work in 1789 in his treatise on artificial teeth,[13,14] but the French Revolution forced him (a man who had been awarded a royal patent giving him the exclusive right to produce removable prostheses in porcelain) to move to England, where he perfected his technique in collaboration with Josiah Wedgwood. During construction of the terminus of the Channel Tunnel Rail Link in London, a denture likely made by de Chemant was discovered in the burial place of the Archbishop Richard Dillon.[15] Each arch of this device consisted of a single piece of porcelain with a glassy finish applied to the teeth and the flange colored to represent the gingival tissues. Giuseppangelo Fonzi, an Italian dentist working in France, later improved this construction in 1806. He constructed single artificial teeth to be fixed in the sockets with metallic hooks.[16] Later on, Fonzi produced complete dentures by welding metallic pins hosting porcelain teeth to a metallic substructure.[17]

Porcelain teeth were introduced in the United States by Planteau in 1817, and S. Wesley Stockton started production of porcelain teeth in 1825. Vulcanized rubber was discovered in 1839 and was subsequently adopted for the bases of dentures with porcelain teeth. In 1844, Samuel Stockton White founded the S.S. White Company in Philadelphia for the industrial production of dental instruments and porcelain denture teeth. By 1867, the company was turning out 4 million teeth per year.[18]

Another step forward was thanks to Dr Charles Henry Land (grandfather of the aviator Charles Lindbergh), who by the end of the 19th century had developed all-porcelain crowns and is thus considered the father of modern metal-free prosthetics. His invention was continuously improved upon and was still in use as late as 1950.[19]

FELDSPATHIC PORCELAIN

Feldspathic porcelain is a potassium aluminosilicate glass obtained by melting feldspar, quartz (15%), kaolin (4%), and other oxides. It is called "porcelain" because it is made of a glassy matrix containing several crystal phases, though *porcelain* really refers to a class of ceramic-based composites made mostly of kaolin (70%) joined to feldspar and quartz (each 14% to 15%). The esthetic properties of feldspathic ceramics are due to their amorphous (glassy) matrix, while their mechanical strength is due to leucite ($K_2O{\cdot}Al_2O_3{\cdot}4SiO_2$) crystals. These porcelains were used in denture teeth and in powder form for inlays and partial dentures.

Although feldspathic ceramics provide excellent esthetics and have good compressive strength, they fracture easily under shear stresses because of their low flexural strength (< 60 MPa).[20] To improve the mechanical reliability of feldspathic porcelain restorations, Weinstein et al[21] developed porcelain-fused-to-metal (PFM) restorations, consisting of porcelain fused to a thin metallic substructure (a crown core or partial denture framework). PFM technology has since been continuously improved, and today it is the standard for crowns and partial denture restorations.

Several types of dental porcelains are currently used, with their applications determined by their melting temperature. High-fusing porcelains (melting temperature 1,250°C–1,350°C) and medium-fusing porcelains (melting temperature 1,100°C–1,250°C) are especially suitable for denture teeth, whereas low-fusing porcelains (melting temperature 850°C–1,100°C) are used for metal-ceramic crowns and partial dentures. Porcelains with a melting point below 850°C (very low-fusing porcelains) can be used with an expanded selection of metal alloys for support.

REINFORCED FELDSPATHIC PORCELAINS

The major limitation of feldspathic porcelains is their low strength. To improve the material strength of feldspathic ceramics, McLean and Hughes[22] proposed the addition of 40% to 50% alumina to the porcelain, increasing strength to between 120 and 150 MPa. The alumina-reinforced porcelain was used for the core of jacket crowns with porcelain veneers to improve their esthetics. Notwithstanding the increase in strength obtained by the introduction of alumina, successful outcomes with these early devices were limited because of the residual porosity of the cores after sintering, and the cores were further reinforced with platinum foils.[23,24] Different reinforcing agents were introduced in the following years, including fibers or leucite crystals added to feldspar glass as a powder or grown in situ during melting of the feldspar.

GLASS-CERAMICS

Dr S.D. Stookey discovered glass-ceramics (GCs) in the late 1950s while working for Corning Glass Works.[25] The discovery was the result of a chain of serendipitous events that occurred while Dr Stookey was developing a different product.[26] The application of GCs are manifold, ranging from household appliances to smartphone screens and from radomes to telescope mirrors. As dental materials, GCs offer both the esthetic properties of glasses and the mechanical properties of crystalline ceramics. Their microstructure is characterized by a fine and homogeneous distribution of ceramic crystals in the glass matrix that are grown directly from the glass through a controlled crystallization process known as *ceraming*.

Ceraming is a two-step thermal treatment to develop the crystalline phase within the glassy matrix. It is achieved by fine-tuning the heating temperature, heating rate, and annealing time. Any crack that eventually develops in the material must follow the contours of the crystals created during ceraming. This results in a longer path and the dissipation of propagation energy as the crack travels through the material. This microstructural feature results in a material with improved fracture strength and hardness.[27–29]

The first dental GC (Dicor, Dentsply International) was developed in 1972 by Grossmann and introduced in 1984 as a GC ingot for castings with a flexural strength of 150 MPa.[30] Dicor was constituted of fluormica (55 vol%), giving the material its high translucency and flexural strength. Dicor was later available as a machinable block (Dicor MGC) for the CEREC system (Dentsply Sirona) and used for inlays, onlays, and crowns.

The application of CAD/CAM technology to dentistry has resulted in the development of an array of processes to obtain ceramic cores for the milling of crowns, partial dentures, and complete dentures. This technologic breakthrough is due to the French dentist François Duret, who patented his "process to obtain a dental prosthesis" in 1982.[31] Unfortunately, the system he developed (Sopha, Hennson SA) was removed from the market in 1993, when the manufacturing company was dissolved.[32] Later, Mörmann et al significantly developed this approach, resulting in the well-known CEREC system that made the success of CAD/CAM in dentistry.[33–36] Today, a number of CAD/CAM systems and machinable materials are available for the production of dental appliances.[37,38]

Difficulties encountered in the lab (eg, long workflow, product inhomogeneity) eventually led to the discontinuation of the early castable GCs and stimulated the development of new ones that were easier to handle in a dental laboratory. The first of these new systems was a GC obtained by the crystallization of leucite in a feldspathic porcelain enriched with K_2O and ceraming performed at a higher temperature. IPS Empress (Ivoclar Vivadent), a well-known leucite GC, is manufactured at a temperature of about 1,050°C to enhance the growth of leucite crystals, resulting in a material with a flexural strength of 160 MPa and excellent esthetics.[26]

LITHIUM DISILICATE GLASS-CERAMICS

Lithium disilicate GCs for dental applications were obtained in the system SiO_2–Li_2O–K_2O–ZnO–P_2O_5–Al_2O_3–La_2O_3 by Höland et al.[39] The material consists of a glassy matrix containing a homogeneous dispersion of randomly oriented rod-like $Li_2Si_2O_5$ crystals. A small fraction of lithium orthophosphate (Li_3PO_4) crystals is present because P_2O_5 is a process additive that promotes the nucleation of lithium silicate phases in the volume of the glass.[40] Two different processing routes are used for the nucleation of crystals of lithium disilicate. A two-stage process is used to obtain pressable ingots with the lost wax hot pressing technique, whereas a three-stage process is used to produce CAD/CAM milling blocks.

The first step to produce pressable ingots is performed at the factory and involves nucleating the glass. The second step is performed in the dental laboratory and involves hot pressing the crystallized ingot in a viscous state at about 920°C into a dental mold shaped like the desired restoration. The elongated $Li_2Si_2O_5$ crystals give the pressable ceramic 400 MPa in strength and a fracture toughness of 2.75 MPa $m^{1/2}$.

For machinable blocks, lithium disilicate is precipitated in a three-stage process. The first stage consists of forming lithium orthophosphate nuclei for the successive crystal growth of metasilicate crystals. In the second stage, the glass block is heated to form lithium metasilicate (Li_2SiO_3) crystals. After cooling, the intermediate metasilicate phase—evenly dispersed small platelet-shaped crystals—accounts for 40 vol%. This material is strong enough to be milled to form the desired restoration. During the third stage, the material undergoes an additional thermal treatment at 850°C for 20 to 31 minutes to precipitate small rod-like and interlocked 1.5-µm-long crystals of lithium disilicate in a volume fraction of up to 70%. The resulting GC has 360 MPa in strength and a fracture toughness of 2.25 MPa $m^{1/2}$. Figure 1-2 shows the microstructure of lithium disilicate.[41]

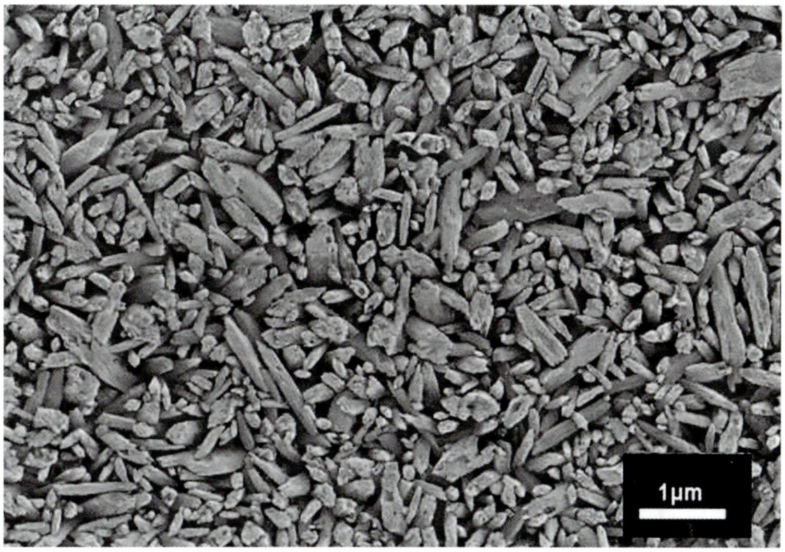

FIG 1-2 › Scanning electron microscopy (SEM) image of the microstructure of a lithium disilicate–type GC (IPS e.max CAD, Ivoclar Vivadent). (Modified with permission from Ritzberger et al.[41])

GLASS-INFILTRATED CERAMICS

VITA Zahnfabrik developed a class of glass-infiltrated dental ceramics (In-Ceram) during the 1980s. In-Ceram crown cores were made in the dental lab by slip casting alumina slurries in porous gypsum dies, followed by sintering of the green body. Sintering process parameters were selected to result in 20% to 25% porosity. After shaping, the alumina porous cores (copings) were infiltrated with molten lanthanum aluminosilicate glass. The composition of the cores may be alumina, magnesium spinel ($MgAl_2O_4$), or a ceramic composite of alumina and zirconia (zirconia-toughened alumina [ZTA]). The ZTA system (In-Ceram Zirconia) is obtained by adding 33 vol% of 12 mol% ceria-stabilized zirconia (12Ce-TZP) to In-Ceram Alumina.

In-Ceram Alumina can be used for three-unit anterior fixed partial dentures (FPDs) and can thus be regarded as the first all-ceramic restorative system.[42,43] In-Ceram Zirconia has a bending strength that is 20% higher than In-Ceram Alumina, and it is recommended for three-unit posterior FPDs.[44] Initially used for ceramic copings, In-Ceram Alumina and In-Ceram Zirconia were later available as presintered porous ceramic blocks for CAD/CAM and prosthetic abutments infiltrated by lanthanum glass. Table 1-1 provides an overview of some basic material properties of glass-containing dental ceramics.

Oxide Ceramics in Dentistry

PURE ALUMINA

Applications of alumina (aluminum oxide, Al_2O_3) as a biomaterial are based on its microstructural properties, which may occur in many metastable phases eventually leading to irreversible transformation into alpha-alumina if heated above 1,200°C. Alpha-alumina is a close-packed hexagonal arrangement of oxygen

TABLE 1-1 › **Properties of glass-containing dental ceramics**

Material	Strength at rupture (MPa)	Fracture toughness (MPa m$^{1/2}$)	Young modulus (GPa)
Feldspathic porcelain	60–70	0.92–1.26	70
Leucite GCs	160	1.4–1.5	65
Lithium disilicate GCs	360–400	2.25–2.75	95
Glass-infiltrated spinel	400	2.7	185
Glass-infiltrated alumina	500	3.9	280
Glass-infiltrated zirconia	600	4.4	260

ions that constitutes a very high thermodynamically stable phase. Known also as *corundum* (or *emery* if containing impurities), alpha-alumina is the alumina material used for biomedical application.

In the lattice of alpha-alumina, each aluminum cation Al^{3+} is surrounded by oxygen anions O^{2-} forming two regular triangles on both sides, twisted by 180 degrees and lying on parallel planes. The surface layer of O^{2-} anions allows the chemisorption on the surface of OH^{+} groups, then the bonding of water molecules or proteins. In other words, the surface has high wettability (higher than several metallic alloys).

One of the physical properties to be controlled to achieve the best clinical outcomes with alumina bioceramics is the residual porosity of the product. The porosity fraction influences the mechanical properties, as explained in the following section. The open porosity fraction especially must be controlled because it allows the permeation of liquids and gases.

Alumina restorations

Andersson and Odén[45] reported the use of high-purity (> 99.9%) alumina ceramic for the manufacture of single crowns (Procera AllCeram, Nobel Biocare) in the early 1990s. Developments in the production system later allowed for the manufacture of partial dentures and abutments. In this ceramic, there is no glassy phase present between the grains, a feature that differentiates it from former dental ceramic materials. Procera Alumina has a flexural strength of about 600 MPa. The Procera AllCeram cores (99.9% polycrystalline alumina) are obtained via an industrial process performed at a centralized manufacturing plant. After milling and sintering, single-crown and multiunit frameworks are veneered with feldspathic ceramics to provide the desired color and form of the restoration.[46]

Alumina dental implants

Alumina was once popular for dental implants worldwide. White, dense, and corrosion and wear resistant, alumina was the most advanced ceramic in the 1970s, ideal for replacing single tooth roots. Already by 1965, Professor Sami Sandhaus, a Ukrainian-born dentist practicing in Lausanne, Switzerland, patented the first ceramic dental implant under the tradename Crystallyne Bone Screw (CBS) (Fig 1-3).[47] Professor Sandhaus developed the entire implant system, including the instruments and an original method for preparing implant sites involving the use of ozone gas.[48]

The CBS implant had a helical shape with a maximum diameter of 5 mm and an external hexagonal termination. There were two implant lengths (15 and 20 mm). CBS implants were manufactured by Rosenthal (now CeramTec) and indicated for use in FPDs connected to natural teeth. By 1984, more than 3,000 patients had received CBS implants. The implants were produced by diamond-milling sintered alumina bars. Later, Sandhaus introduced a second alumina

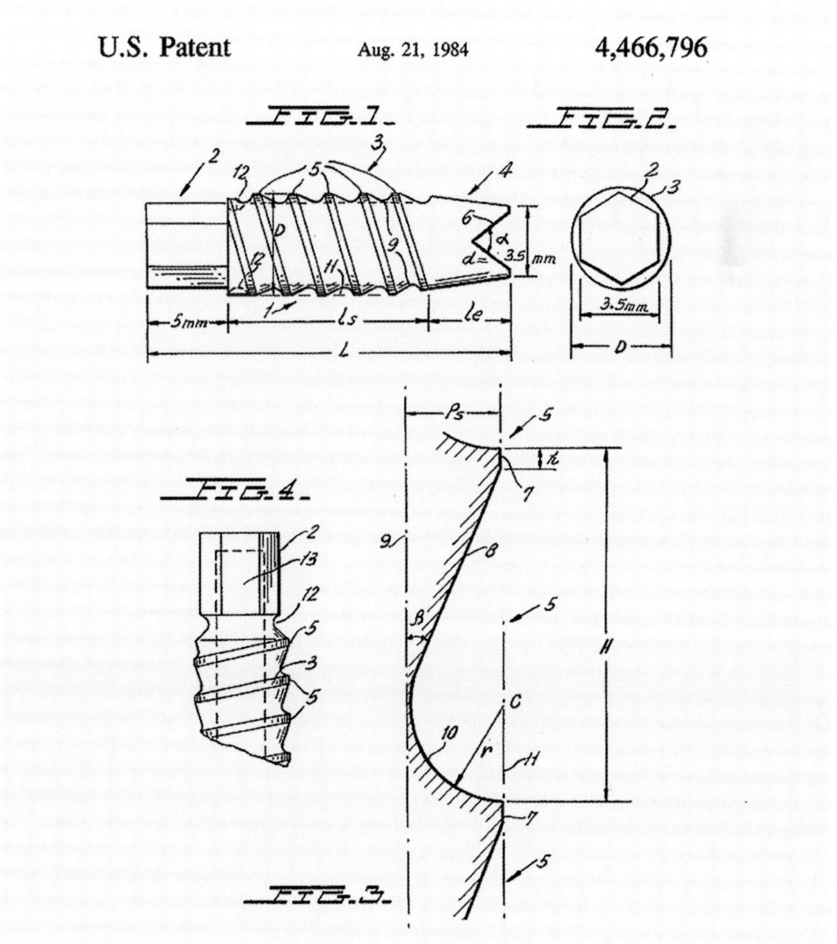

FIG 1-3 › The CBS all-alumina dental implant.[47]

implant (Cerasand) made by slip casting followed by hot isostatic pressing (HIP) to avoid the risk of introducing flaws to the implants during milling.[49] The Cerasand implant had a square abutment and an axial hole to host a metallic post supporting the crown.

Other researchers also developed implant systems from high-purity alumina. One of the most popular was the Tübingen system manufactured by Friedrichsfeld and introduced in 1976 under the Frialit trademark.[50] The Tübingen dental implant was a single-stage tap implant designed in several sizes and shapes for replacing single teeth in either jaw. Initially indicated as an immediate implant, the indication was later extended to delayed implantation. The body of the endosseous implant was characterized by a stepped cylinder with surface gaps to increase the surface area. Because the diameter in the neck area of the implant proved to be too large for implantation in narrow alveolar ridges, the Munich modification of the Tübingen implant was developed. This implant had an asymmetric section.

Other systems with anchor-shaped and screw-shaped alumina dental implants and endodontic dental posts were developed by Münch, Mutshelknaus, and Brinkmann and were manufactured by Feldmühle (now CeramTec). The Münch implant was intended for either immediate or delayed loading. It had a diameter compatible with the slimmer Munich modification of the Tübingen implant but a threaded conical shape to achieve initial stability in the jawbone.[51–53] Another German manufacturer of alumina dental implants was KWH (Keramische Werk Hermsdorf [now Mathys]), which introduced the BIONIT system.[54] Alumina dental implants were still made in Hungary in the second half of the 1980s under the tradename DIAKOR.[55]

A large research program aimed at developing bone substitutes and dental implants from alumina was coordinated in the United States by the Dental Research Division of the US Army Medical Research and Development Command in 1968. T.A. Driskell developed the Synthodont dental implant system, an alumina osseointegrated single-tooth dental implant that achieved significant clinical success in the following years. By 1980, over 3,500 of these implants were in clinical use, either as freestanding individual crowns or along with natural teeth to support a partial denture.[56,57] Studies to develop root-shaped implants to be used in extraction sites were performed using dense alumina molar-shaped implants and porous calcium aluminate replicas, but the results of these investigations did not lead to clinical applications.[58,59]

In Japan, a relevant research effort was focused on single-crystal alumina (artificial sapphire). This option was investigated to overcome the limitations of the polycrystalline ceramics of that time. This solution had significant esthetic advantages because of the clear and transparent gingival part of the implants, which were manufactured by Kyocera.[60] Kyocera manufactured blade-, tap-, and screw-type dental implants that were used in Japan since 1972 and distributed in the United States under the tradename Bioceram.

Outcomes with alumina dental implants have been mixed.[61–63] Today, there are no alumina dental implants on the market. Alumina was abandoned mostly because of its mechanical behavior. The bending strength of high-density alumina in the 1970s (first generation) was about 300 MPa and was paired with low toughness, limiting the design flexibility of implants.[64]

ZIRCONIA

The use of zirconia ceramics in dentistry is well established, and most of this book is devoted to the comprehensive description of the properties of this material, which are only outlined here.

The crystal lattice of zirconia (zirconium dioxide) can take one of three shapes, depending on temperature—the monoclinic phase occurs at room temperature to about 1,170°C, the tetragonal phase occurs at higher temperatures, and finally the cubic phase exists at temperatures above 2,370°C. When cooled, zirconia in the tetragonal phase reverts to the monoclinic phase. This transformation is associated with the expansion of the crystal lattice, and the stress generated by the transformation can lead to fracture of the material.

In the 1930s, Ruff and Passerini each independently demonstrated that the tetragonal and cubic zirconia microstructures formed at high temperatures can be stabilized at room temperature by introducing appropriate oxides (stabilizers) into the zirconia.[65] Cubic zirconia can be either fully stabilized (FSZ) or partially stabilized (PSZ). In 1975, Garvie et al[66] highlighted the relevance of the tetragonal to monoclinic phase transformation during cooling to improve the mechanical behavior of PSZ. Their seminal work, "Ceramic Steel?," paved the way for the structural use of stabilized zirconia ceramics. More important is the discovery by Gupta et al,[67] who demonstrated the feasibility of a material constituted by a solid solution of 3 mol% yttria (Y_2O_3 [yttrium oxide]) in zirconia formed by metastable tetragonal grains at room temperature—yttria-stabilized tetragonal zirconia polycrystal (Y-TZP). The homogeneous and fine-grain microstructure of Y-TZP is illustrated in Fig 1-4.

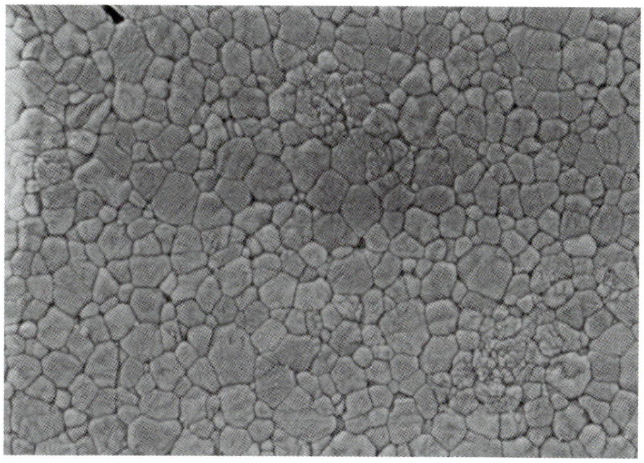

FIG 1-4 › Microstructure of Y-TZP. The microstructure is fine and homogeneous. The two missing grains are artifacts of the specimen processing for SEM examination.

TABLE 1-2 › **Mechanical properties of zirconia and alumina**

Property	Y-TZP	Mg-PSZ	HIP alumina
Density (g/cm^3)	6	5.5	3.97
Average grain size (µm)	0.3–0.5	40–70	1.75
Flexural strength (MPa)	900–1,200	400–650	650
Young modulus (GPa)	210	210	400
Fracture toughness (MPa $m^{1/2}$)	7–9	8–11	4.5
Hardness (GPa)	12.5	12.5	20–21

Other oxides can also be used to stabilize the tetragonal microstructure of zirconia, allowing for the production of several types of zirconia-based ceramics. Ceria (CeO_2 [cerium oxide]) is another tetragonal phase stabilizer for zirconia. Ceria-stabilized tetragonal zirconia polycrystal (Ce-TZP) has potential advantages over Y-TZP in terms of toughness and stability, though it has the drawback of reduced mechanical strength due to the greater grain size. Magnesia (magnesium oxide) is also used as a stabilizer for PSZ. So far, Mg-PSZ has been used in dentistry in only one product (Denzir M, Decim).[68,69] Other stabilizing oxides include calcium oxide (CaO), tantalum oxide (Ta_2O_5), and copper oxide (CuO), sometimes used as minor phases in stabilizing systems based on yttria or ceria.

Yttria is the stabilizer referred to in ISO standards for surgical implants (ISO 13356) and is the material of choice because of its excellent mechanical properties.[70] Y-TZP is the most common form of zirconia used in dental appliances worldwide. It is so popular that the term *zirconia* is commonly accepted in place of Y-TZP even in the scientific literature. It has been in clinical use since 1991, when it was used for dental root pins. It has been available in sintered blanks since 1993 and as presintered blanks for CAD/CAM milling since 1996. Some of the mechanical properties of Y-TZP and Mg-PSZ are summarized in Table 1-2, along with data on alumina as a point of reference.

Zirconia restorations

Two techniques are available for the CAD/CAM production of zirconia dental frameworks: *(1)* soft machining of presintered blanks, which is the most common method, and *(2)* hard machining of full-density sintered zirconia. The world market for zirconia blanks (disks and blocks) reached a value of about US $200 million in 2022, with 62% of that value attributed to zirconia disks to be milled for the production of multiunit frameworks.[71] Hard machining is used only by two CAD/CAM systems, Denzir (Decim) and DC Zirkon (DCS Dental). Milling full-density zirconia is demanding and requires very stiff and powerful milling machines with abrasive diamond burs.[72] Hard machining is a time-consuming process that can trigger subcritical defects in the material and chipping of semifinished parts, resulting in a waste of material and work. The large majority of zirconia dental appliance manufacturers prefer soft machining (ie, milling of presintered blanks that are then fully sintered at a final stage). The characteristics of the blanks (disks and blocks) must be matched with the software controlling the milling process to enlarge the shape of the framework to compensate for shrinkage of the material during sintering (generally about 20% to 25%). Various companies make and distribute Y-TZP blocks for CAD/CAM machining worldwide. A non-exhaustive list of these companies and their products is provided in Table 1-3.

TABLE 1-3 › Sample list of companies manufacturing CAD/CAM zirconia blanks

Manufacturer	Country	Product
Whip Mix	US	Vericore Zr Pro
3M ESPE	US	LAVA Plus Zirconia, LAVA Esthetic
Dentsply Sirona	US	Cercon, inCoris ZTI, Cercon XT
VITA Zahnfabrik	Germany	VITA YZ T/HT
Kuraray Noritake	Japan	Katana HT/ML, ST/STML, UT/UTML
Ivoclar Vivadent	Liechtenstein	ZirCAD MT
Zirkonzahn	Italy	Prettau Zirconia
KaVo Dental	Germany	Everest
Wieland Dental	Germany	Zenostar MO, Zenostar T, Zenostar MT
Glidewell	US	BruxZir, BruxZir Anterior
Tosoh	Japan	Zpex, Zpex 4, Zpex smile
Heany	US	Luxisse, Luxisse +
Dental Direkt	Germany	DD cubeX^2
Straumann	Switzerland	Zerion GI/LT/HTML/UTML

To improve the esthetics of CAD/CAM ceramics, oxides are added to the ceramic powders.[73] Other changes include increasing the translucency of the ceramic by reducing alumina sintering additives from 0.25 wt% to 0.01 wt%. So far, machinable zirconia blocks containing up to 50 wt% cubic FSZ are available on the market. The high concentration of cubic zirconia enhances the translucency of the material, though the reduction in fracture strength and toughness is significant.[38]

Multilayer blanks with shade and translucency gradients are also available. The first one was Katana (Kuraray Noritake). This product is obtained by adding layers of different pigments to provide a graded shade (but not translucency) between the cervical and incisal portions of the restoration to mimic a natural tooth. Later, blanks with gradients of pigments and cubic phase were developed (eg, e.max ZirCAD Multi, Ivoclar Vivadent), thus allowing for restorations graded in shade and translucency in the gingival and incisal regions.

Zirconia dental implants

The first application of zirconia in dentistry reported in the literature (1975) is related to the testing of ceramic coatings on vitallium anchor implants to protect them from corrosion and improve their biocompatibility.[74] The fabrication of zirconia blade implants by slip casting followed by Nd:YAG laser surface treatment to improve bone apposition was described in 1990 by Minamizato.[75] These first studies were followed by others demonstrating the osseointegration of zirconia. In 1993, Miani et al[76] evaluated ceramic cylinders implanted in beagles, and Akagawa et al[77] studied experimental screw-shaped implants. Shortly thereafter, Sandhaus and Pasche[78] reported the results obtained with Sigma Implants (Fig 1-5), a two-step zirconia (Y-TZP) dental implant system consisting of implants with an internal hexagonal connection housing a cemented zirconia post and core. The fabrication and characterization of zirconia posts was reported in 1997 by Meyenberg et al.[79]

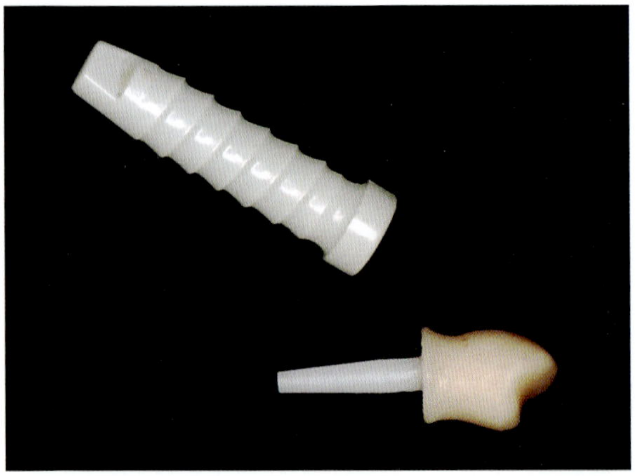

FIG 1-5 › The Sigma zirconia dental implant. (Courtesy of Prof Sami Sandhaus.)

TABLE 1-4 › Sample list of various zirconia dental implant systems

Product	Country	Manufacturer
Axis Implant	Switzerland	Axis Biodental
whiteSKY	Germany	bredent medical
Zirconium Oxyde Implant	US	Ceradyne
Zirconium Root	Hungary	Denti System
Zeramex	Switzerland	Dentalpoint
Easy Kon	Germany	General Implants
Sigma Quatro	Switzerland	Incermed
Omnis	Germany	Maxon Dental
Ziraldent	Switzerland	Metoxit
CeraRoot	Germany	Oral Iceberg
ZIR ROC	France	Paris Implants
Pure	Switzerland	Straumann
Neodent	Switzerland	Straumann
SDS1.1, SDS2.0	Switzerland	Swiss Dental Solutions
One- and two-piece zirconia implants	Israel	TAV Dental
ZV3	Germany	Zircon Vision
Z5-BL	Switzerland	Z-Systems

The real starting point for metal-free implantology with zirconia was in 2004, when Volz patented his zirconia implant system.[80,81] Since then, various zirconia dental implant systems have been introduced to the market (Table 1-4).

The work of Dubruille et al[82] in 1999 showed that there was no statistical difference between the osseointegration of titanium, zirconia, and alumina implants.[82] Today, the osseointegration of zirconia is a clinically established behavior, with kinetics that can be enhanced by treatments to increase the cleanliness and hydrophilicity of the endosseous surfaces of the implant.[83–90]

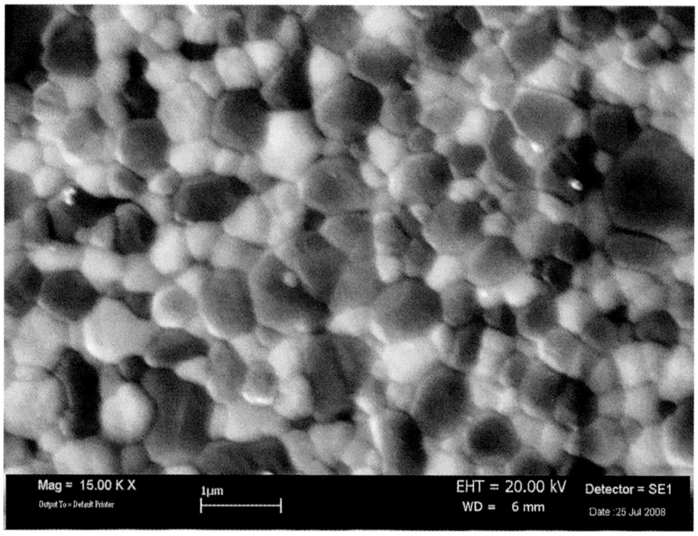

FIG 1-6 › ZTA microstructure. Zirconia grains appear white in the SEM image. (Courtesy of ENEA Laboratory.)

Zirconia-alumina composites

Since the 1990s, ceramists have been strongly focused on developing zirconia-based composites with binary or ternary structures for use in medical devices with improved mechanical properties over those made with Y-TZP. These are essentially zirconia-alumina composites that can be classified according to the main constituent: ZTA if alumina is containing a zirconia dispersion (Fig 1-6) or alumina-toughened zirconia (ATZ) if zirconia is the matrix of the composite. The energy threshold for the tetragonal to monoclinic phase transition is increased both by the increased stiffness of the alumina grains (E_{Al2O3} = 380 GPa; E_{YTZP} = 200 GPa), which counteracts the expansion of the zirconia grains during phase transformation, and by the internal compressive stresses that occur during cooling.

An ATZ with established use in dental implantology is ATZ BIO-HIP (Metoxit), which has been used for the manufacture of dental implants since 2012.[91,92] It consists of a submicron-sized Y-TZP matrix containing a fine and homogeneous dispersion (20 wt%) of alumina grains. The tetragonal zirconia phase is stabilized with 3 mol% yttrium, as for standard monolithic zirconia (3Y-TZP). The average grain diameter approaches 0.4 μm for both zirconia and alumina.[93,94] ATZ may appear to be a relatively simple material. However, the properties of these specialty materials depend significantly on the manufacturing steps and conditions. In an additional ATZ produced by the same company (Ziraldent), the alumina content is increased to 25%, resulting in a reinforced material that due to its high strength and toughness is used to produce ceramic dental drilling tools.[72]

Nawa et al[95] and Ban et al[96] reported on the development of an ATZ composite constituted of Ce-TZP matrix (10 mol% ceria) with 30 vol% alumina and 0.05 mol% titania. This material has a duplex intergranular-type nanostructure in which several 10- to 100-nm alumina particles are trapped within the zirconia grains and several 10-nm zirconia particles are trapped within the alumina grains. The mechanical behavior of this composite promises to offer some advantages in comparison with alumina and Y-TZP. This ATZ is designed for dental application with clinical use for CAD/CAM milling blanks for dental restorations under the tradename NANOZR (Matsushita/Panasonic). Studies considering its use for dental implants have not given rise to products so far.[97–99]

Elongated phases (eg, $SrAl_{12}O_{19}$, $LaAl_{11}O_{18}$) were incorporated into ceramics to increase toughness and strength. This concept was further developed by Burger, with a focus on ZTA composites.[100,101] The ZTA material he developed is an alumina matrix composite containing Y-TZP (17 vol%) and strontium exaluminate ($SrAl_{12}O_{19}$ [SHA]) elongated crystals with a length-to-diameter ratio of about 10:1. The material has a bending strength above 1,350 MPa. The process is proprietary of CeramTec, which is using this material (BIOLOX delta) to manufacture ceramic components for joint replacements.[102] CeramTec has also recently disclosed a new ZTA with remarkable mechanical properties.[103,104] Identified as HTZ500, it consists of a Y-TZP matrix (particle size 0.27 mm) containing a 5 vol% dispersion of SHA. The SHA crystals that nucleate in the material during sintering have an elongated shape (length-to-diameter ratio of 10:1) and behave like short fibers to reinforce the material, which has high resistance to damage during milling operations and a flexural strength about 1.6 times greater than that of Y-TZP.

Other composites under development today are based on Ce-TZP, although the mechanical strength of Ce-TZPs is inferior to that of Y-TZP. Innovative Ce-TZP–based triphasic composites have recently been developed.[105] Ce-TZP/8 vol% alumina/8 vol% SHA composites (referred to as *ZA8Sr8*) are obtained by a process that allows for a highly homogeneous distribution of second phases in the zirconia matrix, adaptation of particle size and morphology, tight control of stoichiometry, and purity of all phases.[106]

Another material exploiting Ce-TZP behavior is the ZCA10P (Oxymatec) constituted by 90 wt% Ce-TZP with alumina/lanthanum oxide. A third platelet-like phase is obtained during sintering. This material is optimized to maximize toughness while maintaining reasonable mechanical strength, giving it a fracture toughness of 15 MPa $m^{1/2}$ and a strength of 760 MPa, measured in four-point bending configuration.[107] Table 1-5 summarizes the properties of some composite zirconia–based ceramics.

TABLE 1-5 › **Properties of zirconia composite ceramics**

Material	Stress at rupture (MPa)	Fracture toughness (MPa m$^{1/2}$)	Young modulus (GPa)
ATZ Bio-HIP	> 1,300	6	–
Y-TZP	900–1,000	6–8	210
Alumina matrix composite (BIOLOX delta)	1,360	7.5	300
Ce-TZP/$LaAl_{11}O_{18}$ composite	950	10.5	–
HTZ500	1,630	8.6	–
Ce-TZP/Al_2O_3/$SrAl_{12}O_{19}$	1,200	10.2	–

Natural Ceramics

Three implants made of a natural ceramic (nacre) dating back to the 7th century AD were found in a jaw fragment discovered in 1931 by Dr Wilson Popenoe and his wife Dorothy in a grave in Playa de Los Muertos in Ulua Valley, Honduras. This jaw fragment is now in the Peabody Museum of Archaeology and Ethnology at Harvard University. The jaw and implants were studied by Amedeo Bobbio, who demonstrated osseointegration of two of the implants with radiographic controls.[108]

Dental implants made of mother-of-pearl (Bioracine) were in clinical use during the 1990s in France,[109] but these devices are no longer on the market.

Carbon

Experimental studies on porous carbon implants have been carried out in the United States since the early 1970s.[110] At 6 months postoperatively, experimental implants in mongrel dogs exhibited direct contact between the bone and the pyrolytic carbon without fibrous tissue interposition.[111] A pyrolytic carbon dental implant system (Root Replacement System, Vitredent) was distributed in the United States during the 1970s and implanted in several hundred patients.[112] In an overview on pyrolytic carbon biomaterials, Bokros[113] reported that 89 implants showed a success rate of 88% at the 4-year follow-up. This system was intended for two-stage implantation. It consisted of a polycrystalline carbon body with an upper collar of polished carbon for soft tissue adaptation and a stainless steel pin extending about two-thirds of the way through the center of the implant, with a stainless steel abutment insert for attachment of the intraoral crown or partial denture. This implant system is no longer on the market.[114] Carbon fiber–reinforced carbon (CFRC) blade and tap implants have been investigated in Japan and tested in monkeys up to 2 years, but this research has not resulted in clinical applications so far.[115]

Conclusion

The ceramics currently used in dentistry are the results of research performed over the course of more than two centuries. Since the second half of the 18th century, porcelain has been improved continuously for use in dentistry, leading to the feldspathic porcelains in use today. Additional developments led to the use of GC materials, though their properties limit their use to metallic structures. Today, zirconia has proved to be the breakthrough ceramic in dentistry, with its use in dental applications now widespread throughout the world.

References

1. Kingery WD, Bowen HK, Uhlmann DR. Introduction to Ceramics, ed 2. Wiley, 1976.
2. Griffith AA. The phenomena of rupture and flow in solids. Phil Trans Roy Soc 1920;A221:163–198.
3. Tai Y, De Long R, Goodkind RJ, Douglas WH. Leaching of nickel, chromium, and beryllium ions from base metal alloy in an artificial oral environment. J Prosthet Dent 1992;68:692–697.
4. Upadhyay D, Manoj A, Panchal A, Dubey RS, Srivastava VK. Corrosion of alloys used in dentistry: A review. Mater Science Eng A 2006;432:1–11.
5. Chaturvedi TP. Corrosive behaviour of implant biomaterials in oral environment. Mater Technol 2016;31:1–7.
6. Matusiewicz H. Potential release of in vivo trace metals from metallic medical implants in the human body: From ions to nanoparticles—A systematic analytical review. Acta Biomater 2014;10:2379–2403.
7. Muris J, Kleverlaan CJ. Hypersensitivity to dental alloys. In: Chen JK, Thyssen JP (eds). Metal Allergy: From Dermatitis to Implant and Device Failure. Springer, 2018:285–300.
8. Biological Responses to Metal Implants: September 2019. U.S. Food and Drug Administration Center for Devices and Radiological Health, 2019. https://www.fda.gov/media/131150/download. Accessed 19 April 2024.
9. Berglundh T, Armitage G, Araujo MG, et al. Peri-implant diseases and conditions: Consensus report of workgroup 4 of the 2017 World Workshop on the Classification of Periodontal and Peri-Implant Diseases and Conditions. J Periodontol 2018;89(suppl 1):S313–S318.
10. Rimondini L, Cerroni L, Carrassi A, Torricelli P. Bacterial colonization of zirconia ceramic surfaces: An in vitro and in vivo study. Int J Oral Maxillofac Implants 2002;17:793–798.
11. Gleeson J. Arcanum. Bantam, 1998.
12. Verchére L. Alexis Duchateau, pharmacist, inventor of porcelain teeth [in French]. Rev Odontostomatol (Paris) 1974;5:423–426.
13. De Chemant N. Dissertation sur les advantages des nouvelles dents et râteliers artificiels incorruptibles et sans odeur. Gattey, 1789.
14. Menzies CJ. Nicolas Dubois de Chemant—A contribution to dental history. Dent Pract Dent Rec 1960;10:6.
15. Powers N. Archaeological evidence for dental innovation: An eighteenth century porcelain dental prosthesis belonging to Archbishop Arthur Richard Dillon. Br Dent J 2006;201:459–463.
16. Pasqualini U, Pasqualini ME. Treatise of Implant Dentistry: The Italian Tribute to Modern Implantology. Ariesdue, 2009.
17. Guerini V. The life and works of Giuseppangelo Fonzi. Lea & Febiger, 1925.
18. Obituary Dr. Samuel Stockton White. Am J Dent Sci 1880;13:429–432.
19. Ring ME. Geschichte der Zahnmedizin. Könemann, 1997.
20. Anusavice KJ. Dental ceramics. In: Anusavice KJ, Shen C, Rawls HR (eds). Phillip's Science of Dental Materials, ed 12. Elsevier, 2013:418–473.
21. Weinstein M, Weinstein LK, Katz S, Weinstein AB [inventors]. Fused porcelain-to-metal teeth. US patent 3,052,982. 11 September 1962.

22. McLean JW, Hughes TH. The reinforcement of dental porcelain with ceramic oxides. Br Dent J 1965;119:251–267.
23. McLean JW, Sced IR. The bonded alumina crown. 1. The bonding of platinum to aluminous dental porcelain using tin oxide coatings. Aust Dent J 1976;21:119–127.
24. McLean JW, Kedge MI, Hubbard JR. The bonded alumina crown. 2. Construction using the twin foil technique. Aust Dent J 1976;21:262–267.
25. Stookey SD [inventor]. Method of making ceramics and product thereof. US patent 2,920,971. 4 June 1956.
26. Höland W, Beall GH. Glass-Ceramic Technology. Wiley/American Ceramic Society, 2020.
27. Tinschert J, Zwez D, Marx R, Anusavice KJ. Structural reliability of alumina-, feldspar-, leucite-, mica- and zirconia-based ceramics. J Dent 2000;28:529–535.
28. Cattell MJ, Chadwick TC, Knowles JC, Clarke RL, Lynch E. Flexural strength optimisation of a leucite reinforced glass ceramic. Dent Mater 2001;17:21–33.
29. Rekow ED, Silva NRFA, Coelho PG, Zhang Y, Guess P, Thompson VP. Performance of dental ceramics: Challenges for improvements. J Dent Res 2011;90:937–952.
30. Grossman DG [inventor]. Tetrasilicic mica glass-ceramic method. US patent 3,732,087. 8 May 1973.
31. Duret F [inventor]. Method for producing a dental prosthesis [in French]. French patent 2536654. 1 Jan 1982.
32. Duret F, Preston J, Duret B. Performance of CAD/CAM crown restorations. J Calif Dent Assoc 1996;24:64–71.
33. Mörmann WH, Brandestini M, Lutz F. The Cerec system: Computer-assisted preparation of direct ceramic inlays in 1 setting. Quintessenz 1987;38:457–470.
34. Mörmann WH, Brandestini M, Lutz F, Barbakow F. Chairside computer-aided direct ceramic inlays. Quintessence Int 1989;20:329–339.
35. Russell MM, Andersson M, Dahlmo K, Razzoog ME, Lang BR. A new computer-assisted method for fabrication of crowns and fixed partial dentures. Quintessence Int 1995;26:757–763.
36. Willer J, Rossbach A, Weber HP. Computer-assisted milling of dental restorations using a new CAD/CAM data acquisition system. J Prosthet Dent 1998;80:346–353.
37. Stawarcyk B, Keul C, Eichberger M, Figge D, Edelhoff D, Lümkermann N. Three generations of zirconia: From veneered to monolithic. Part II. Quintessence Int 2017;48:441–450.
38. Zhang Y, Lawn BR. Novel zirconia materials in dentistry. J Dent Res 2018;97:140–147.
39. Höland W, Schweiger M, Watzke R, Peschke A, Kappert H. Ceramics as biomaterials for dental restoration. Expert Rev Med Devices 2008;5:729–745.
40. Höland W, Rheinberger V, Van't Hoen C, Apel E. P2O5 as an effective nucleating agent of lithium disilicate glass-ceramics. Phosphorus Res Bull 2005;19:36–41.
41. Ritzberger C, Apel E, Holand W, Peschle A, Rheinberger V. Properties and clinical application of three types of dental glass-ceramics and ceramics for CAD-CAM technologies. Materials (Basel) 2010;3:3700–3713.
42. Claus H. Vita In-Ceram, a new procedure for preparation of oxide-ceramic crown and bridge framework [in German]. Quintessenz Zahntech 1990;16:35–46.
43. Della Bona A, Mecholsky JJ, Barrett AA, Griggs JA. Characterization of glass-infiltrated alumina-based ceramics. Dent Mater 2008;24:1568–1574.
44. McLaren EA, White SN. Glass-infiltrated zirconia/alumina-based ceramic for crowns and fixed partial dentures: Clinical and laboratory guidelines. Quintessence Dent Technol 2000;23:63–76.
45. Andersson M, Odén A. A new all-ceramic crown: A dense-sintered, high-purity alumina coping with porcelain. Acta Odontol Scand 1993;51:59–64.
46. Odman P, Andersson B. Procera AllCeram crowns followed for 5 to 10.5 years: A prospective clinical study. Int J Prosthodont 2001;14:504–509.
47. Sandhaus S [inventor]. JSB DENTAL SUPPLY SA, CBS Biotechnic SA, assignees. Dental implant for use as a pillar in a mouth. US patent 4,466,796. 21 August 1984.
48. Sandhaus S. New Aspects of Implantology: The CBS Implant [in French]. Sandhaus, 1969.
49. Sandhaus S. The Cerasand endosseous implant [in French]. Actual Odontostomatol (Paris) 1987;41:607–626.
50. Heimke G, Schulte W [inventors]. Friatec AG, assignee. Dental implants having a biocompatible surface. US patent 4,185,383. 29 January 1980.
51. Mutshelknaus E, Dörre E. Extension implants of aluminum oxide ceramic (I) [in German]. Quintessenz 1977;28:21–25.
52. Brinkmann E. Endosseous implants of aluminum oxide ceramic [in German]. Zahnarztl Prax 1980;31:328–330.

53. Brinkmann E, Dörre E. Biolox screw implants [in German]. Zahnarztl Prax 1981;32:528–534.
54. Piesold JU, Müller W. Tooth replacement by BIONIT implants. Dtsch Stomatol 1991;41:128–132.
55. Vajadovich I, Fazekas A, Divinyi T. Principles and practical questions of oral endosseous implantation of DIAKOR aluminum bioceramics. I. The implant [in German]. Forgov Sz 1989;82:7–12.
56. Chess JT, Babbush CA. Restoration of lost dentition using aluminum oxide endosteal implants. Dent Clin North Am 1980;24:521–533.
57. Driskell TD, Heller AL, Koenigs JF [inventors]. Miter Enterprises, assignee. Dental prosthetic implants. US patent 3,950,850. 22 March 1983.
58. Driskell TD, O'Hara MJ, Sheets HD, Greene GW, Natiella JR, Armitage J. Development of ceramic and ceramic composite devices for maxillofacial applications. J Biomed Mater Res Symp 1972;6:345–361.
59. Young FA Jr. Ceramic tooth implants. J Biomed Mater Res 1972;6:281–296.
60. Kawahara H, Hirabajashi M, Shikita T. Single crystal alumina for dental implants and bone screws. J Biomed Mater Res 1980;14:597–605.
61. Fartash B, Tangerud T, Silness J, Arvidson K. Rehabilitation of mandibular edentulism by single crystal sapphire implants and overdentures: 3–12 year results in 86 patients. A dual center international study. Clin Oral Implants Res 1996;7:220–229.
62. Berge TI, Grøningsæter AG. Survival of single crystal sapphire implants supporting mandibular overdentures. Clin Oral Implants Res 2000;11:154–162.
63. Andreiotelli M, Wenz HJ, Kohal R-J. Are ceramic implants a viable alternative to titanium implants? A systematic literature review. Clin Oral Implants Res 2009;20(suppl 4):32–47.
64. Piconi C. Alumina. In: Ducheyne P, Grainger DW, Healy KE, Hutmacher DW, Kirkpatrick CJ (eds). Comprehensive Biomaterials II, vol. 1. Elsevier, 2017:92–121.
65. Lughi V, Sergo W. Low temperature degradation—aging—of zirconia: A critical review of the relevant aspects in dentistry. Dent Mater 2010;26:807–820.
66. Garvie RC, Hannink RHJ, Pascoe RT. Ceramic steel? Nature 1975;258:703–704.
67. Gupta TK, Lange FF, Bechtold JH. Effect of stress-induced phase transformation on the properties of polycrystalline zirconia containing metastable tetragonal phase. J Mater Sci 1978;13:1464–1470.
68. Denry I, Kelly R. State of the art of zirconia for dental applications. Dent Mater 2008;24:299–307.
69. Sundh A, Sjögren G. Fracture resistance of all-ceramic zirconia bridges with differing phase stabilizers and quality of sintering. Dent Mater 2006;22:778–784.
70. Implants for surgery: Ceramic materials based on yttria-stabilized tetragonal zirconia (Y-TZP), ISO13356. International Organization for Standardization, 2015.
71. Coherent Market Insights. Zirconia based dental materials market size by 2030. https://www.coherentmarketinsights.com/market-insight/zirconia-based-dental-materials-market-4997. Accessed 6 May 2024.
72. Weber W, Rieger W. ZrO2-TZP in dentistry: Materials, properties and applications. Key Eng Mater 2000;192:922–932.
73. Calés B. Colored zirconia ceramics for dental applications. In: LeGeros LZ, LeGeros JP (eds). Bioceramics, vol 11. World Scientific Publishing, 1998:591–594.
74. Cranin AN, Schnitman PA, Rabkin SM, Onesto EJ. Alumina and zirconia coated vitallium oral endosteal implants in beagles. J Biomed Mater Res 1975;9:257–262.
75. Minamizato T. Slip-cast zirconia dental roots with tunnels drilled by laser process. J Prosthet Dent 1990;6:677–684.
76. Miani C, Piconi C, Piselli D, Ponti M. Experimental in vivo studies on zirconia in oral implantology. Italian Osseoint J 1993:3:23–34.
77. Akagawa Y, Ichikawa Y, Nikai H, Tsuru H. Interface histology of unloaded and early loaded partially stabilized zirconia endosseous implant in initial bone healing. J Prosthet Dent 1993:69:599–604.
78. Sandhaus S, Pasche K. Tenon radiculaire en zircone pour la realisation d'inlays-cores tout ceramique. Tribune Dentaire 1994;2:17–24.
79. Meyenberg KH, Lüthy H, Schärer P. Zirconia posts: A new all-ceramic concept for nonvital abutment teeth. J Esthet Dent 1995;7:73–80.
80. Volz U. Zirconia implants with zirconium oxide crowns. Metal-free reconstruction [in German]. Z Zahnarzt Impl 2003;19:176–180.
81. Volz U, Blaschke CH. Metal-free reconstruction with zirconia implants and zirconia crowns. Quintessence Int 2004;2:324–330.

82. Dubruille JH, Viguier E, Le Naour G, Dubruille MT, Auriol M, Yves Le Charpentier Y. Evaluation of combinations of titanium, zirconia, and alumina implants with 2 bone fillers in the dog. Int J Oral Maxillofac implants 1999;14:271–277.
83. Depprich R, Zipprich H, Ommerborn M, et al. Osseointegration of zirconia implants compared with titanium: An in vivo study. Head Face Med 2008;11:30.
84. Gahlert M, Roehling S, Sprecher CM, Kniha H, Milz S, Bormann K. In vivo performance of zirconia and titanium implants: A histomorphometric study in mini pig maxillae. Clin Oral Implants Res 2012;23:281–286.
85. Pieralli S, Kohal RJ, Jung RE, Vach K, Spies BC. Clinical outcomes of zirconia dental implants: A systematic review. J Dent Res 2017;96:38–46.
86. Han JM, Hong G, Lin H, et al. Biomechanical and histological evaluation of the osseointegration capacity of two types of zirconia implant. Int J Nanomedicine 2016:11:6507–6516.
87. Rupp F, Liang L, Geis-Gerstorfer J, Scheideler L, Hüttig F. Surface characteristics of dental implants: A review. Dent Mater 2018;34:40–57.
88. Saulacic N, Erdösi R, Bosshardt DD, Gruber R, Buser D. Acid and alkaline etching of sandblasted zirconia implants: A histomorphometric study in miniature pigs. Clin Implant Dent Relat Res 2014;6:313–322.
89. Altmann B, Kohal RJ, Steinberg T, et al. Distinct cell functions of osteoblasts on UV-functionalized titanium- and zirconia-based implant materials are modulated by surface topography. Tissue Eng Part C Methods 2013;19:850–863.
90. Watanabe H, Saito K, Kokubo K, et al. Change in surface properties of zirconia and initial attachment of osteoblast-like cells with hydrophilic treatment. Dent Mater 2012;31:806–814.
91. Spies BC, Balmer M, Patzelt SBM, Vach K, Kohal RJ. Clinical and patient-reported outcomes of a zirconia oral implant: Three-year results of a prospective cohort investigation. J Dent Res 2015:94:1385–1391.
92. Jank S, Hochgattener G. Succes rate of two-piece zirconia implants: A retrospective statistical analysis. Implant Dent 2016:25:193.
93. Magnani G, Fabbri P, Leoni E, Salernitano E. New perspectives on zirconia composites as biomaterials. J Compos Sci 2021;5:244.
94. Rieger W, Leyen S, Weber W. The use of bioceramics in dental and medical applications. Digital Dental News 2009:3:6–13.
95. Nawa M, Nakamoto S, Sekino T, Niihara K. Tough and strong Ce-TZP/alumina nanocomposite doped with titania. Ceram Int 1998:24:497–506.
96. Ban S, Sato H, Suehiro Y, Nakanishi H, Nawa M. Biaxial flexure strength and low temperature degradation of Ce-TZP/Al2O3 nanocomposite and Y-TZP as dental restoratives. J Biomed Mater Res B: Appl Biomater 2008:87B:492–498.
97. Kim DG, Kwon HJ, Jeong YH, et al. Mechanical properties of bone tissues surrounding dental implant systems with different treatments and healing periods. Clin Oral Investig 2016:20:2211–2220.
98. Oshima Y, Iwasa F, Tachi K, Baba K. Effect of nanofeatured topography on ceria-stabilized zirconia/alumina nanocomposite on osteogenesis and osseointegration. Int J Oral Maxillofac Implants 2017:32:81–91.
99. Han J, Zhao J, Shen Z. Zirconia ceramics in metal-free dentistry. Adv Appl Ceram 2017;116:138–150.
100. Burger W. Wrap and platelet-reinforced aluminum oxide matrix materials (part 1) [in German]. Keram Z 1997;49:1067–1070.
101. Burger W. Wrap- and platelet-reinforced aluminum oxide matrix materials (part 1) [in German]. Keram Z 1998;50:18–22.
102. Burger W, Richter HG. High strength and toughness alumina matrix composites by transformation toughening and "in situ" platelet reinforcement (ZPTA). Key Eng Mater 2000;192–195:545–548.
103. Gottwik L, Wippermann A, Kuntz M, Denkena B. Effect of strontium hexaluminate on the damage tolerance of yttria-stabilized zirconia. Ceram Int 2017:43:15891–15898.
104. Denkena B, Wippermann A, Busemann S, Kuntz M, Gottwik L. Comparison of residual strength behavior after indentation, scratching and grinding of zirconia-based ceramics for medical-technical applications. J Eur Ceram Soc 2018;38:1760–1768.
105. Reveron H, Fornabaio M, Palmero P, et al. Towards long lasting zirconia-based composites for dental implants: Transformation induced plasticity and its consequence on ceramic reliability. Acta Biomater 2017:48:423–432.

106. Fornabaio M, Reveron H, Adolfsson E, Montanaro L, Chevalier J, Palmero P. Design and development of dental ceramics: Examples of current innovations and future concepts. In: Palmero P, Cambier F, de Barra E (eds). Advances in Ceramic Biomaterials. Woodhead, 2017.
107. Burger W, Kiefer G. Alumina, zirconia and their composite ceramics with properties tailored for medical applications. J Compos Sci 2021;5:306.
108. Bobbio A. Maya il primo autentico impianto dentario alloplastico endosseo. Rass Trimest Odontoiatr 1973;54:5–15.
109. Camprasse S, Camprasse G, Pouzol M, Lopez E. Artificial dental root made out natural calcium carbonate (Bioracine). Clin Mater 1990;5:235–250.
110. Hucke EE, Fuys RA, Craig RG. Glassy carbon: A potential dental implant material. J Biomed Mater Res 1973;4:263–274.
111. Weinstein AM, Cook SB, Anderson RC. An evaluation of LTI carbon, carbon coated and uncoated porous titanium implants. In: Vincenzini P (ed). Ceramics in Surgery. Elsevier, 1983:373–385.
112. Dumas M, Myers HM. The vitreous carbon tooth root replacement system: A surgical discipline. Int J Oral Surg 1974;3:273–277.
113. Bokros JC. New material concepts in orthopedics. In: Lee SM (ed). Advances in Biomaterials. Technomic, 1987:79–89.
114. Lemons JE. Applied electrochemical studies of surgical implants. In: Kovacs P, Istephanous NS (eds). Proceedings on the Compatibility of Biomedical Implants. The Electrochemical Society, 1994:27–34.
115. Yanashigawa S. Carbon implants with fine rahmen surface layer. In: Lin OCC, Chao EYS (eds). Perspectives on Biomaterials. Elsevier, 1986:333–358.

02 ZIRCONIA IN DENTISTRY

Alessandro Alan Porporati

The use of ceramics in medicine continues to grow in popularity, especially in the field of orthopedics. For example, the high wear resistance[1] and excellent biologic behavior of ceramic particles[2] have made ceramic femoral heads the preferred choice in total hip replacement in many countries.[3–6] Ceramics are also gaining great momentum within dentistry, thanks to their favorable esthetic outcomes[7] and high resistance to corrosion in the aggressive oral environment, which is characterized by extensive fluctuations in pH and temperature.[8] Ceramic dental implants are unlikely to trigger immune reactions caused by particle and ion release after implantation, which can be a problem with metal restorations.[9]

Garvie, Hannink, and Pascoe's discovery of the phase transformation toughening of zirconia[10] has played a key role in the expansion of ceramic use in medicine. The martensitic-like properties of zirconia led Garvie et al[10] to refer to it as "ceramic steel." There is no doubt that the discovery of the increased toughening in zirconia paved the way for the use of ceramics in many applications from which it had been barred due to a lack of plasticity. Not least of these new applications was the use of ceramics in dental implantology, a field in which alumina had been used to a limited extent due to its relatively low fracture resistance and toughness. Perhaps the most important discovery for the purposes of this chapter is that of Gupta et al,[11] who demonstrated the synthesis of a zirconia composed of metastable tetragonal grains at room temperature with the addition of 3 mol% yttria, or yttria-stabilized tetragonal zirconia polycrystal (Y-TZP or 3Y-TZP). This is the representative zirconia material used in dental implantology today. In this chapter, we share the story of these discoveries and describe the physics behind zirconia phase transformation and its applications in dentistry.

A Brief History of Zirconia Phase Transformation Discovery

The name *zirkonerde* was first used by Martin Heinrich Klaproth, a German chemist studying mineral composition and the characterization of chemical elements. While studying the composition of jargon or hyacinth mineral (zircon) from the island of Sri Lanka in 1789, Klaproth found an unknown "erde" (earth), which was later found to have the chemical formula $ZrSiO_4$ (zirconium silicate). Through a reaction with sodium hydroxide, Klaproth was able to produce the oxide now known as *zirconium dioxide* (ZrO_2), or alternatively *zirconia*. Although the metal element of this formula is zirconium, Klaproth was never successful in obtaining it in its pure metallic state. Only later in 1824 was Jöns Jacob Berzelius able to extract crude zirconium powder. The difficulty in isolation was due to the coexistence of zirconium and hafnium in the zirconium ore. The world had to wait until 1925 for van Arkel and de Boer to produce a high-purity zirconium.[12]

Today, most zirconium is extracted from the mineral sources of zirconium silicate and baddeleyite. Zirconium metal is used in the nuclear energy industry because of its high transparency to neutrons and in the chemical and medical industry because of its high resistance to corrosion.[12] At room temperature, zirconia in its natural form is distinguished by its monoclinic lattice. At the beginning of the last century, it became popular for use as a refractory due to its high melting temperature, low thermal conductivity, and small expansion coefficient. Audley first proposed it for this application in 1917.[13]

However, the reversible transformation of zirconia from the high-temperature tetragonal phase to the room-temperature monoclinic phase results in lattice

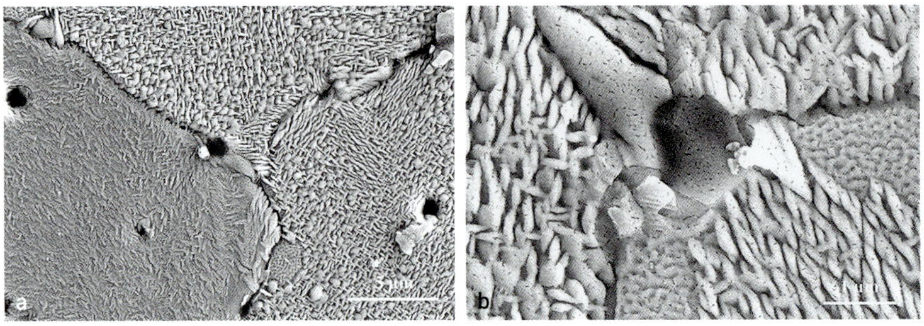

FIG 2-1 › Scanning electron micrographs (SEMs) of PSZ with magnesia after thermal etching at 5,000× *(a)* and 20,000× *(b)* magnification. Mg-PSZ consists of a cubic matrix with transformable tetragonal zirconia precipitates. The tetragonal precipitates are influenced by multiple factors, which makes the production process very sensitive. (Courtesy of CeramTec.)

expansion, which leads to macroscopic shattering of sintered products made of pure zirconia. This phenomenon restricted the large-scale use of zirconia as a refractory material until the late 1920s, when Ruff et al[14] and Passerini[15] demonstrated how to maintain the high-temperature phases of zirconia (tetragonal and cubic) at room temperature to prevent brick breakage during cooling. This achievement was made possible by alloying zirconia with other oxides, later called *stabilizers*.

Additional applications of this ceramic material were rather limited due to its low mechanical strength until Garvie's revolutionary discovery in the mid-1970s. It was partially stabilized zirconia (PSZ), with its transformable tetragonal zirconia grains in a cubic zirconia matrix,[10] that finally opened up the possibility of using zirconia in a wide range of applications. The microstructure of PSZ with magnesia (MgO), Mg-PSZ, is depicted in Fig 2-1 and is formed by large grains (diameter: 40–50 µm) containing nanometric lenticular tetragonal precipitates that nucleate during cooling. The microstructure of a ceramic material can be revealed by thermal etching. A temperature of 50°C to 100°C below sintering temperature is typically effective for microstructure analysis. Because the peculiar sintering process for Mg-PSZ demands strict time and temperature control to obtain the intragranular precipitates and it has overall poor mechanical properties in comparison with Y-TZP, Mg-PSZ had limited applications as a biomaterial.

In the 1980s, new developments allowed for the possibility of changing the microstructural design of zirconia by stabilizing the polycrystals of the tetragonal phase at room temperature with the addition of yttrium oxide (Y_2O_3) (Fig 2-2). This discovery by Gupta et al[11] was made shortly after Rieth et al[16] made it possible to create a ceramic material with very high mechanical strength and toughness by taking advantage of the change in lattice volume from the tetragonal to the monoclinic phase. This phase transformation takes place in a martensitic manner, as in

FIG 2-2 › SEM after thermal etching of 3Y-TZP. 3 mol% yttria is the most common stabilizing oxide concentration to obtain the tetragonal shape. (Courtesy of CeramTec.)

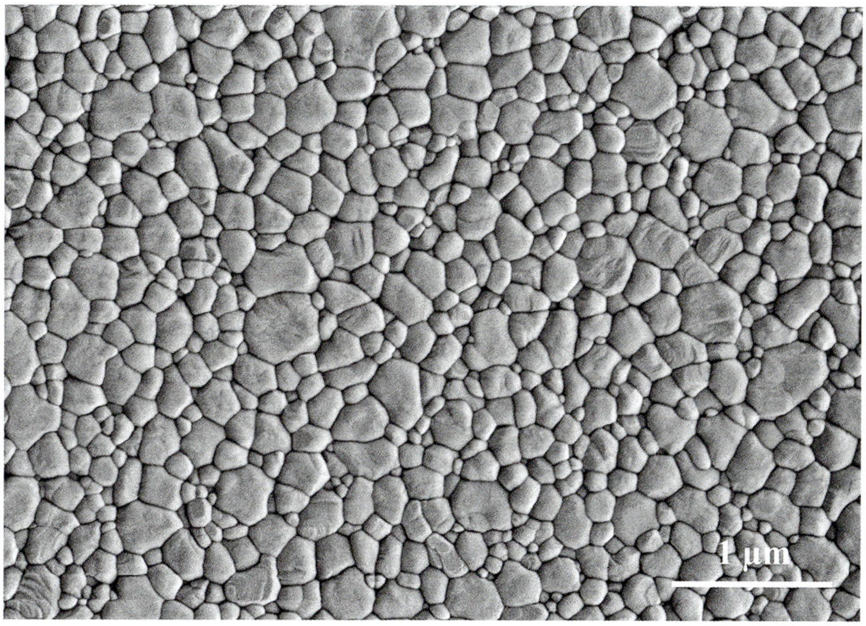

some steels. It manages to dissipate fracture energy by putting the crack under compression, stopping its propagation and thus preventing fracture of the ceramic component. There are several very accurate reviews of the models proposed to explain the mechanisms of transformation toughening in zirconia-containing ceramics, to which the reader may refer for details.[17–19]

Y-TZP is characterized by its white color, high strength, and toughness, making it the most suitable zirconia material for medical applications to date. The processing of Y-TZP also meets the industrial requirements of medical devices, and ZrO_2-Y_2O_3 has reached the status of having a dedicated ISO standard for surgical application.[20] Y-TZP was introduced to the medical market in 1990 for hip replacement femoral heads with the goal of reducing the fracture rate of the second-generation alumina femoral heads then in use.[21] That was also the first structural use of zirconia in medical devices. However, in the early 2000s, the orthopedic market moved toward a better solution, favoring ceramic composites of alumina with yttria-stabilized zirconia as a reinforcing phase.[22] Monolithic zirconia, on the other hand, is gaining ground in dental implantology. According to studies from the early 1990s, direct apposition of bone to zirconia is likely to occur without the interposition of fibrous tissue.[23]

Physics of Zirconia Phase Transformation Toughening

In nature, zirconia exists with three crystal structures—monoclinic, tetragonal, and cubic—depending on the temperature. Phase transition is diffusionless, meaning that it does not involve any transport of matter, and it is athermal, meaning that it does not occur at a specific temperature but takes place over a temperature range. Up to 1,170°C, the crystal lattice of zirconia is in the monoclinic phase. At higher temperatures but below 2,370°C, this oxide has the tetragonal structure. This is followed by the cubic form, which is maintained up to the melting temperature of 2,680°C. The phase transformations are reversible and involve a change in volume and shape based on differences in the crystal lattice. Thus, the cubic to tetragonal phase transition results in a volume change of 2.5% during cooling when the crystals are not constrained, whereas the phase transformation of technologic interest (ie, from the tetragonal to the monoclinic phase) occurs with a volume change of about 4% in a temperature range between 1,000°C and 1,200°C[24] (Fig 2-3). Both tetragonal and cubic grains can be maintained at room temperature with appropriate chemical stabilization. Many oxides have been studied as stabilizers for zirconia, but in biomedical applications, studies have focused on calcia (CaO), magnesia, ceria (CeO_2), and yttria. However, it is only the latter that has reached industrialization in medical technology.

The cause of tetragonal to monoclinic phase transformation toughening is the metastable nature of the chemically stabilized tetragonal grains at room temperature. When a crack advances in the material, the grains at the crack tip change from the tetragonal to the monoclinic phase due to a lack of constraint from adjacent grains. It follows that the grains in direct contact deform to accommodate the increase in volume of the transformed grain and the shear deformation. These microstructural changes then dissipate mechanical energy by slowing

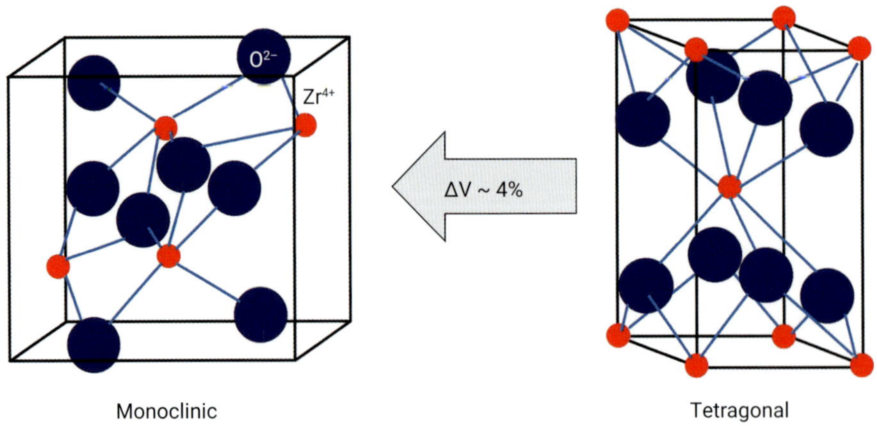

FIG 2-3 › The zirconia tetragonal to monoclinic phase transformation involves a reorientation of the ions within the crystal, with a density change from 6.1 g/cm^3 to 5.85 g/cm^3. The volume increase is about 4%, with about 7% shear distortion.

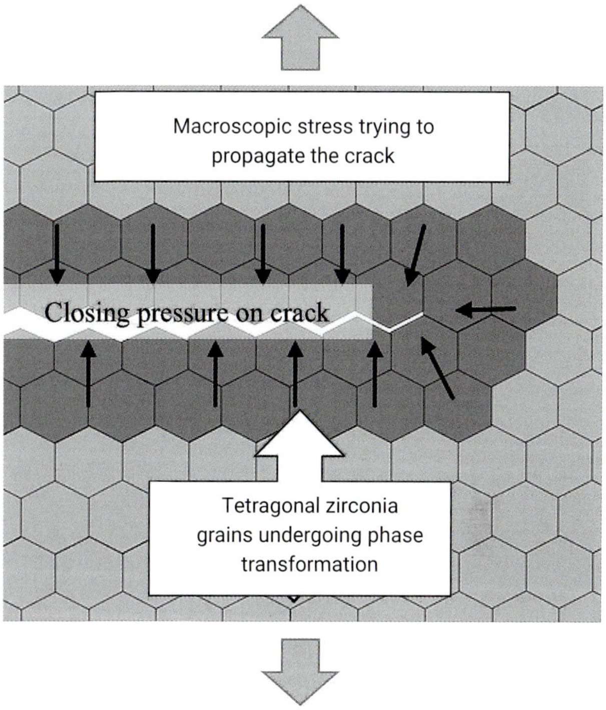

FIG 2-4 › Schematic representation of phase transformation toughening of zirconia. The metastable tetragonal grains of zirconia are transformed in the presence of stresses surrounding the crack tip. The volumetric expansion resulting from the lattice change sets the process zone on both sides of the crack under compressive stresses that impede crack propagation.

down the advance of the crack, which must overcome the compressive stress field due to volume expansion to advance further. At the microscopic level, this mechanism results in an increase in toughness at the macroscopic level (Fig 2-4).

Phase transformation effectiveness is conditioned by the maintenance of the metastable state of the tetragonal grains at room temperature. The contribution of phase transformation to mechanical properties depends on three main factors related to the design of the material, which therefore contribute to its ability to dissipate crack propagation energy[25]:

1. The concentration of the stabilizing oxide
2. The constraint exerted by the matrix on the grains
3. The size and shape of the grains and their homogeneous distribution

It follows that the balance between these characteristics must be carefully tailored during the material design phase. To achieve the desired "transformability" and mechanical properties, appropriate maintenance of the metastable nature of the material is required at the microstructural level. It should also be borne in mind that the same low-temperature degradation (LTD)—the spontaneous phase transformation that occurs over time at low temperatures and is not triggered mechanically—underlies the aging of tetragonal zirconia.[26] A balance must be struck between the best mechanical performance for clinical use and the avoidance of zirconia aging becoming clinically relevant over the lifetime of the medical product. Obviously, this balance must be engineered according to the requirements of the specific medical application. For example, it is pointless to overstabilize zirconia for fear of surface roughening if the latter does not play a role in the medical application under consideration, whereas an increase in toughness would allow for thinner geometries, which could benefit the patient. The best balance exploits the possibility of phase transformation toughening without exposing the material to the risks of aging. It follows that not only the design of the material must be optimized but also that the production process must be carefully monitored to ensure that the zirconia always behaves within the desired parameters.

Zirconia Processing for Medical Use

Just as we have seen that the zirconia material must be carefully tailored to take advantage of the tetragonal stabilized zirconia's metastable nature, it follows that meticulous control of the manufacturing process is equally important. History shows us that blunders in zirconia production can lead to extremely negative consequences.[26] In 1997, the United States Food and Drug Administration cautioned about the roughening of zirconia femoral heads after sterilization in an autoclave, which could potentially lead to increased wear of the polyethylene acetabular component.[27] The best-known case of poorly controlled zirconia metastability is the change in the sintering process of Saint Gobain Desmarquest femoral heads, which effectively brought an end to the use of monolithic zirconia in hip arthroplasty.[28,29] Between 1999 and 2000, a consistent number of patients required retreatment due to femoral head failure.[24–26,30] This event helped reinforce the critical role of manufacturing in the transformability of zirconia.

EFFECT OF SINTERING ON ZIRCONIA TRANSFORMABILITY

Sintering, also called *firing*, is the process of consolidating pressed ceramic powder into a single piece, resulting in a single solid mass of material. This process involves applying pressure and heat below the melting point of the material and is generally used for materials with high melting points. The transformability of tetragonal grains is linked closely to the sintering process, which is a critical step in producing yttria-stabilized zirconia because the sintering temperature influences the distribution of yttria, creating a gradient in the stabilization of the material and thus affecting its transformability. A local increase in yttria can lead to the formation of large cubic grains, whereas an yttria deficiency can lead to grains that are poorly stabilized and prone to aging. As might be expected, sintering also affects the kinetics of phase transformation.[31]

Because sintering plays a cardinal role in zirconia processing, it is logical to assume that the selection of raw materials and the preparation of the powders for shaping are important for the quality of the final ceramic component. Indeed, to achieve a homogeneous distribution of grain size and shape, the preparation of well-dispersed ceramic slurries with high powder purity and precise particle size distribution is crucial. Clearly, reproducibility of the process is vital, and all production of medical ceramic implants must be conducted in a controlled environment. First and foremost, it is necessary to avoid any kind of contamination that could affect the mechanical performance of the zirconia implant.

CRITICAL GRAIN SIZE

The optimal grain size for which the balance between the phase transformation and aging can be achieved is difficult to predict due to the various processing conditions employed to prepare Y-TZP and the amount of yttria stabilizer added during powder preparation. Indeed, it is possible to suppress phase transformation by reducing the grain size sufficiently. The grain size at which phase transformation is suppressed has been defined as the *critical grain size*[25,26,31] and is dependent on the properties of the starting powders (or *precursors*) and their processing.

The properties of the starting powders define their behavior along the processing routes, which allows for the achievement of the desired grain size distribution and homogeneity, as well as the avoidance of aggregates. The colloidal route is the most popular powder production method for ceramics in medicine at the industrial scale. The key to the colloidal process lies in the rheologic properties of the colloidal suspension. A colloidal suspension consists of microscopically dispersed insoluble particles suspended in a medium. Thus, the colloidal suspension must be kept homogeneous, well dispersed, and without agglomerates by controlling process parameters. For further details, refer to more technical reading.[32]

Sintering of ceramic powders at full density and obtaining the desired grain size is a technologic challenge. The full densification of ceramic powders requires high sintering temperatures, which usually result in large grain sizes. Several techniques have been proposed to overcome this problem. The most popular industrial-level technique is hot isostatic pressing (HIP), in which the material is subjected to both high temperature and isostatic gas pressure. This method is currently performed after sintering to produce both dental implants and ceramic bearings for arthroplasty. Obtaining fully dense pieces with preserved grain size improves the mechanical properties and reliability of ceramic implants.

Alumina-Toughened Zirconia

The phase transformation of yttria-stabilized zirconia can also be modulated with the help of alumina (Al_2O_3). Only a small amount, in the range of 0.15 wt% to 0.3 wt%, is useful to significantly improve resistance to aging. The anti-aging effect is thought to be due to the presence of alumina at the boundaries of the zirconia grains. Nevertheless, alumina and zirconia are immiscible, and consequently, two distinct phases are created when they are mixed together. In fact, increasing the alumina fraction above 10 vol% results in alumina-toughened zirconia (ATZ) ceramic composite.[31] However, the most common commercial composition includes 20 vol% of fine

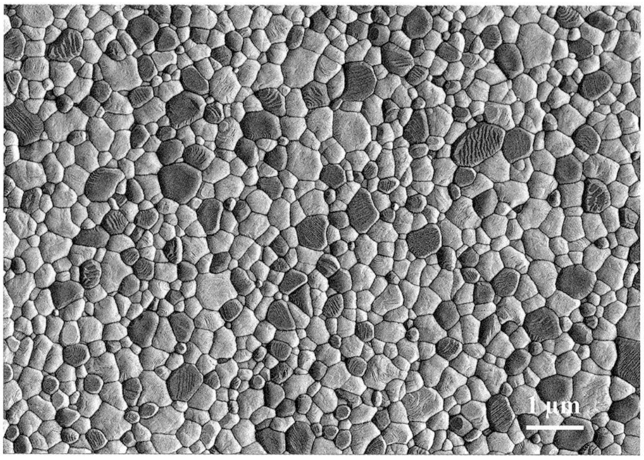

FIG 2-5 › SEM of ATZ after thermal etching. The fine alumina grains are dispersed in the yttria-stabilized zirconia matrix (3Y-TZP). (Courtesy of CeramTec.)

and homogeneously dispersed alumina grains in the zirconia matrix (Fig 2-5). The addition of the alumina phase results in a clear improvement in mechanical behavior when compared with pure yttria-stabilized zirconia, especially in terms of mechanical strength. This makes it advantageous for the production of two-piece dental implants and/or dental implants with small diameters. In addition, the high elastic modulus of alumina (about 380 GPa) increases the elastic stiffness of the ceramic matrix, further improving the material's resistance to aging. Toughness, on the other hand, is only marginally reduced.[24]

Zirconia Materials for CAD/CAM

Several changes have been introduced in the formulation of zirconia for CAD/CAM to improve its esthetics. Materials have been developed that consist of multiple layers with different pigments, a shade gradient, and translucency like that of natural teeth. Now CAD/CAM disks are available with layered composition and microstructure, giving the frameworks a gradual progression of shade and translucency. Colored zirconia is obtained by adding oxides to the ceramic powders or soaking the porous frameworks in salt solutions before firing to full density.[33] The concentration of alumina sintering additives has also been decreased while increasing the ceramic bulk density to improve material translucency.

To further enhance the optical properties of zirconia CAD/CAM materials for frameworks, the composition of Y-TZP was slightly changed to obtain the formation of cubic fully stabilized zirconia (FSZ) in the ceramic. High-purity forms of FSZ are used as gemstones because of their transparency, making them almost as bright as diamonds but with a much lower cost. Increasing the amount of yttria up to 5 mol% allows for obtaining the precipitation of a high amount (up to 50 wt%) of the non-birefringent cubic phase in 5Y-TZP ceramics, thus enhancing the translucency of the ceramic but with detrimental effects on mechanical properties. Namely, zirconia ceramics containing 50 wt% of cubic phase may have a strength much lower than that of 3Y-TZP.[34]

Conclusion

The expanded use of ceramics from bricks and tableware to medical applications took a century, and only discoveries in ceramic science and ceramic processing technology made it possible. After a brief appearance in orthopedics, zirconia has found its place in dental implantology, where its properties better meet the requirements of the application and it has achieved clinical results comparable with titanium implants, which are still considered the standard of care. Today, ceramic bearings are commonly used in everyday clinical practice in arthroplasty, and ceramic implants are gaining ground in dental implantology. The main player in this impressive technologic progress is zirconia. The phase transformation toughening of zirconia has radically changed the way we look at ceramics and has enabled its use in ways that were once unimaginable. The industrial use of zirconia has been possible only with advances in ceramic processing technology, the ability to precisely control the phase transformation of zirconia, and all the process variables that affect it. Maintaining the reproducibility of the process requires an in-depth knowledge of all the processing routes and production variables. It has taken some time, but zirconia is now ready for wider use in dentistry, and it is easy to imagine the presence of this material in all dental practices in the not-so-distant future.

References

1. Grupp TM, Holderied M, Mulliez MA, et al. Biotribology of a vitamin E-stabilized polyethylene for hip arthroplasty—Influence of artificial ageing and third-body particles on wear. Acta Biomater 2014;10:3068–3078.
2. Asif IM. Characterisation and biological impact of wear particles from composite ceramic hip replacements [thesis]. University of Leeds, 2018.
3. The National Joint Registry 18th Annual Report 2021. Surgical Data to 31 December 2020. National Joint Registry, 2021:1–376.
4. Australian Orthopaedic Association National Joint Replacement Registry: Hip, Knee & Shoulder Arthroplasty: 2021 Annual Report. https://aoanjrr.sahmri.com/en-US/annual-reports-2021. Accessed 16 May 2024.
5. American Joint Replacement Registry: 2021 Annual Report. American Academy of Orthopaedic Surgeons, 2021.
6. The German Arthroplasty Registry (EPRD): Annual Report 2021. German Society for Orthopaedics and Orthopaedic Surgery, 2021:1–193.
7. de Medeiros RA, Vechiato-Filho AJ, Pellizzer EP, Mazaro JV, dos Santos DM, Goiato MC. Analysis of the peri-implant soft tissues in contact with zirconia abutments: An evidence-based literature review. J Contemp Dent Pract 2013;14:567–572.
8. Oshida Y, Tuna EB, Aktören O, Gençay K. Dental implant systems. Int J Mol Sci 2010;11:1580–1678.
9. Cionca N, Hashim D, Mombelli A. Zirconia dental implants: Where are we now, and where are we heading? Periodontol 2000 2017;73:241–258.
10. Garvie RC, Hannink RHJ, Pascoe RT. Ceramic steel? Nature 1975;258:703–704.
11. Gupta TK, Bechtold JH, Kuznicki RC, Cadoff LH, Rossing BR. Stabilization of tetragonal phase in polycrystalline zirconia. J Mater Sci 1977;12:2421–2426.
12. Nielsen RH, Schlewitz JH, Nielsen H. Zirconium and zirconium compounds. In: Kirk-Othmer (ed). Encyclopedia of Chemical Technology, vol 26. Wiley, 2013:621–664.
13. Audley JA. The use of zirconia as a refractory material. Nature 1917;99:375–376.
14. Ruff O, Ebert F, Stephen E. Contributions to the ceramics of highly refractory materials: II, System Zirconia-Lime. Z Anorg Allg Chem 1929;180:215–224.
15. Passerini L. Isomorphism among oxides of different tetravalent metals: CeO2-ThO2; CeO2-ZrO2; CeO2-HfO2. Gazz Chim Ital 1939;60:762–776.
16. Rieth PH, Reed JS, Naumann AW. Fabrication and flexural strength of ultra-fine grained yttria-stabilised zirconia. Bull Am Ceram Soc 1976;55:717.

17. Lange FF. Transformation toughening—Part 1-4. J Mater Sci 1982;17:225–263.
18. Becher PF, Francis Rose LR. Toughening mechanisms in ceramic systems. In: Swain MV (ed). Structure and Properties of Ceramics. Materials Science and Technology, vol 11. VCH, 1994:409–461.
19. Hannink RHJ, Kelly PM, Muddle BC. Transformation toughening in zirconia-containing ceramics. J Am Ceram Soc 2000;83:461–487.
20. ISO 13356:2015 Implants for surgery—Ceramic materials based on yttria-stabilized tetragonal zirconia (Y-TZP), ed 3. International Organization for Standardization, 2015.
21. Christel P, Meunier A, Dorlot JM, et al. Biomechanical compatibility and design of ceramic implants for orthopedic surgery. Bioceramics: Material characteristics versus in vivo behavior. Ann N Y Acad Sci 1988;523:234–256.
22. Porporati AA, Piconi C, Mettang M, Deisinger U, Reinhardt C, Pitto R. Ceramics for artificial joints: The relevance of material biocompatibility. In: Osaka A, Narayan R (eds). Bioceramics: From Macro to Nanoscale. Elsevier, 2021:263–295.
23. Miani C, Piconi C, Piselli D, Ponti M. Prove sperimentali in vivo della zirconia in implantologia orale. Riv Ital Osseoint 1994;106:605–614.
24. Piconi C, Porporati AA. Bioinert ceramics: Zirconia and alumina. In: Antoniac I (ed.) Handbook of Bioceramics and Biocomposites, vol 1. Springer, 2016:59–90.
25. Lughi V, Sergo V. Low temperature degradation—aging—of zirconia: A critical review of the relevant aspects in dentistry. Dent Mater 2010;26:807–820.
26. Chevalier J, Gremillard L, Deville S. Low-temperature degradation of zirconia and implications for biomedical implants. Annu Rev Mater Res 2007;37:1–32.
27. Steam re-sterilization causes deterioration of zirconia ceramic heads of total hip prostheses. US Food and Drug Administration, 1997.
28. Recall of zirconia ceramic femoral heads for hip implants. US Food and Drug Administration, 2001.
29. Piconi C, Maccauro G, Pilloni L, Burger W, Muratori F, Richter HG. On the fracture of a zirconia ball head. J Mater Sci Mater Med 2006;17:289–300.
30. Chevalier J. What future for zirconia as a biomaterial? Biomaterials 2006;27:535–543.
31. Ramesh S, Sara Lee KY, Tan CY. A review on the hydrothermal ageing behaviour of Y-TZP ceramics. Ceram Int 2018;44:20620–20634.
32. Pugh RJ, Bergström L. Surface and Colloid Chemistry in Advanced Ceramics Processing. CRC Press, 2019:1–376.
33. Calés B. Colored zirconia ceramics for dental applications. In: LeGeros LZ, LeGeros JP (eds). Bioceramics, vol 11. World Scientific Publishing, 1998:591–594.
34. Zhang Y, Lawn BR. Novel zirconia materials in dentistry. J Dent Res 2018;97:140–147.

03

RELIABILITY, LONG-TERM BEHAVIOR, AND MECHANICAL PROPERTIES OF ZIRCONIA CERAMICS

Jérôme Chevalier and Corrado Piconi

Ceramics are brittle at room temperature, generally failing under high stresses and low strains before any signs of plasticity. They also exhibit a much greater scatter in strength values than is found with metals. Therefore, statistical approaches to failure analysis and the careful control of processing defects are required to avoid premature fractures. The principles of fracture mechanics are generally employed when dealing with the mechanical behavior of brittle materials such as glasses, ceramics, and even some metals. Although the foundations of fracture mechanics are outside the scope of this chapter, we describe some of the basics, and curious readers can consult the key references.[1–3] In addition to helping us understand the mechanical behavior of ceramics, fracture mechanics explain the benefits of phase transformation toughening and transformation-induced plasticity in zirconia, which place these materials at the forefront of damage tolerance and crack resistance.

When dealing with implants, the risk of both immediate and delayed failure must be considered. Ceramics are less sensitive to fatigue than metals because fatigue is generally associated with dislocation-related plasticity and crack growth at stresses lower than the apparent (ie, macroscopic) elastic limit. (In a crystal lattice structure, *dislocation activity* refers to a row of misaligned atoms [ie, a line defect] that glides in response to shear stresses, resulting in plasticity.) Oxide ceramics, however, are sensitive to slow crack propagation caused by water-induced stress corrosion. Tetragonal to monoclinic phase transformation increases the toughness and reliability of zirconia, making it one of the most attractive ceramic materials for use in dental implantology. However, it has been shown that yttria-stabilized zirconia—the preferred zirconia ceramic for dental applications because of its high strength—is susceptible to spontaneous slow phase transformation at its surface in the presence of water. This phenomenon is often referred to as *aging* or *low-temperature degradation* (LTD), and it can lead to progressive surface degradation, including roughening and microcracking. In the worst cases, it will lead to failure. It is noteworthy, however, that the only cases in which LTD has caused problems with biomedical implants were associated with insufficient control of factors related to microstructural aging resistance during the ceramic production process.

In this chapter the basics of fracture mechanics are presented to help the reader understand the meaning of fracture toughness and the need for controlling defects throughout the processing of ceramic implants. The physical mechanisms behind slow crack growth (SCG), which are important for avoiding delayed failure in zirconia implants, are explained, along with the main features of LTD and how it can occur even at body temperature. The execution and analysis of the mechanical tests typically conducted in ceramic materials are discussed, and the chapter concludes with several case studies to underscore the key role of ceramic processing parameters in extending the life of zirconia implants.

Crack Propagation in Ceramics

Ceramics are sensitive to stress concentrations around preexisting small defects, including pores, scratches, and cracks. Under an applied macroscopic tensile stress, the local stresses around a preexisting defect or crack can be much higher than the applied macroscopic stress. Figure 3-1 shows a finite element analysis (FEA) simulation of stress concentrations around a spherical defect and crack, showing that preexisting internal cracks are much more detrimental than inclusions or pores and exhibit higher local stresses. The stress field at the tip of a crack of size *c* can be well described by the stress intensity factor K_I, which is given by the following equation, where s represents the applied tensile stress[1–3]:

$$K_I = \sigma \times \sqrt{\pi \times c}$$

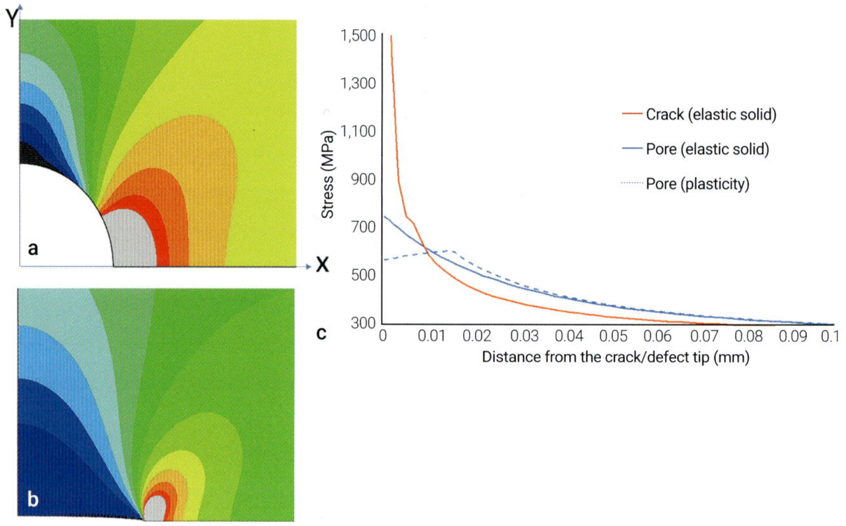

FIG 3-1 › FEA simulations of the local stresses around a spherical pore with a diameter of 200 microns *(a)* and a crack of the same length *(b)* in a purely elastic solid. For calculation purposes, only a quarter of the system is modeled. *(c)* Stress evolution as a function of the distance to the crack tip in the case of a spherical pore and a crack in a purely elastic (ceramic) material and a pore in the case of an elastic-plastic (metallic) material exhibiting an elastic limit of 500 MPa (von Mises criteria used for plasticity in the simulation). It is shown that stresses are more concentrated in the case of a crack and reach higher values. Thus, a crack is more critical than a spherical defect. It is also evident that plasticity limits stresses in metallic materials, leading to a reduced risk of brittle fracture.

K_I represents the intensity of the local stresses at the crack tip. When K_I reaches a critical value (K_{IC}), crack propagation and failure occur. The fracture strength (σ_R) of a brittle material in the presence of a defect of size *c* is given by the following equation:

$$\sigma_R = \frac{K_{IC}}{\sqrt{\pi \times c}}$$

Thus, fracture strength can be increased by increasing K_{IC} (toughness) and decreasing defect size.

The K_{IC} of ceramics is generally lower than that of metals because there is little to no plasticity occurring at the crack tip to dissipate the mechanical energy exerted by external forces. Plasticity also helps limit the local stresses at the crack tip, leading to reduced stress concentration (see Fig 3-1). The extent of plastic deformation (d_y), often called the *process zone*, is related to the yield stress (σ_y), or *elastic limit*, and the toughness of the material according to the following equation[4]:

$$d_y = \frac{{K_{IC}}^2}{\pi \times {\sigma_Y}^2}$$

This equation is logical; the lower the yield stress of a material is, the greater is its propensity to plasticity and the larger the size of the plastic zone. In other words, because ceramics have a much higher yield stress than most metals due to their ionic/covalent nature, they exhibit far less plasticity at the crack tip and

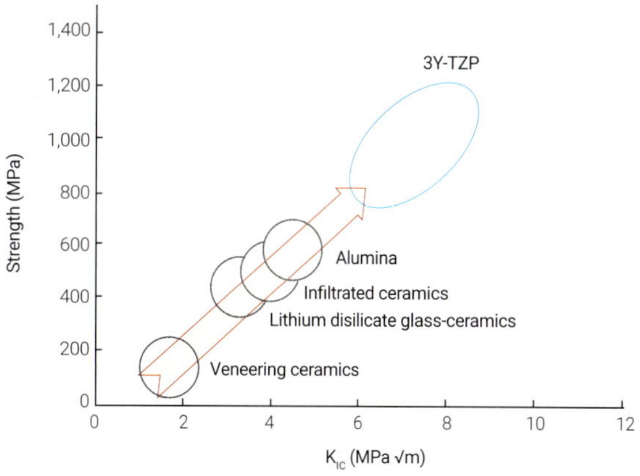

FIG 3-2 › Fracture toughness and strength values (maximum reachable stress) for different ceramics used in the dental field.

thus reduced toughness. On the other hand, stress concentration occurring at the crack tip has the capacity to trigger tetragonal to monoclinic phase transformation (see chapter 2), which can function as a mechanism to hinder crack propagation and increase toughness. Figure 3-2 shows that zirconia ceramics are indeed the ceramic materials used in dentistry with the highest value of K_{IC}—and thus the highest strength.

The size of the transformation zone depends on alloying (determined by the type and content of the stabilizer that is used) and grain size, as shown in Fig 3-3, where the size of the transformation zone is highlighted for different zirconia-based ceramics.[5,6] Some zirconia ceramics with a high yttria content (up to 6 mol% yttria instead of 3 mol%) are used for dental restorations because of their translucency. These zirconia grades do not demonstrate any phase transformation at the crack tip and thus exhibit reduced toughness. Thus, not all zirconia ceramics are the same, and zirconia must be considered as a large family of materials with varying properties that can answer different needs (eg, high resistance to loads, translucency) depending on the application. Only zirconia grades that show transformation at the crack tip can exhibit high toughness, which is necessary for dental implants and abutments.[5]

Because ceramics have little plasticity, they tend to exhibit scattered strength values. Fractures occur due to preexisting defects (eg, pores, cracks, inclusions) of varying size, orientation, and location within the material, resulting in variations in measured strengths. Metals, on the other hand, generally exhibit far less strength dispersion, with the maximum sustainable stress related to the onset and propagation of plasticity (ie, yield stress). Thus, scatter in strength values must absolutely be reported when testing ceramic materials because it gives hints about the dispersion of defects and thus the robustness of the production process. The Weibull distribution is the best statistical tool for describing strength

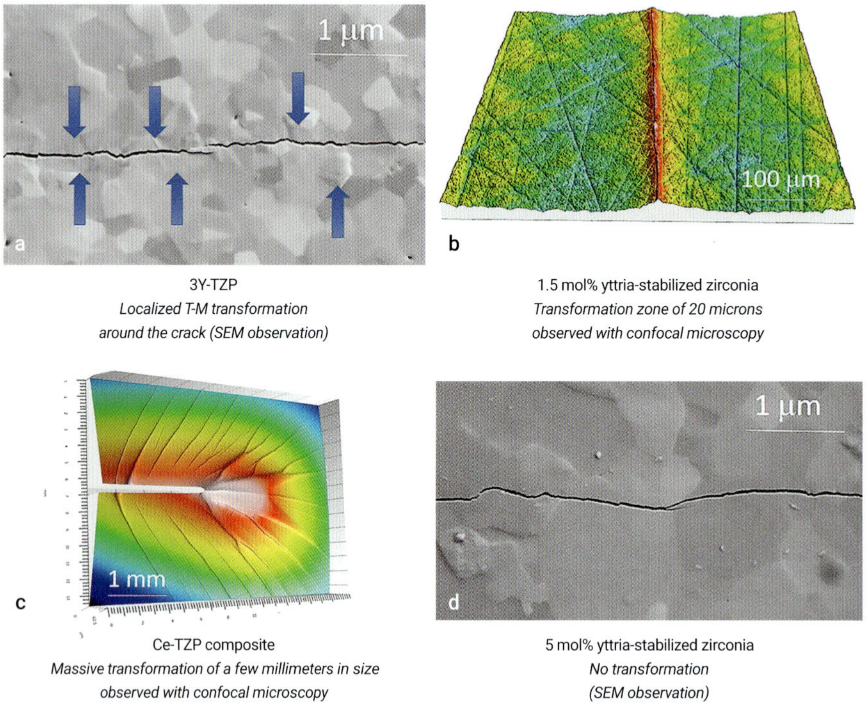

FIG 3-3 › Transformation zones in three zirconia ceramics. *(a)* In 3 mol% yttria-stabilized zirconia polycrystal (3Y-TZP), which is generally used for dental restorations and implants, there are few grains transformed near the crack tip. *(b)* Transformation zone of 20 microns in 1.5 mol% yttria-stabilized zirconia. *(c)* A transformation zone reaching several millimeters in a ceria-stabilized tetragonal zirconia polycrystal (Ce-TZP) composite. *(d)* Crack propagation in a 5 mol% yttria-stabilized zirconia used for dental restoration with no transformation toughening.

dispersion in ceramics[7] through the Weibull modulus (*m*), as described later in this chapter. Briefly, the larger the Weibull modulus is, the lower the dispersion in strength and the lower the effect of material volume on strength.

The value of the Weibull modulus is not characteristic of any particular type of ceramic. Instead, it provides a picture of the manufacturing process–related defect variations in the specific sample or product. It can range from values as low as 5 to values exceeding 15 for 3 mol% yttria-stabilized zirconia polycrystal (3Y-TZP), depending on the manufacturing process. Additive manufacturing, for example, still presents a challenge and results in lower values than those achieved with conventional ceramic technologies.[8,9] Extremely high Weibull modulus values have been obtained with zirconia ceramics that exhibit macroscopic and generalized transformation-induced plasticity before failure, like in metals, because the maximum sustainable stress is linked to the onset of transformation (ie, the elastic limit in metals).[6]

Slow Crack Growth, Fatigue, and Delayed Failure

K_{IC} is the basis of theories on fracture mechanics in brittle materials. However, it is now widely recognized that failure of ceramics and glasses can occur even when stresses are under K_{IC} (or σ_R). K_{IC} actually represents a critical level for fast crack growth, but ceramic materials may also be susceptible to slow crack propagation at stress intensity values less than K_{IC}. In terms of applied stresses, this means there is potential for delayed failure at stress values lower than that required for fast fracture. This phenomenon is often referred as *slow crack growth* (SCG) or *subcritical crack growth*. SCG is notable for its sensitivity to applied loads, and it tends to depend on the concentration of environmental chemical species, temperature, and other environmental variables.[1,2] Under the appropriate conditions, cracks can continue growing slowly for some time before eventually causing fracture.

As a general trend, SCG is described based on a crack velocity (V) versus stress intensity factor (K_I) diagram. SCG in ceramics is attributed to stress and corrosion at the crack tip or any preexisting defect in the ceramic. This is the combined effect of high stresses at the crack tip and the presence of water molecules that induce slow crack propagation. Figure 3-4 demonstrates the mechanism of stress-assisted corrosion by water molecules in zirconia. As is true of all oxide ceramics, zirconia is prone to reactions with polar water molecules because of its ionic bonding nature. This is in contrast with covalent ceramics such as silicon carbide (SiC) or silicon nitride (Si_3N_4), which are not sensitive to stress-assisted water corrosion.

The threshold of the stress intensity factor under which no crack propagation occurs (K_{I0}) has been the subject of important research in ceramics, especially for applications in which delayed failure must be absolutely avoided, as is the case with biomedical implants.[10] For ceramic implants, this threshold determines

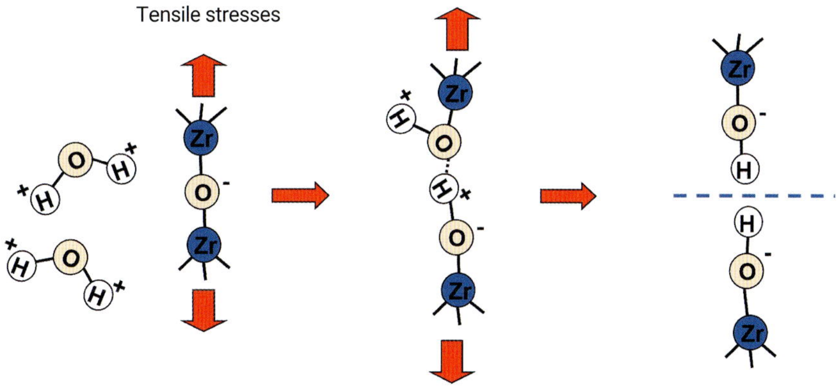

FIG 3-4 › Schematic representation of the proposed reaction between water and a strained Zr–O–Zr bond at the crack tip, which explains SCG. Reaction steps involve *(1)* adsorption of water to the Zr–O bond, *(2)* a reaction involving simultaneous proton and electron transfers, and *(3)* formation of surface hydroxyls.

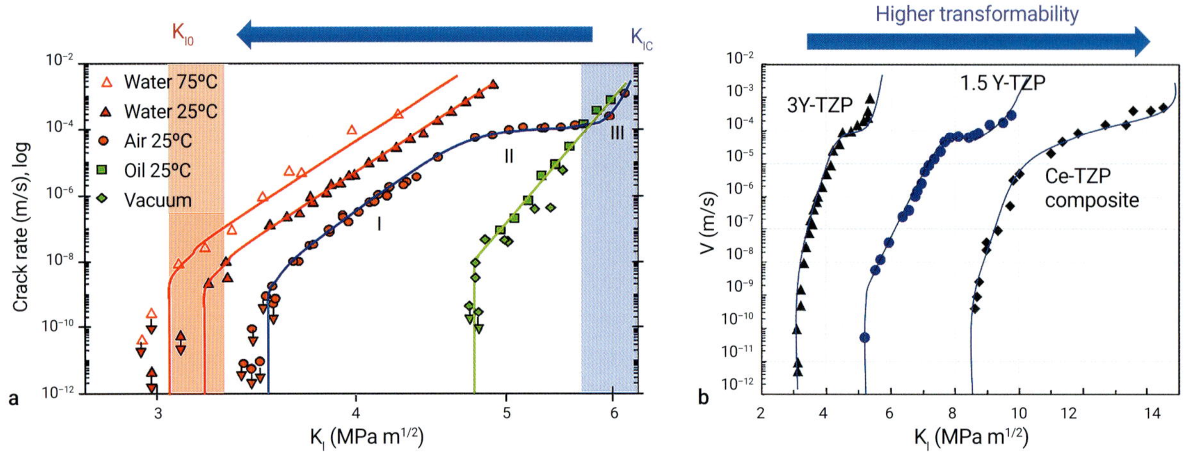

FIG 3-5 › *(a)* Overall *V* to K_I curves for 3Y-TZP ceramics in different environments. *(b)* The *V* to K_I curves of three zirconia-based materials with various transformation toughening capacities.

the safe range of use. The higher this threshold is, the higher the reliability of the ceramic and the longer its lifetime.

Figure 3-5 shows the overall crack velocity (*V*) versus K_I curve in 3Y-TZP in different environments, including the three propagation stages and the stress intensity threshold. The three propagation stages are linked to *(1)* limitation of the crack growth rate by the reaction rate between water and the zirconia bonds at the crack tip (the higher K_I is, the faster the reaction rate); *(2)* the diffusion of water-derived chemical species toward the crack tip (when the crack rate is rapid [in air, for example], the diffusion of water becomes the limiting mechanism); and *(3)* propagation without the need for stress-assisted corrosion (fast propagation for K_I reaching K_{IC}).

Figure 3-5 also shows the beneficial effect of transformation toughening in shifting the overall *V to* K_I curves to higher K_I values. For example, decreasing the yttria content in Y-TZP (or alternatively increasing the grain size) leads to greater K_{IC} and K_{I0} values. The case of ceria-stabilized zirconia is again interesting because the resulting transformation zones can be very large, leading to threshold stress intensity factors greater than those of Y-TZP ceramics. Biocomponents should be designed to work at stresses under the threshold stress intensity factor, because at stress values within the range of zones I to III (see Fig 3-5a), delayed fracture will eventually occur, generally in less than 1 month. A crack rate of 10^{-9} m/s might seem slow but correlates to a propagation rate of almost 90 microns a day!

The curves presented in Fig 3-5 were obtained under constant loading. Fatigue due to alternate loading was thought to be irrelevant in ceramics before the 1990s, and its significance was brought to light mainly thanks to the works of Ritchie and Dauskardt.[11] It was once thought that fatigue crack growth could be

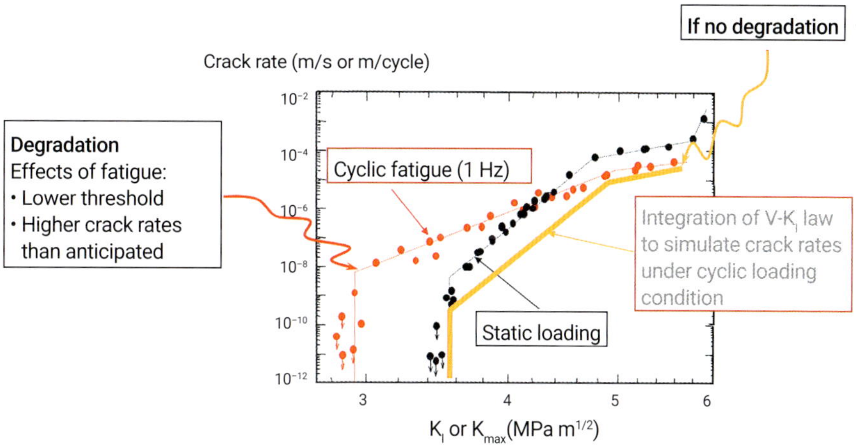

FIG 3-6 › Fatigue crack growth of zirconia. Note the lower threshold and the higher crack rates under cyclic conditions compared with the values calculated based on SCG curves obtained under static loading.

directly extrapolated from SCG laws obtained under static loading conditions. In fact, although the relevance of fatigue is limited in ceramics and glasses because there is little to no plasticity at ambient temperature, there is a slight but measurable increase in crack growth rate under fatigue conditions compared with conditions of constant stress. Thus in practical terms, under the same maximal stresses, the K_{I0} threshold under fatigue is generally lower than the one measured under constant stress. This is illustrated in Fig 3-6, where the fatigue threshold is significantly lower for a 3Y-TZP than the constant loading threshold (and the crack rates are higher for a given K_I above K_{I0}).[10]

The reasons for reduced crack resistance under fatigue have been discussed in a series of papers and are related to the degradation of transformation toughening under fatigue. In any case, this phenomenon means that zirconia ceramics must be tested in the presence of water and under fatigue to capture all the features of SCG that could occur in the presence of body fluids and under varying stress conditions.

Low-Temperature Degradation

Water can trigger tetragonal to monoclinic phase transformation at the surface of zirconia. This is especially true and well documented in the case of Y-TZP.[12–15] In contrast with the beneficial tetragonal to monoclinic transformation in the vicinity of a propagating crack, tetragonal to monoclinic transformation at the surface in the presence of water may lead to degradation of the material's properties. The mechanism by which the presence of moisture leads to a transformation of Y-TZP is not yet fully understood. The favored hypothesis is that the filling of oxygen vacancies by water-derived species (hydroxyl, oxygen, or hydrogen ions) probably leads to destabilization of the tetragonal structure—initially stabilized by yttrium ions in the case of Y-TZP—and an accumulation of internal tensile stresses in the grains in contact with the water, caused by a decrease in lattice parameters. The diffusion of water-derived chemical species from the surface thus leads to a progressive change in the stability of the tetragonal grains. Metastable tetragonal grains at the surface become unstable and transform to the monoclinic phase after a certain exposure time. The increase in volume that accompanies phase transformation results in a surface uplift and large stresses that can promote crack formation along the grain boundaries, as well as the transformation of surrounding grains. The main features of this hypothesis are illustrated in Fig 3-7.

The nucleation and growth of monoclinic spots on tetragonal zirconia surfaces exposed to water can be observed with techniques such as optical interferometry and atomic force microscopy (AFM). Scanning electron microscopy (SEM) shows that the phase transformation starts at the surface and then extends further into the material.[13] Aging kinetics can be characterized by quantifying the extent of monoclinic phase transformation at the zirconia surface versus time, using techniques such as x-ray diffraction or Raman spectroscopy.

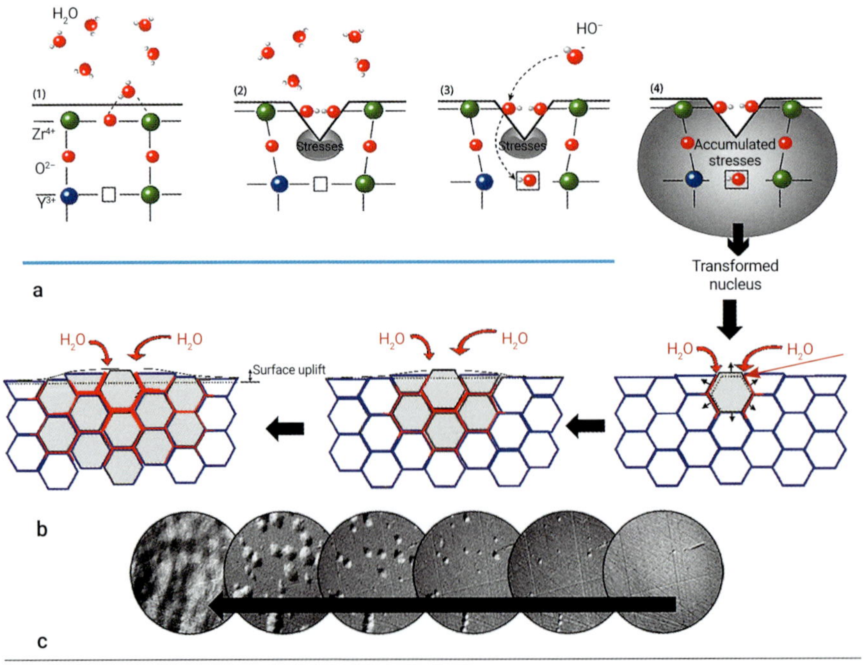

FIG 3-7 › Main features of the aging mechanism, often referred to as *LTD*, in Y-TZP. *(a)* Filling of oxygen vacancies by water-derived chemical species and destabilization of the tetragonal phase. *(b)* Transformation extension from grain to grain by a nucleation-growth mechanism. *(c)* Sequence of optical microscopy images taken at the surface of polished samples after aging in an autoclave, showing progressive surface roughening.

LTD KINETICS IN Y-TZP

Results obtained to date show that LTD kinetics in Y-TZP can often be fit with the standard Mehl-Avrami-Johnson (MAJ) equation for a nucleation and growth process, where f_m is the fraction of tetragonal phase that has transformed to the monoclinic phase; t is the time of exposure to moisture; n is a value between 0.5 and 4, depending on the microstructural features of the material; and b is a constant depending on the microstructural features of the material and the temperature[13,16]:

$$f_m = 1 - \exp(-(bt)^n)$$

The nucleation-growth mechanism of LTD is related to the fact that it starts sporadically at grains that are depleted in yttrium, and/or larger than average, and/or under stresses and then propagates to neighboring grains, as was shown in Fig 3-7.

For 3Y-TZP, aging occurs most quickly at temperatures around 250°C. At temperatures that are sufficiently lower (say below 150°C), the phenomenon is thermally activated, and the value of b in the following equation follows the Arrhenius law, where b_0 is a constant, Q is the apparent activation energy, R is the gas constant, and T is the absolute temperature (in K):

$$b = b_0 \exp\left(-\frac{Q}{RT}\right)$$

The reported activation energies are approximately 100 kJ/mol, which is similar to the activation energy for oxygen vacancy diffusion extrapolated from higher temperatures. Values of activation energies reported in the literature can differ significantly (from 60 to 110 kJ/mol). This makes it difficult to extrapolate data on aging performed at high temperatures (eg, in an autoclave) to aging processes that occur at body temperature.[14] It is widely considered that 1 hour of autoclaving at 134°C in steam is roughly equivalent to 1 to 4 years of aging at 37°C (based on research performed on a particular 3Y-TZP[13]). This can be used as a tool for obtaining rough estimates of the aging sensibility of a given zirconia material in an in vivo situation. However, activation energy should be measured for any Y-TZP–containing material under consideration to obtain more precise estimates. Kinetics extrapolated from high-temperature treatments are highly dependent on the accuracy of the measured activation energy and may differ from one material to another.[14]

Again, aging kinetics are the most rapid at around 250°C. Time-temperature plots of experimental data obtained at different temperatures show that transformation kinetics form C-shaped curves. This behavior is interpreted in terms of a balance between the driving force for tetragonal to monoclinic phase transformation, which is increased at lower temperatures, and the growth rate, which is decreased at lower temperatures due to reduced water-diffusion kinetics.[17] At sufficiently low temperatures (well below 250°C), the Arrhenius law allows us to make rough predictions about kinetics at 37°C based on values obtained at higher temperatures (eg, via autoclaving at 134°C).

Although hydrothermal aging was discovered in the early 1980s, its influence on the durability of biomedical implants was neglected until the early 2000s, when a series of fractures in zirconia orthopedic ball heads occurred several months after implantation. These failures were later determined to have been caused by accelerated aging of balls that were not sufficiently densified during sintering due to a change in furnace technology.[13,17,18] There is less documentation on the processing of dental devices, but there is evidence that specific processing or surface modifications might promote aging in dental-grade zirconia.[19] Aging has also been reported in implants and restorations processed under "normal" conditions.[20,21]

Mechanical Tests on Zirconia

The elastic modulus and tensile strength of a ceramic device are undoubtedly among its most important mechanical properties. It is these two factors that are often considered and compared when various materials are available.

The tensile strength tests used for metallic materials are not suitable for ceramics. Machining on hourglass-shaped specimens, as is done when testing metal alloys, would be a complex operation with ceramic specimens. Thus, mechanical tests on ceramics are carried out with specimens shaped like bars or disks of various geometries. The tests are classified as uniaxial or biaxial depending on the way loading is applied to the specimen, and the stresses are calculated by algorithms depending on the specific test.

Remember, fracture in ceramics is caused by the propagation of preexisting defects—pores, inclusions, and intrinsic microdefects—within the crystalline structure of the material. Ceramics are tested in tension because tensile stress is the most critical parameter in these materials. The tensile stress that leads to failure in ceramics is about 10 times lower than the fracture stress measured in compression. The fracture stress value is dependent on the probability that there is a defect within the mass of the tested specimen that can propagate applied stresses and lead to failure. Thus, the larger the volume of material under stress, the higher the probability of it having a defect and the lower its strength. Consequently, data must be obtained via a suitable number of tests on the same material to increase the total volume tested and then undergo statistical analysis using Weibull algorithms.

UNIAXIAL BENDING TESTS

Uniaxial bending tests are carried out using beam-shaped specimens with a rectangular cross section that are tested in either a three-point or four-point bending configuration (Fig 3-8). The European reference standard for both tests is EN 843.[23] A tensile stress is applied to the bottom surface of the beam, which activates the propagation of defects on the surface, eventually resulting in failure. The four-point bending test is more severe because a greater volume of material is subjected to the maximum stress. In other words, the probability that the applied

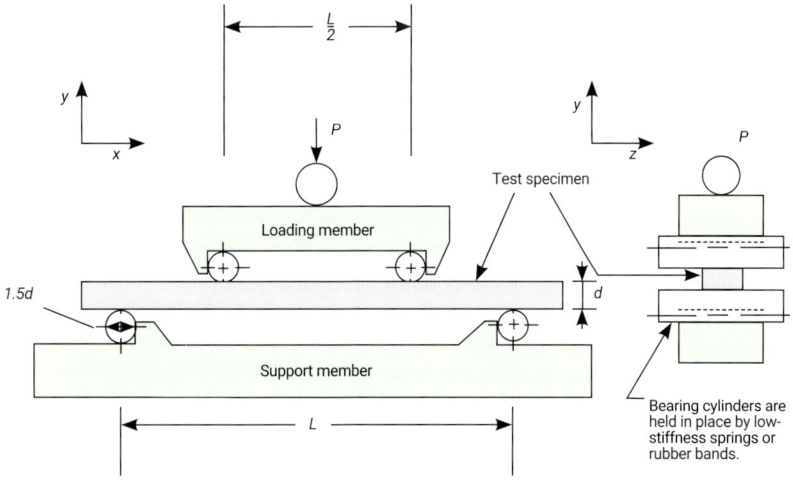

FIG 3-8 › The test rig configuration for a four-point bending test.[22]

stress will activate a defect is higher because the probability that a defect is present in the stressed volume is higher. For this reason, bending strength values measured with the four-point test are systematically lower than those measured with the three-point test. The strength value that is measured is thus influenced by the dimensions of the specimen (ie, the volume under tension). If test results are to be compared, the mode of testing, whether three-point or four-point, and the dimensions of the test specimens must be considered.

BIAXIAL BENDING TESTS

Biaxial bending tests can be carried out under various configurations: piston-on-three balls, piston-on-ring, ball-on-ring, and ring-on-ring tests. The piston-on-three balls configuration is common for ceramics used in dentistry because the flat disk specimens used in this test are much easier and cheaper to produce than the bars used in uniaxial bending tests. In addition, this test configuration is reported in ISO 6872[24] for materials used to fabricate crowns, veneers, and inlays and onlays. Finally, the main tensile stress is found at the center of the tensile side. Thus, the quality of machining at the disk border does not affect the measured strength value.

ISO 6872 prescribes the use of ceramic disks with a diameter of 12 to 16 mm and a thickness of 1.2 mm placed on three 3.2-mm-diameter spheres at 120 degrees to each other on a 10- to 12-mm-diameter circumference. The load is applied in a central position by means of a flat punch with a diameter of 1.2 to 1.6 mm. Because the volume of the specimen that is under tensile stress is very small in comparison to the volume that is stressed in four-point flexural tests, greater strengths are measured.

CAUSES OF ERROR IN BENDING TESTS

The results of bending tests can be affected by several variables, including how the test is conducted and the preparation of the specimens. Testing machines induce deformation in the specimen via mutual displacement of the loading beams, and the strain rate is an important testing parameter. Increasing strain rates gives rise to increasing values of flexural strength, and therefore the test must be performed according to the parameters set by the technical standards for the chosen test geometry.

The way the specimen is connected to the machine is also an element that must be given the utmost consideration. The design and construction of support systems is critical because these components ensure the proper transfer of loads from the testing machine to the specimen being tested. Errors in the design or construction of support systems can cause systematic errors in the test. Friction between the components of support systems is a frequent source of error in stress measurement.

Another critical element is the fabrication of the specimens, particularly the surface finish that is used. The surface finish is relevant because the maximum tensile stress that causes failure of the specimen is localized to its surface. Only if machining is performed carefully is it possible for the fracture to be triggered by natural defects in the material. Special care is required when machining specimens of metastable materials, such as zirconia, because if performed improperly, the surface state of the material could be altered due to tetragonal to monoclinic phase transformation. The measured results would be affected by surface compressive stresses that could abnormally increase flexural strength. Moreover, chipping of the specimen edges affects the fracture stress.

Statistical Distribution of Flexural Strength in Ceramics

Ceramics generally fracture before any sign of plasticity, which leads to a statistical dispersion of strength. This is the case for most ceramics. Fracture occurs due to preexisting defects in the ceramic material that vary in size, orientation, and location, and activating one of these defects (ie, the “critical defect”) is much like breaking a chain by fracturing its weakest link. This means that the strength values measured throughout a specific ceramic will vary, whereas metals generally exhibit far less dispersion in strength values because the maximum sustainable stress is related to the onset and propagation of plasticity. The scattering in strength values when testing ceramic materials must be reported because it gives hints about the dispersion of defects and thus the robustness of the process.

Because the distribution of defects in the structure of a ceramic is not random as in metallic materials but asymmetric because it depends on the manufacturing process, there is a probability that ceramic pieces can fracture even at stresses much lower than the average fracture stress. In other words, there is a finite probability that for each test stress a given number of pieces will survive. This concept was developed mathematically by Weibull,[7] who devised a method that allows for determining the probability that a part of a given volume will fail when subjected to a given level of stress.[25] This method treats the breaking strength of a set of specimens of well-defined geometry brought to failure with uniaxial stress as a random variable.

The practical value of data processing with Weibull statistics is the capacity to determine the value of bending strength that corresponds with a determined probability of failure. Its fundamental assumption is the weakest link hypothesis: The sample fails if its weakest volume element breaks.

Weibull statistics defines the *survival probability* $P_S(V_0)$ as the number of samples of equal volume (V_0) that survive a stress (σ), which can be represented by the following equation, where P_f is the fracture probability:

$$P_S(V_0) = 1 - P_f$$

Obviously, when the stress is zero ($\sigma = 0$), 100% of the samples will pass the test ($P_f = 0$), and thus the probability of survival is total [$P_S(V_0) = 1$].

In its simplest form, for a uniaxial homogenous tensile stress (σ) and volume (V), the Weibull cumulative probability function can be written as follows:

$$P_f = 1 - exp\left[-\frac{V}{V_0} \times \left(\frac{\sigma - \sigma_S}{\sigma_0}\right)^m\right]$$

P_f is thus the probability of fracture for a given applied stress σ. In this equation (often called the *three-parameter strength distribution*), σ_s represents the threshold strength below which there is no risk of failure at all, σ_0 is the Weibull characteristic strength (for which the probability of failure is 63%), and m is the Weibull modulus. V is the volume of the material, and V_0 is a scale parameter.

The greater the Weibull modulus is, the lower the strength dispersion in a material is, which makes this parameter an important figure to consider when evaluating the process quality. It is quite straightforward that the larger the sample or product dimensions are, the more defects are likely to be present in the ceramic and the higher the risk of failure under a given stress.

The no-risk of failure (σ_s) is generally considered null in ceramics. This gives a two-parameter Weibull expression and the possibility to highlight the effect of the volume tested on measured strength. For example, for the same probability of failure of 50%, the ratio of mean strength of two samples of volumes V_1 and V_2 is given by the following equation:

$$\frac{\sigma_{R1}}{\sigma_{R2}} = \left(\frac{V_2}{V_1}\right)^{1/m}$$

Case Studies on Implant Failure

Zirconia is a very reliable ceramic for dental implant applications because it can provide high toughness and strength along with biocompatibility and good tissue integration. It is also resistant to the aggressive oral environment, with no risk of corrosion as it is already an oxide. The main risks for dental implants made of zirconia include the following:

- Large processing flaws in an implant region under high tensile stresses
- Sensitivity to LTD for some grades of zirconia, especially if the production process/microstructure of the material was not fully controlled

Here we show examples of implant failure, either fracture or loss of osseointegration, that occurred due to a change in processing that led to large flaws at the surface of the material or to increased aging sensitivity. These two examples have been only partially disclosed in the literature and should not be considered the "fault" of the manufacturers. Instead, they show how seemingly subtle modifications in processing can lead to unexpected events that could have been prevented had they been thoroughly assessed before launching the product.

FAILURE OF DENTAL IMPLANTS DUE TO SURFACE FLAWS

In early 2006, the Swiss company AXIS biodental undertook the development of high-performance zirconia implants in connection with the ceramic injection molding (IM) process. Clinical trials started in 2007, with 3Y-TZP implants created via ceramic IM and with surface roughness obtained with one of the injection molds. The first implants marketed were all one piece. By 2012, two-piece Ceralog Hexalobe implants were successfully developed by the company, which is now integrated as BioHorizons Camlog.

Between 2007 and 2012, however, AXIS was seeking to develop a novel alveolar implant surface to enhance bone growth and osseointegration over their standard implants made via IM with a rough mold. An alveolar surface was obtained after deposition and sintering of a mixture of zirconia powder and polymer beads onto ceramic IM implants. Unfortunately, preclinical studies showed an unacceptably high failure rate (15%) after a few months, associated with fracture of the implant at bone level after short periods of loading. Figure 3-9 illustrates the fracture of one of these AXIS alveolar implants after only 2 weeks of real loading. It was clear that the porous coating led to large surface pores and cracks, which were the causes of the high failure rate. Figure 3-10 illustrates the surface features of the two types of implants. If the surface roughness of the standard "rough" implants was acceptable in terms of failure risk, craters of up to 80 to 100 microns distributed in the valleys of the threads in the AXIS alveolar implant surfaces could easily be considered potential critical defects. Their dimensions were related to the size of the pore formers (polymer beads) used during the production process. Surface cracks were also detected in the valleys of the threads of the implant prototypes. The results are partially reported in the outstanding paper from Scherrer et al,[26] which analyzes the cause of failure of several implants in vivo.

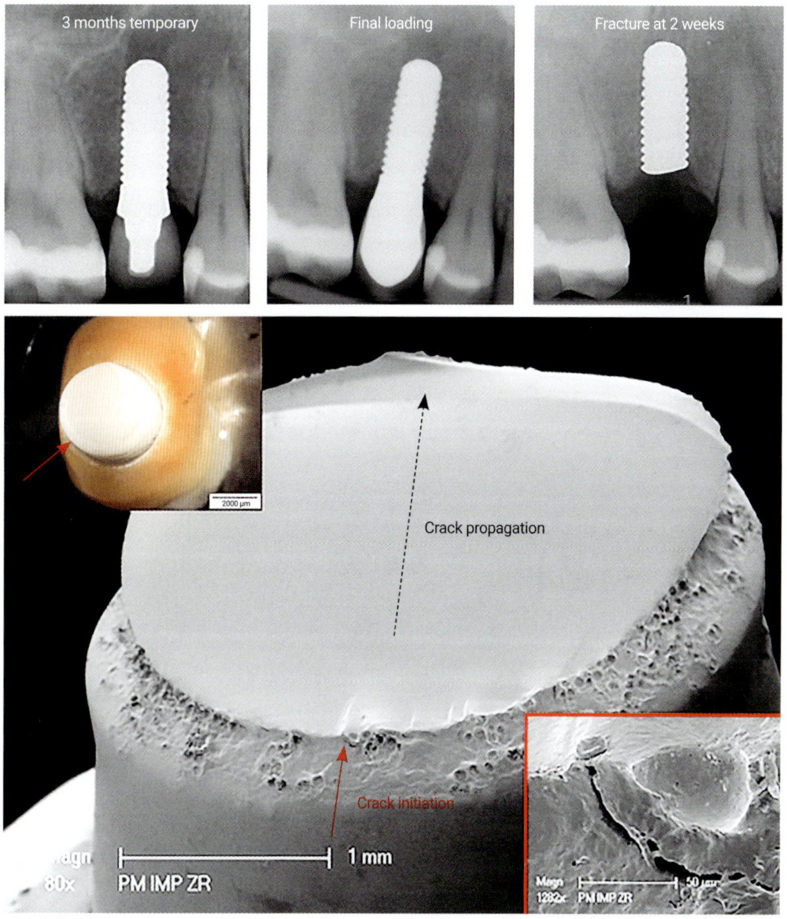

FIG 3-9 › Fracture of an AXIS implant 2 weeks after final loading. The implant broke in a brittle manner at the bone level. Fractography showed that the fracture origin was a defect at the surface resulting from the porous coating (see bottom right image). The area was placed under tension during the bending that occurs during mastication. (Courtesy of Susanne Scherrer, University of Geneva.)

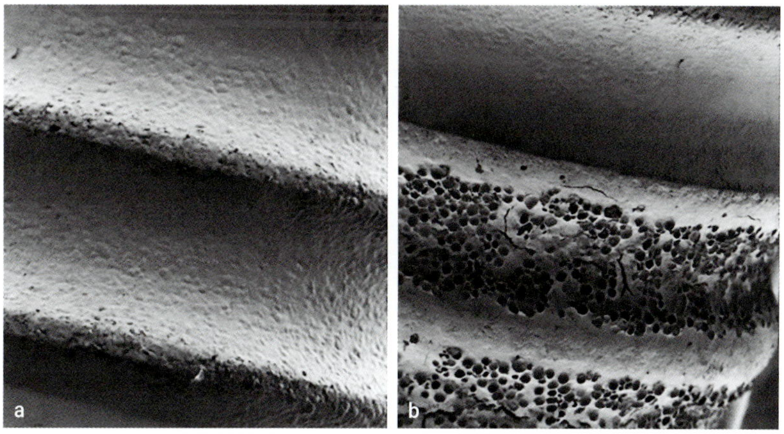

FIG 3-10 › Surface features of AXIS implants with a standard rough surface resulting from the injection mold *(a)* and with an alveolar surface *(b)* observed at the same magnification.

Sanon et al[27] showed that critical fractures like these could have been avoided by applying a simple in vitro protocol adapted from ISO 14801,[28] in which the ceramic implants are tested monotonically under a high loading rate. The authors tested 15 of the rough AXIS implants and 15 of the alveolar AXIS implants by embedding them in a stiff epoxy resin to avoid any viscoelastic deformation during loading. They were embedded up to 3 mm below the nominal level to simulate bone resorption. They were then loaded to failure at a crosshead speed of 1 mm/min to limit SCG during loading. The rough and alveolar implants broke at an average of 596 N (deviation of 74 N) and 392 N (standard deviation of 27 N), respectively, which shows the critical effect of the porous coating.

The value of K_{IC} and K_{I0} of 3Y-TZP (which has a grain size similar to the materials tested in this work) are K_{IC} = 6.0 MPa and K_{I0} = 3.0 MPa (under fatigue), respectively (see Fig 3-6). The fatigue limit (P_0) of an implant could therefore be roughly anticipated from the load to failure (P_f) by the following equation, in which P_0 and σ_0 refer to the fatigue load and stress limit, respectively, and P_f and σ_f are the load and stress to failure during fast fracture tests, respectively:

$$\frac{P_0}{P_C} = \frac{\sigma_0}{\sigma_C} = \frac{K_{I0}}{K_{IC}}$$

In the case of the AXIS prototypes, the average value of the load to failure was 392 N, which would mean that roughly 50% of the implants would resist to 196 N without delayed failure (and thus 50% would fail), this load value being in the order of the reported average mastication forces.

Obviously, based on the analysis above, the manufacturer abandoned this type of implant design. This example shows that an understanding of simple fracture mechanics and testing are useful to avoid an embarrassing situation. It also shows that even though 3Y-TZP is a tough bioceramic, it remains sensitive to large defects, especially if they are at the surface of the region and placed under tension during in vivo situations. In ceramics, "large" defects are in the range of some dozens of microns.

LTD OF IMPLANTS DUE TO PROCESSING CONDITIONS

In 2005, Nobel Biocare developed one-piece dental implants made of 3Y-TZP (ZiUnite). The implant design was similar to the Nobel Direct titanium implants. To improve osseointegration, Nobel Biocare introduced a porous surface achieved by sintering the implants with a zirconia slurry and burnable pore former. Two processes were then implemented based on this overall strategy, with just a change in the fabrication steps, summarized in Table 3-1 (Fig 3-11):

- In the first process (P_1), the zirconia coating was applied to fully sintered bulk implants and then sintered to achieve sufficient adhesion and mechanical properties. The implant itself was thus sintered twice, with the coating sintered on an already fully dense zirconia ceramic.
- In the second process (P_2), the coating was deposited on presintered zirconia implants and then sintered to achieve full density. Both the coating and the ceramic body of the implant were thus sintered simultaneously.

TABLE 3-1 › Processing steps used by Nobel Biocare to fabricate ZiUnite implants

Step	Process 1 (P_1)	Process 2 (P_2)
1	Cold isostatic press of 3Y-TZP powder	Cold isostatic press of 3Y-TZP powder
2	Mill into cylindrical shape	Mill into cylindrical shape
3	Presinter	Presinter
4	Mill into final shape	Mill into final shape
5	Sintering to full density	Spray of the porous coating
6	Hot isostatic press	Sintering of both bulk and coating
7	Reoxidation	Hot isostatic press
8	Spray of the porous coating	Reoxidation
9	Sintering of the porous coating	Packaging
10	Packaging	

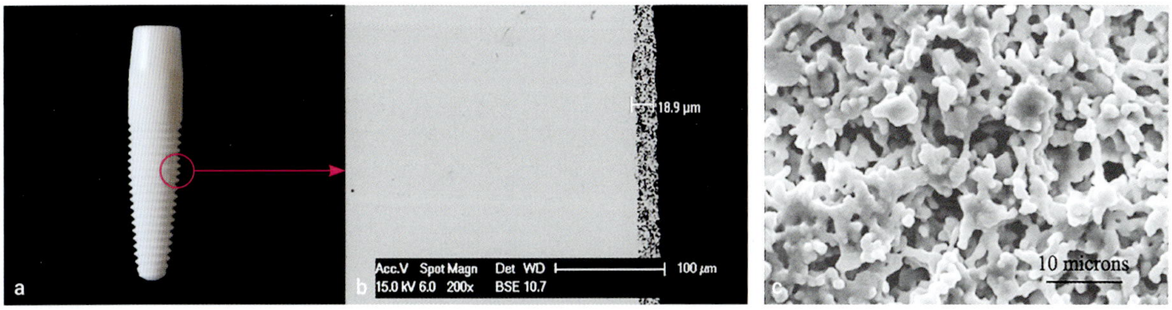

FIG 3-11 › *(a to c)* Concept of the ZiUnite coating, sprayed and sintered at the surface of zirconia implants.

Preclinical trials were launched, with a quite high failure rate for implants processed according to the first technique. These implants showed a loss of integration after unacceptably short durations. Figure 3-12 shows the surface analysis of one of these implants after 3 years in vivo. The porous coating was almost fully transformed to monoclinic symmetry and showed extensive microcracking. X-ray diffraction analysis of the surface revealed a monoclinic content of more than 50%, confirming that the coating was heavily transformed after a short period of time. Such transformation-induced microcracking is likely the cause of the loss of the implants, due to progressive degradation of osseointegration.

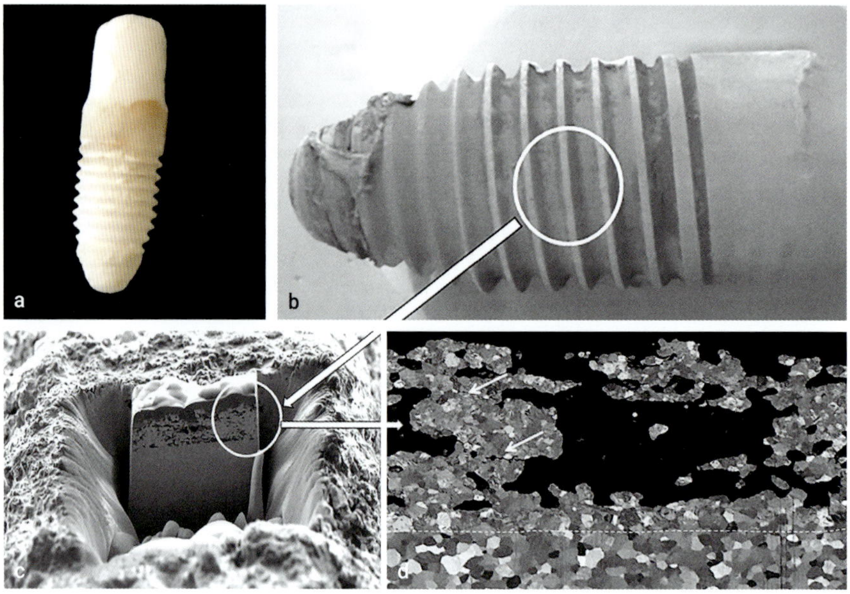

FIG 3-12 › Degradation of the ZiUnite coating by LTD in vivo, eventually leading to a loss of osseointegration and clinical failure. *(a)* The retrieved implant. *(b)* SEM image of the thread obtained with a focused ion beam (FIB) technique to observe a cross section of the coating and the bulk underneath. *(c and d)* Cross sections obtained with SEM showing that the surface coating is transformed (the contrast of the tetragonal grains is lost) and that microcracks are present in the coating *(arrows)*. The monoclinic phase content measured by X-ray diffraction was 50%, which is in agreement with full transformation of the coating.

Nobel Biocare began collaborating with INSA-Lyon to perform an in vitro study on both types of implants to understand the causes of accelerated degradation of the P_1 implants. The LTD kinetics of P_1 and P_2 implants were found to be profoundly different (in the range 90°C to 140°C), with P_1 implants aging 20 times faster than P_2 implants (Fig 3-13). The following facts were also discovered:

- The aging kinetics of P_1 implants recorded directly on the surface of interest were different from those measured on polished samples representative of the bulk of the implants when following the ISO 13356 standard.[29]
- The aging kinetics observed at 37°C on the implants in vivo were in agreement with extrapolations from the high-temperature tests at 90°C to 140°C.

In-depth investigation showed that the coating on P_1 implants exhibited quite high tensile residual stresses after the process. This may be explained by the fact that sintering of the coating was conducted on an already fully dense zirconia core. Shrinkage of the coating was thus constrained, leading to tensile stresses and triggering LTD.

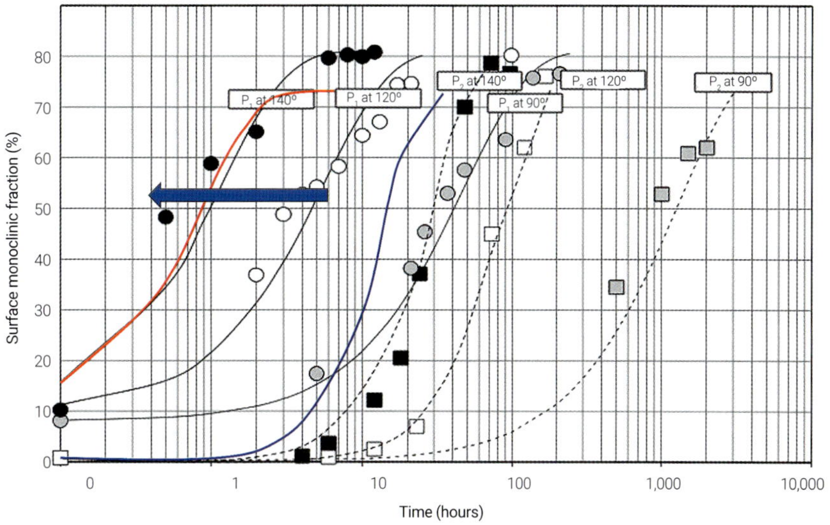

FIG 3-13 › Drastic change of LTD kinetics obtained at different temperatures between P_1 and P_2 implants. Aging kinetics at 140°C are shown for P_1 implants *(red)* and P_2 implants *(blue)*. Subtle changes in processing steps may lead to a significant effect on LTD resistance. In this case, differences in processing led to a 20-fold increase in aging kinetics.

ZiUnite implants were abandoned due to unsatisfactory clinical success. This negative story shows that even if 3Y-TZP is generally sufficiently resistant to LTD, changes in processing may lead to accelerated aging. Fortunately, there are tools to monitor aging and predict the aging performance of a given zirconia processed under a particular condition. These tools are described later in the book and are based on accelerated tests in autoclaves, time-temperature equivalence, and structural (X-ray diffraction) and microstructural (SEM) analyses. This event also shows that ISO standards can give insight into the aging kinetics of a given zirconia but that testing should be done on the real surface of interest, not on polished samples, which are inevitably different.

Conclusion

This chapter covered the concepts of brittle failure and crack resistance, which are of great importance when dealing with ceramics. Even though zirconia is tougher than many other oxides, it is still less tough than metals like titanium. Understanding the effects of stress concentrations and processing defects on strength and fatigue resistance can help avoid implant fracture. Beyond toughness and strength parameters, the long-term performance and lifetime of a zirconia implant can be linked to its resistance to SCG and LTD, both of which must be evaluated prior to clinical use to avoid critical situations.

References

1. Munz D, Fett T. Ceramics: Mechanical Properties, Failure Behavior, Materials Selection. Springer, 1999.
2. Lawn B. Fracture of Brittle Solids, ed 2. Cambridge Solid State Science Series. Cambridge University Press, 1993.
3. Danzer R, Lube T, Supancic P, Damani R. Fracture of ceramics. Adv Eng Mater 2008;10:275–298.
4. Ashby MF. Materials Selection in Mechanical Design, ed 4. Butterworth-Heinemann, 2011.
5. Zhang F, Reveron H, Spies BC, Van Meerbeek B, Chevalier J. Trade-off between fracture resistance and translucency of zirconia and lithium-disilicate glass ceramics for monolithic restorations. Acta Biomater 2019;91:24–34.
6. Chevalier J, Liens A, Reveron H, et al. Forty years after the promise of "ceramic steel?": Zirconia-based composites with a metal-like mechanical behavior. J Am Ceram Soc 2020;103:1482–1513.
7. Danzer R, Supancic P, Pascual J, Lube T. Fracture statistics of ceramics—Weibull statistics and deviations from Weibull statistics. Eng Fracture Mech 2007;74:2919–2932.
8. Revilla-León M, Al-Haj Husain N, Ceballos L, Özcan M. Flexural strength and Weibull characteristics of stereolithography additive manufactured versus milled zirconia. J Prosthet Dent 2021;125:685–690.
9. Saâdaoui M, Khaldoun F, Adrien J, Reveron H, Chevalier J. X-ray tomography of additive-manufactured zirconia: Processing defects—Strength relations. J Eur Ceram Soc 2020;40:3200–3207.
10. Chevalier J, Olagnon C, Fantozzi G. Subcritical crack propagation in 3Y-TZP ceramics: Static and cyclic fatigue. J Am Ceram Soc 1999;82:3129–3138.
11. Ritchie RO, Dauskardt RH. Cyclic fatigue of ceramics. J Ceram Soc Jap 1991;99:1047–1062.
12. Lawson S. Environment degradation of zirconia ceramics. J Eur Ceram Soc 1995;15:485–502.
13. Chevalier J, Gremillard L. Low-temperature degradation of zirconia and implications for biomedical implants. Annu Rev Mater Res 2007;37:1–32.
14. Lughi V, Sergo V. Low temperature degradation—aging—of zirconia: A critical review of the relevant aspects in dentistry. Dent Mater 2010;26:807–820.
15. Chevalier J, Grémillard L. Zirconia as a biomaterial. Comprehensive Biomaterials 2017;1:122–144.
16. Chevalier J, Cales B, Drouin JM. Low-temperature aging of Y-TZP ceramics. J Am Ceram Soc 1999;82:2150–2154.
17. Chevalier J, Gremillard L, Virkar AV, Clarke DR. The tetragonal-monoclinic transformation in zirconia: Lessons learned and future trends. J Am Ceram Soc 2009;92:1901–1920.
18. Maccauro G, Piconi C, Burger W, et al. Fracture of a Y-TZP ceramic femoral head. J Bone Joint Surg Br 2004;86:1192–1196.
19. Sanon C, Chevalier J, Douillard T, et al. Low temperature degradation and reliability of one-piece ceramic oral implants with a porous surface. Dent Mater 2013;29:389–397.
20. Kocjan A, Cotič J, Kosmač T, Jevnikar P. In vivo aging of zirconia dental ceramics—Part I: Biomedical grade 3Y-TZP. Dent Mater 2021;37:443–453.
21. Koenig V, Wulfman C, Bekaert S, et al. Clinical behavior of second-generation zirconia monolithic posterior restorations: Two-year results of a prospective study with ex vivo analyses including patients with clinical signs of bruxism. J Dent 2019;91:103229.
22. ISO 14704:2016 Fine ceramics (advanced ceramics, advanced technical ceramics)—Test method for flexural strength of monolithic ceramics at room temperature, ed 3. International Standard for Organization, 2016.
23. EN 843-1:2006 Advanced technical ceramics—Mechanical properties of monolithic ceramics at room temperature—Part 1: Determination of flexural strength. European Committee for Standardization, 2006.
24. ISO 6872:2015 Dentistry—Ceramic materials. International Organization for Standardization, 2015.
25. ISO/TC 20501 Fine ceramics (advanced ceramics, advanced technical ceramics)—Weibull statistics for strength data. International Standard for Organization, 2003.
26. Scherrer SS, Mekki M, Crottaz C, et al. Translational research on clinically failed zirconia implants. Dent Mater 2019;35:368–388.
27. Sanon C, Chevalier J, Douillard T, Cattani-Lorente M, Scherrer SS, Gremillard L. A new testing protocol for zirconia dental implants. Dent Mater 2015;31:15–25.
28. ISO 14801:2016 Dentistry—Implants. Dynamic loading test for endosseous dental implants, ed 3. International Organization for Standardization, 2016.
29. ISO 13356:2015 Implants for surgery—Ceramic materials based on yttria-stabilized tetragonal zirconia (Y-TZP), ed 3. International Organization for Standardization, 2015.

04

PROCESSING ZIRCONIA DENTAL IMPLANTS

Corrado Piconi, Claudia Angela Maziero Volpato, Bruno Freitas Mello, and Mutlu Özcan

Ceramic dental implants and other advanced ceramic products are produced from powders used as starting materials. The whole process consists of the consolidation of these powders through various treatments and can be summarized in five main steps: *(1)* powder processing before firing (the product of this step is called the *batch*, and the powder is termed *ready-to-press powder*), *(2)* shaping the body (the body is referred to as the *green body*), *(3)* binder removal, *(4)* sintering, and *(5)* machining. This chapter provides an overview of these five steps as related to dental implant production, as well as touching on some of the various implant designs and surface treatments. A detailed discussion of the science of ceramic production is outside the scope of this book. For deeper analysis, readers may refer to the works of Kingery et al[1] or Trunec and Maca.[2]

FIG 4-1 › Defect size and frequency according to origin.

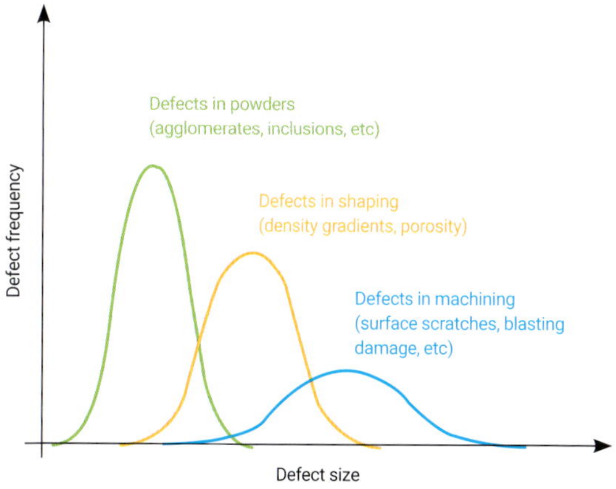

Ceramic Processing and Its Effects on Strength

In addition to consolidating the powders, the production process determines the microstructural characteristics of the material, which subsequently determine the macroscopic properties of the finished product. Defects in the microstructure, including discontinuities such as pores, inclusions, and larger-than-average grains, can result in stress concentrations when loads are applied. Thus, microstructural defects limit the strength of the material. Although generally the strength of ceramic materials is determined and limited by defect size, defect frequency (ie, the number of defects per volume unit) in the material is also relevant to material strength. In addition to defects in the material based on powder characteristics and the consolidation route, defects of different sizes can be introduced in the material during any step of the production process (Fig 4-1). Thus, the strength of a ceramic product is a statistical, process-dependent property, as described in detail in chapter 3.

Powder Processing Before Firing

Powders used to produce advanced ceramics (called *ceramic precursors*) are not immediately ready for use upon receipt from the manufacturer. This is because different batches of powder, even from the same manufacturer, can exhibit small deviations from nominal characteristics such as grain size distribution, particle shape and structure, and homogeneity of the chemical composition. Another relevant parameter is the specific surface area (surface-to-mass ratio) that gives a rough indication about the reactivity of the powder. Current values for ceramic precursors are in the order of some square meters per gram. Flowability of the powder is also relevant for processing, as it indicates a powder's capacity to flow freely during feeding and filling of the dies used for powder consolidation without forming coarse agglomerates due to moisture or Van der Waals forces. The shape of raw powder grains is irregular, and although grain size is characterized as "grain diameter," a grain's shape may be far from spherical.

Powders should be treated to homogenize the particle size and improve packing efficiency during compaction. Two treatments can be used to obtain homogeneous granulates from raw powders: *(1)* milling in a ball or in an attrition mill (either in dry or, more commonly, wet conditions) or *(2)* spray drying, which is a process more frequently used at an industrial scale.

Spray drying consists of dispersing the powders in a slurry containing process additives and then spraying the mixture in a cyclone in the presence of hot air. Some of the additives that determine the final characteristics of the ceramic can be introduced to the powder at this time, for example, yttria (Y_2O_3) in yttria-stabilized tetragonal zirconia polycrystal (Y-TZP) precursors and magnesia (MgO) in partially stabilized zirconia (PSZ) precursors. Depending on the shaping process, additives such as binders, lubricants, and sintering aids may also be joined to the powders. In this way, a ready-to-press granulate is obtained with homogeneous size distribution containing the process additives that are optimal for the chosen shaping route. The ready-to-press product is also termed *feedstock*.

Shaping

There are several shaping methods for ceramics. Shaping methods relevant to zirconia include the following:

- Dry shaping processes
- Uniaxial pressing
- Isostatic pressing
- Plastic shaping processes
- Injection molding (IM)
- Extrusion
- Wet shaping processes
- Colloidal shaping
- Slip casting
- Free-form shaping

The shaping process selected by manufacturers depends on the projected number of parts that will be produced and their size and design, as well as the optimization of production costs. When the production volume is small (up to 1,000 parts per year), the most common process consists in milling semifinished sintered or presintered parts (for example, cylindrical bars). The initial investment is limited, and this process is especially suitable for the development of new designs because of its flexibility. For medium production volumes (1,000 to 5,000 parts per year), the IM process combined with hard machining may be the best choice for managing machining costs. The feedstock is injected into a mold to obtain a near net shape green body. This is sintered and then machined according to the planned design. Although the cost of the molds can be high, especially for complex designs, this process minimizes ceramic machining and eliminates the cost of finished lots that must be discarded due to defects introduced during milling. Finally, for larger production volumes, IM is the process of choice. The internal and external characteristics of the implant are defined in a mold and produced during a single operation that requires only minimal finishing after sintering.

So far, the popular shaping process for producing zirconia dental implants involves dry shaping green bodies that are sintered and then machined close to the intended shape, with consideration for the shrinkage that occurs during sintering. Alternatively, IM has also been used. A satisfactory wet shaping process has not been found so far, whereas free-form shaping (ie, 3D printing) processes are showing promising results, as described later in this chapter. Regardless of the process selected, a strict control of material shrinkage during subsequent sintering is mandatory.

UNIAXIAL PRESSING

Uniaxial pressing is the most common method for shaping a ceramic *green body*—a term for shaped precursors before firing. The green body may contain a certain amount of organic components used as binders or lubricants to ease extraction from the die. Uniaxial pressing can be easily automated, and it is very suitable for industrial production. However, it can be used to obtain only simple shapes, usually either short cylinders with a maximum length-to-diameter ratio of 1:3 or flat disks. The process consists of pressing feedstock into a rigid die under a pressure of some tons. When performed in optimal conditions, uniaxial pressing crushes the particles and leaves minimal porosity in the green body. If conditions are not optimized, the green body may show density gradients because of the elastic behavior of the granulate and die. This should be avoided because it will cause shrinkage gradients and internal stresses in the sintered body during firing. In the most severe cases, this can result in fracture. Density gradients can be minimized by double-action uniaxial pressing, in which pressure is applied to the granulate by two coaxial pistons moving inward from the two sides of the die (Fig 4-2).

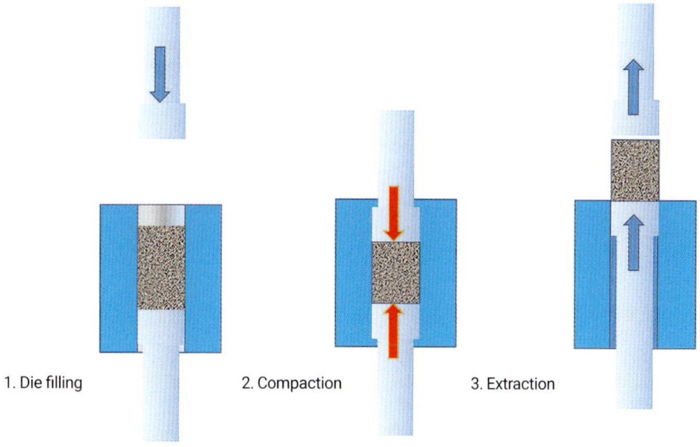

FIG 4-2 › Double-action uniaxial pressing.

ISOSTATIC PRESSING

In isostatic pressing, a uniform hydrostatic pressure is applied to a flexible mold containing the granulate. The green body has uniform density, but its shape is not as accurate as that which is achievable with uniaxial pressing because of the elastic deformation of the mold, meaning machining is required after shaping.

INJECTION MOLDING

IM can be used to shape ceramic green bodies, especially if they are small and complex in shape, like ceramic dental implants. Because IM can be automated, it is especially suitable for mass production. In addition, IM makes it possible to obtain near net shape green bodies, avoiding the need for costly machining of ceramic products. Nevertheless, molds are very expensive, as is the injection apparatus (Fig 4-3).

The IM process consists of several steps, the first one being preparation of the IM feedstock. The ceramic precursors should be integrated in a polymeric binder system to give the feedstock plasticity and flow behavior suitable for optimal filling of the mold. To reach this goal, spray drying is performed and the granulate is treated in a kneader with low-molecular-weight polymers, waxes, and solvents to obtain a paste containing 50 vol% to 60 vol% binder. A screw injector is then used to transform this paste into pellets containing the binder system that is the IM feedstock. The feedstock is warmed to 100°C to 250°C and injected as a paste into a mold, from which the shaped parts are extracted after cooling. Figure 4-4 depicts a dental implant before extraction from the mold.

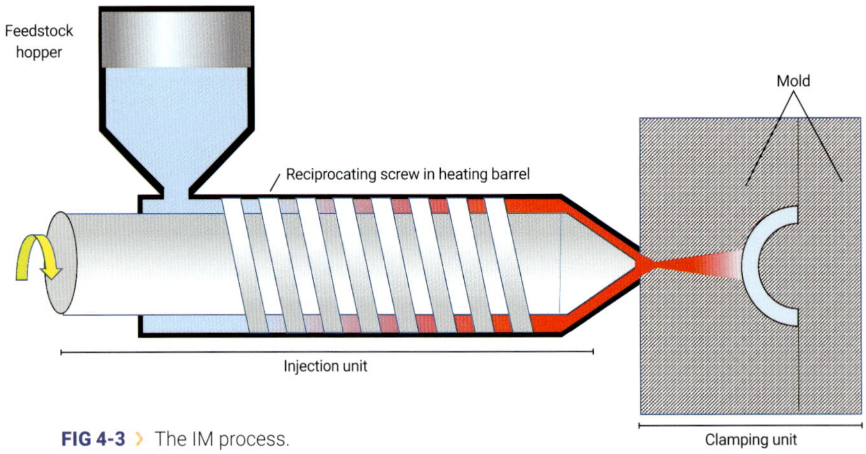

FIG 4-3 › The IM process.

FIG 4-4 › Open mold showing a ceramic implant during the extraction phase. Note the retracted plug that is used to shape the connection of this two-piece implant. (Courtesy of CeramTec.)

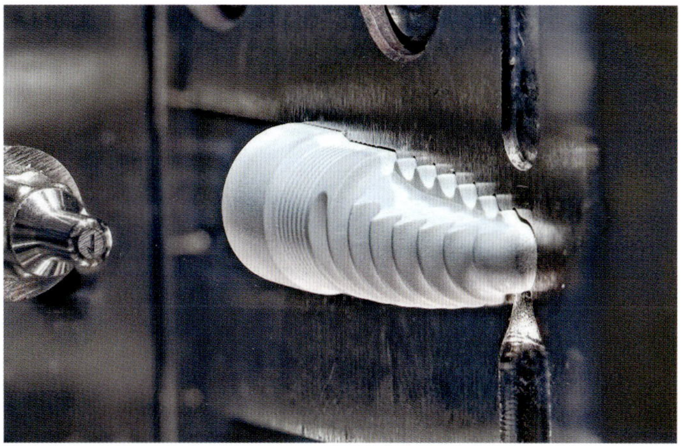

All the process additives should be removed from the green bodies before final consolidation by sintering. In the case of uniaxial or isostatically shaped parts, this can be performed at an intermediate temperature during the sintering cycle to allow for extraction of the melted binder through the porous green body. In the case of injection-molded green bodies, binder removal (or *debinding*) is one of the most critical steps due to the high volume of binder that must be removed. Thermal debinding is the most common process and is performed in an inert atmosphere at medium/high temperature, depending on the composition of the binder system. It involves the fusion and evaporation of the binder from the surface of the green body. High-molecular-weight fractions are thermally degraded into low-molecular-weight products before extraction. The debinding temperature must be kept under the boiling point of the binder system to avoid the formation of gas bubbles within the green body and, in the worst cases, binder burnout. Both situations would result in large defects in the green body. An alternative process involves thermal debinding with the green bodies kept in an inert powder bed. The molten binder is extracted by capillarity from the green body. A further variation consists in binder extraction from the green bodies with a suitable solvent.

ADDITIVE MANUFACTURING OF ZIRCONIA DENTAL IMPLANTS

Digital workflow in dentistry originated from the invention of French dentist Francois Duret[3] and the successive improvements introduced by Mörmann et al.[4] Today it is typical practice to produce crowns, fixed partial dentures (FPDs), and complete dentures using digital workflows. In 1989, Hull was granted a United States patent for the first system for creating a solid product via stereolithography.[5] Since then, stereolithographic processes have evolved and are identified collectively as *rapid*

TABLE 4-1 › AM processes for producing zirconia products[9]

	How it works	Material	Energy source	Postprocessing
SLS/SLM	Powder bed fusion	Powder	Laser	Cleaning of unbound powder, sintering
BJ	Powder bed fusion	Powder	Laser	Cleaning of unbound powder, sintering
DLP	Photopolymerization	Slurry	Light	Curing, cleaning, sintering
FDM	Extrusion	Feedstock	Heat, pressure	Debinding, cleaning, sintering

SLS/SLM = selective laser sintering/melting; BJ = binder jetting; DLP = digital light processing; FDM = fused deposition modeling.

prototyping, *3D printing*, or *additive manufacturing* (AM), which is the official term acknowledged by the International Organization for Standardization as "the process of joining materials to make objects from 3D model data, usually layer upon layer, as opposite to subtractive manufacturing technologies."[6]

The applications of AM in biomedical engineering are manifold, and new applications continue to be developed.[7,8] Applications range from the deposition of polymeric droplets to form 3D scaffolds to the selective melting of titanium powders via laser and the use of an electron beam for the selective melting of cobalt alloys. The common basis of various AM processes is the deposition and joining of layers of a material to create the final product. The layered nature of additively manufactured products influences their mechanical properties, including anisotropy. These properties can either be exploited to endow the product with specific behavior, or they must be compensated for to avoid residual stresses that could result in mechanical failure of the device. The basic steps of the various AM processes (Table 4-1)[9] are as follows:

1. Creation of a computer-aided design (CAD) file of the desired product, including the appropriate supports
2. Decomposition of the CAD file into layers that are oriented according to the direction of deposition by means of computer-aided manufacturing (CAM) slicer software that converts the CAD and model into files suitable for the machine (eg, .stl, .obj, or .amf)
3. Construction of the product layer by layer
4. Removal of the product from the machine
5. Removal of any supports
6. Postprocessing treatments (cleaning, sintering, etc)

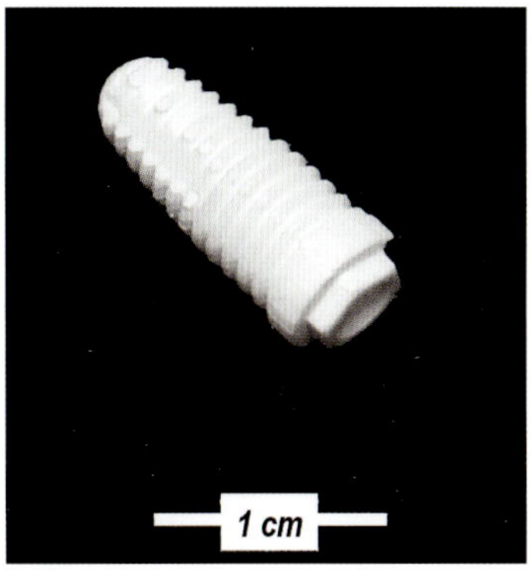

FIG 4-5 › An alumina-toughened zirconia (ATZ) dental implant made via DLP. (Reprinted with permission from Magnani et al.[11])

Although several AM processes have been investigated for zirconia (see Table 4-2), there is not yet a clear role for AM in the production of zirconia dental appliances.[10] Vat photopolymerization, or *digital light processing* (DLP), has been demonstrated to result in zirconia with good dimensional accuracy and sufficient flexural strength and microstructure—close to that of conventional subtractively manufactured zirconia (Fig 4-5).[11] However, the cost of this technology limits its applications in dentistry. Subtractive manufacturing is still standard for production of both patient-specific devices in dental laboratories and industrially mass-produced dental implants. Research on 3D printing zirconia ceramics is in progress to improve dimensional tolerances, homogenize residual stresses, and improve microstructural homogeneity and the impact of building alignment, which are all factors that can alter the mechanical properties of additively manufactured zirconia.[12–16]

Today, AM is being investigated for its potential use in the production of root analog implants (RAIs). RAIs are patient-specific devices designed to fit the anatomy of the natural alveolus and be inserted just after extraction of the native tooth.[17] Potential advantages of RAIs are the reduction of bone and soft tissue trauma and improved primary stability coupled with a less invasive procedure (ie, no bone drilling, sinus elevation, etc). The first implant of this type, made from polymethyl methacrylate (PMMA), was created by Hodosh et al in 1969.[18] A similar device was described by Driskell et al.[19] The outcomes of zirconia RAIs were analyzed recently in some excellent reviews[8,20–23] (Table 4-2).

TABLE 4-2 › Select results obtained in the experimental additive manufacture of zirconia dental implants

Study	Type of device	Material	Process	Mechanical properties
Osman et al[24] (2017)	Dental implants	Yttria-stabilized zirconia	DLP	943 MPa flexural strength
Cheng et al[25] (2017)	Dental implants	Yttria-stabilized zirconia	DLP	632.1 MPa flexural strength; VH: 14.72 GPa
Anssari Moin et al[26] (2017)	RAIs	Yttria-stabilized zirconia	DLP	3.5 Weibull modulus; 6.7 MPa $m^{1/2}$ fracture toughness
Magnani et al[11] (2021)	Dental implants	ATZ 60/40/2Y	DLP	872 MPa flexural strength
Nakai et al[27] (2021)	Square-shaped specimen	Commercial slurries: LithaCon 3Y 230 (Lithoz), 3DMix Zirconia (3DCeram), and 3D Mix ATZ (3DCeram)	SLA	3D Mix ATZ: 11.1 Weibull modulus

ATZ = alumina-toughened zirconia; DLP = digital light processing; VH = Vicker's hardness; SLA = stereolithography.

Sintering

Although sintering has been used by ceramists for thousands of years, there is still no unified theory to explain this phenomenon.[28,29] There are several sintering processes and a very wide body of scientific literature to which the reader can refer.[1,30,31] Sintering is an irreversible thermal process that minimizes the surface energy of the green body. As the temperature increases, porosity disappears and the volume of the green body shrinks while density increases to values near theoretical one. The typical density of Y-TZP dental implants is > 99.5% theoretical density (TD).

Sintering takes place in three stages (Fig 4-6). During the first stage, necks form between the powder particles, with little shrinkage of the body. As the temperature increases, sintering begins in the second stage. Mass transport then creates a continuous and interconnected system of pore channels communicating with the surface like a sponge (ie, *open porosity*). In the case of advanced ceramics, mass transport is mainly due to diffusion of particles from the necks into the pores. This

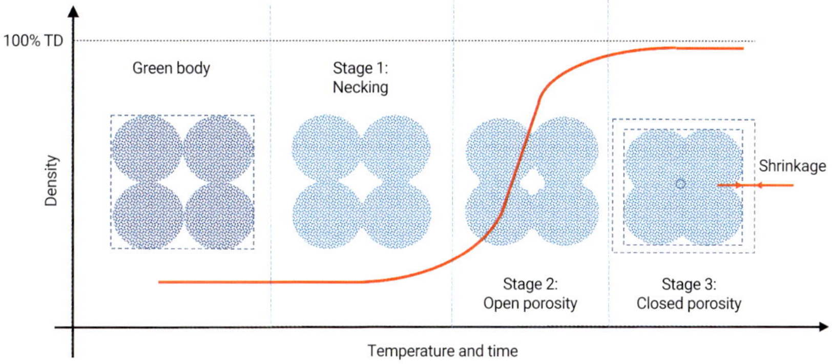

FIG 4-6 › Illustration of the sintering process, showing the transition of the green body to its final density during thermal treatment.

causes shrinkage of the green body while the porosity progressively disappears. The process takes place at temperatures ranging from 50% to 70% of the material's melting temperature. The progressive shrinkage of the pores continues until pores account for only a small percentage of the material's mass. Then the green body enters the third sintering phase, the *closed porosity stage*, when the pores are isolated from the outer surface of the ceramic and the density is close to TD. The decrease in surface energy during sintering is due not only to the decrease in porosity but also to the growth of grains in the microstructure of the ceramic (ie, *grain coarsening*). Because this behavior affects the mechanical properties of hardness and flexural strength, it should be carefully controlled by limiting the temperature at which the ceramic reaches full density.

Zirconia for dental appliances is usually sintered in air at atmospheric pressure, a process known as *pressureless sintering*. Key parameters include the heating ratio, the final temperature (usually below 1,500°C), and dwell time. A variation of this sintering route involves stopping sintering once sufficient mechanical resistance is achieved. Stopping sintering during this stage can be used to obtain blanks, which can be used to produce crowns, partial dentures, and implants that reach full density by sintering after shaping. Figure 4-7 in the next section depicts the milling of a cylindrical blank that will be sintered to the desired shape after tooling.

Machined blanks for dental implants can reach full density by high-temperature pressureless sintering. However, it is preferable that full density is obtained by hot isostatic pressing (HIP). HIP consists of heating the parts in a pressurized chamber (800–1,000 MPa) in inert atmosphere to a temperature lower than that to obtain full density by pressureless sintering. The concurrent effects of temperature and high pressure lead to the high final density of the ceramic part without grain growth thanks to the relatively low temperature of the HIP process. In addition, the isostatic (ie, homogeneous) pressure and thermal treatment can repair defects in ceramics caused by machining in the blank state.

Milling

Milling of zirconia during implant production may be done using presintered zirconia blanks at about 80% TD or full-density ceramic. Milling presintered zirconia blanks is currently used for zirconia restorative applications (crowns, partial dentures, etc), whereas dental implants can be made by machining full-density ceramic or, more commonly, by milling presintered blanks.

Milling presintered blanks is common in dentistry and has been done since the end of the 1980s for the production of dental restorations and frameworks with CAD/CAM.[3,4] The working time and wear of tools is limited because of the high porosity fraction of the blanks (usually about 20 vol%). This implies that shrinkage during sintering should be carefully considered during milling.

Milling hard materials such as full-density zirconia is a rather complex task, and the final results depend on numerous factors, including the characteristics of the milling machine, the tools, the material itself, and operational factors, as summarized in Table 4-3. Milling of full-density zirconia ceramics demands accurate

TABLE 4-3 › **Some of the parameters that influence zirconia milling**

Machine-related factors	Design	Rigidity, absence of vibration
	Operation	Positioning accuracy, positioning repeatability, spindle speed
	Coolant system	Type, pressure, temperature, coolant access to the workpiece
Tool-related factors	Design	Shape, material, cutting profile
	Abrasive	Type, particle size, distribution, hardness
	Bonding agent	Stiffness, thermal conductivity
Material-related factors	Properties	Hardness, fracture strength, toughness, elongation at rupture, thermal conductivity, abrasion resistance, chemical stability in the working conditions
	Product geometry	Machine compatibility, coolant access
	Product quality	Production tolerances, surface characteristics
Operational factors	Working process	Milling cycle design, system balancing and stiffness, workpiece fixture design, spindle speed

control of the cutting parameters to avoid creating subsurface flaws that can lead to fracture during clinical use. Moreover, tool wear during milling must be monitored to maintain machining efficiency. The cutting edges of a traditional tungsten carbide tool may not possess the hardness and abrasive resistance necessary for machining hard ceramics, which requires tools coated by harder materials, such as cubic boron nitride (CBN) or diamond. In the case of machining by abrasive wheels, the grain of the abrasive and bonding medium are important because of their dampening effect on tool vibrations. Furthermore, accurate cooling of the zirconia under milling is mandatory to avoid triggering a tetragonal to monoclinic phase transition that will shorten the life of the product.[32–34] Figures 4-7 to 4-9 depict some of the steps of milling zirconia dental implants.

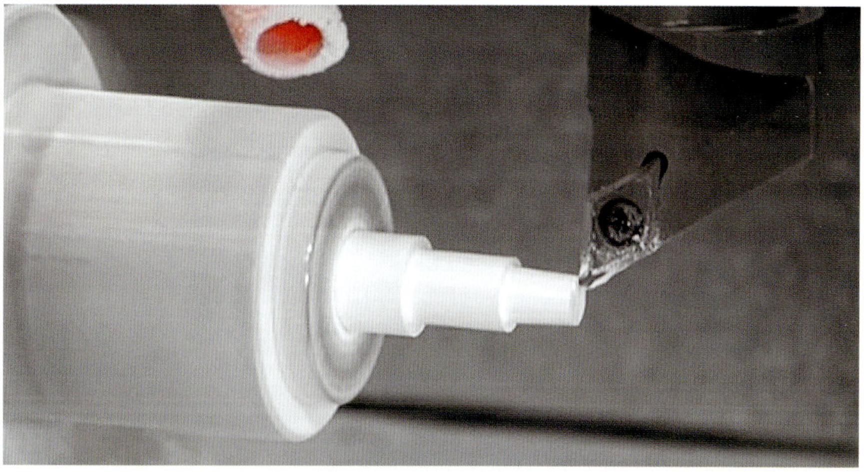

FIG 4-7 > Milling of a zirconia blank for the production of a dental implant. (Courtesy of CeramTec.)

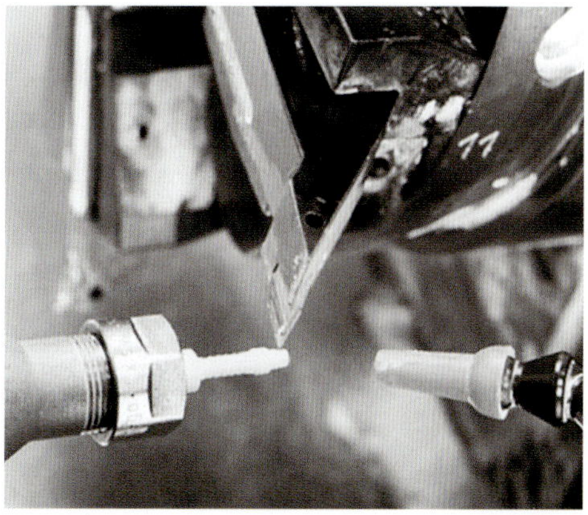

FIG 4-8 > Milling of a semifinished zirconia implant. (Courtesy of CeramTec.)

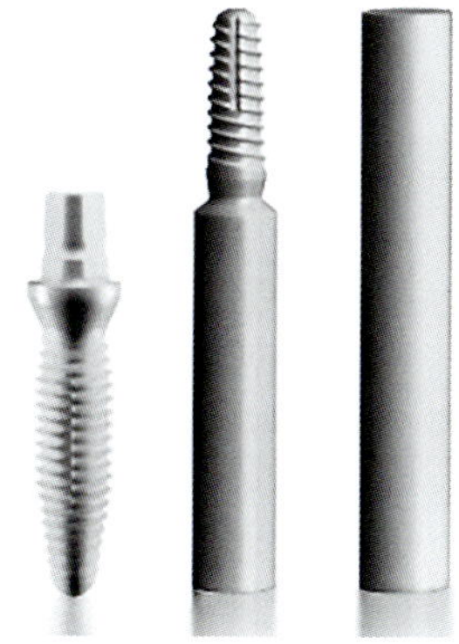

FIG 4-9 > Zirconia implants at different steps of the production process. (Courtesy of Metoxit.)

Specifics of Dental Implant Design and Production

Zirconia implants were introduced for clinical use in 1993 by Professor Sami Sandhaus, who had formerly developed the alumina CBS (Crystalline Bone Screw) implant system—the first ceramic dental implant,[35] manufactured by Rosenthal (now CeramTec) using high-alumina precursors. The SIGMA zirconia implant system (Incermed)[36] was very innovative and possessed a two-piece design with an internal hexagonal connection hosting a zirconia abutment fixed by cementation (Fig 4-10).

The modern era of zirconia dental implants was ushered in by Volz, who introduced the first modern zirconia implant system (Z-System) in 2003.[37] Since then, implant manufacturers have been continuously developing zirconia implants, aiming to improve implant reliability and macro- and microdesign. In fact, the number of innovations taking place has been so high and so fast that assessing their clinical advantages is sometimes difficult.

At the micro level, implant surface treatments have been used successfully to enhance osseointegration. Today it is widely acknowledged that the integration of zirconia and titanium dental implants is similar. At the macro level, implant design has evolved from one-piece implants to two-piece implants, allowing for the use of angled abutments, patient-specific abutments, and screw-retained prosthetic reconstructions. Some of the implants available today are shown in Fig 4-11.

IMPLANT SHAPE AND THREAD DESIGN

At a glance, zirconia and titanium dental implant designs do not differ much. In both cases, the shape of the implant can be classified as cylindrical or almost conical (Table 4-4). The endosseous surface is threaded to ensure implant stability and a good distribution of occlusal forces to the bone. The thread design may be the first macroscopic difference between titanium and zirconia implants. In the first series of zirconia implants, the thread design was like that of titanium implants. Later, different thread profiles were developed (Fig 4-12). These new thread designs are aimed to avoid sharp corners that can lead to stress concentrations in the implant.

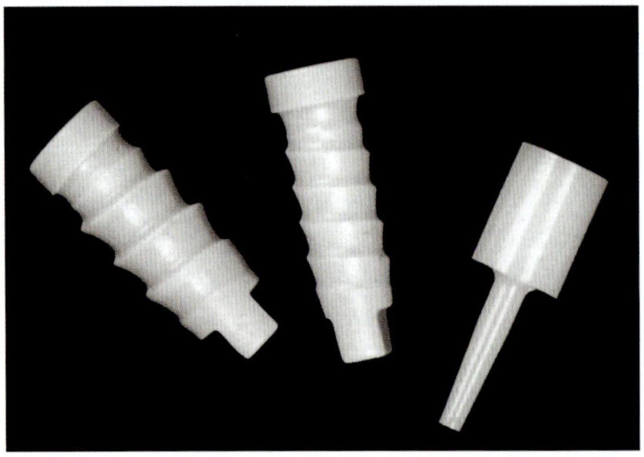

FIG 4-10 › SIGMA dental implants and abutment. (Courtesy of Prof Sami Sandhaus.)

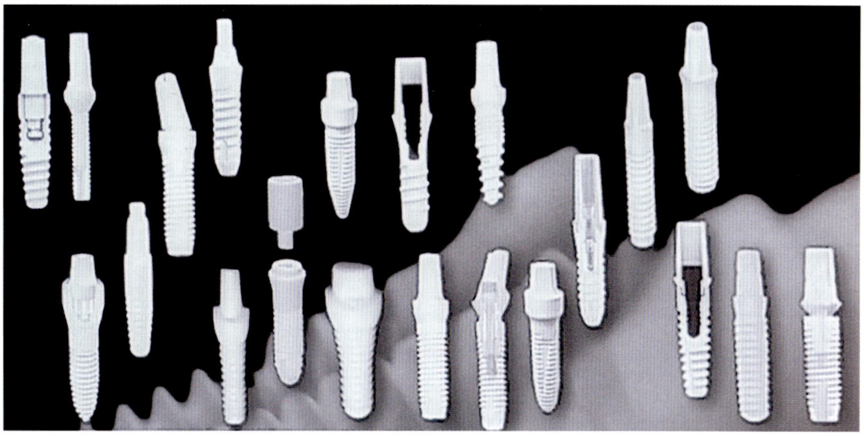

FIG 4-11 › Examples of zirconia implants. (Courtesy of Dr Stefan Roehling.)

TABLE 4-4 › Examples of implant geometries

Type	Model	Manufacturer
Cylindrical, one-piece	ZiBone	COHO Biomedical Technology
	PURE Ceramic	Straumann
	Zircasso	Zircosol
	Z5m	Z-Systems
	W One Piece Zirconia Implant	TAV Medical
Cylindrical, two-piece	PURE Ceramic	Straumann
	Z5c	Z-Systems
	Zeramex P6	Dentalpoint
	Patent	Zircon Medical
	W Two Piece Zirconia Implant	TAV Medical
	Ceralog	BioHorizons Camlog
Conical, one-piece	whiteSKY	bredent medical
	Z5m(t)	Z-Systems
	SDS1.2	Swiss Dental Solutions
Conical, two-piece	Zeramex XT	Dentalpoint
	Ceralog Hexalobe	BioHorizons Camlog
	SDS2.2.0	Swiss Dental Solutions

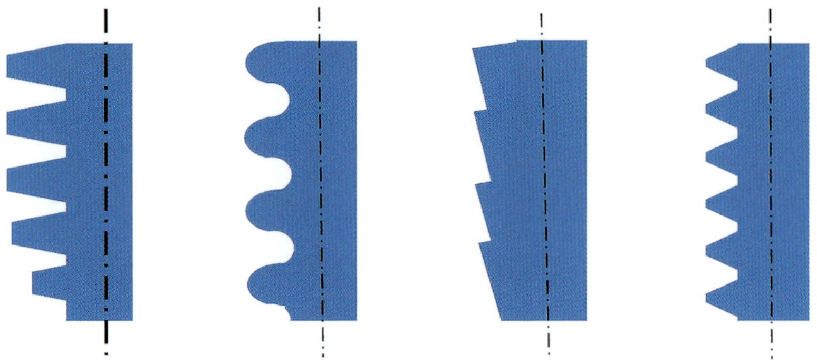

FIG 4-12 › Examples of thread profiles used in zirconia dental implants.

IMPLANT ABUTMENT CONNECTION

The design of two-piece implants raises the issue of the implant abutment connection. This element of the implant system is relevant to the strength and stability of the implant, as well as the supported restorations. The implant abutment connection should be designed to avoid the relative rotation of the two components of the implant, and the dimensional tolerance of the junction should be leakproof to protect against bacterial penetration. A common feature of two-piece implants on the market today are internal connections of various shapes (hexagon, octagon, spline, trichannel, etc) with geometric antirotational features (Fig 4-13). Some designs use an internal tapered connection that works on the self-locking principle of the Morse taper.

Implant abutment connections are secured by screws made of titanium, gold, carbon fiber–reinforced composite (CFRC), or zirconia. Screw design is a critical factor for the stability of the system. The recommended tightening torque ranges from 10 to 15 Ncm, which generates the elastic strain–derived compressive forces (preload) between the abutment and the implant that gives initial stability to the junction. Elastic stress relaxation can undermine the implant abutment stability, and the screw is designed to maximize preload and reduce the loss of elastic recovery, which must be compensated for by retightening the screw.

ENDOSSEOUS SURFACE TREATMENTS

Aside from the various thread designs, the endosseous surface of implants can be treated to improve surface properties and enhance osseointegration. This can be achieved by optimizing the surface roughness via either physical or biochemical approaches.[38–46]

Studies suggest that zirconia implants are not able to stimulate an initial reaction with the surrounding tissues after implantation because zirconia is a bioinert material.[38] Thus, surface treatments have been recommended to improve the

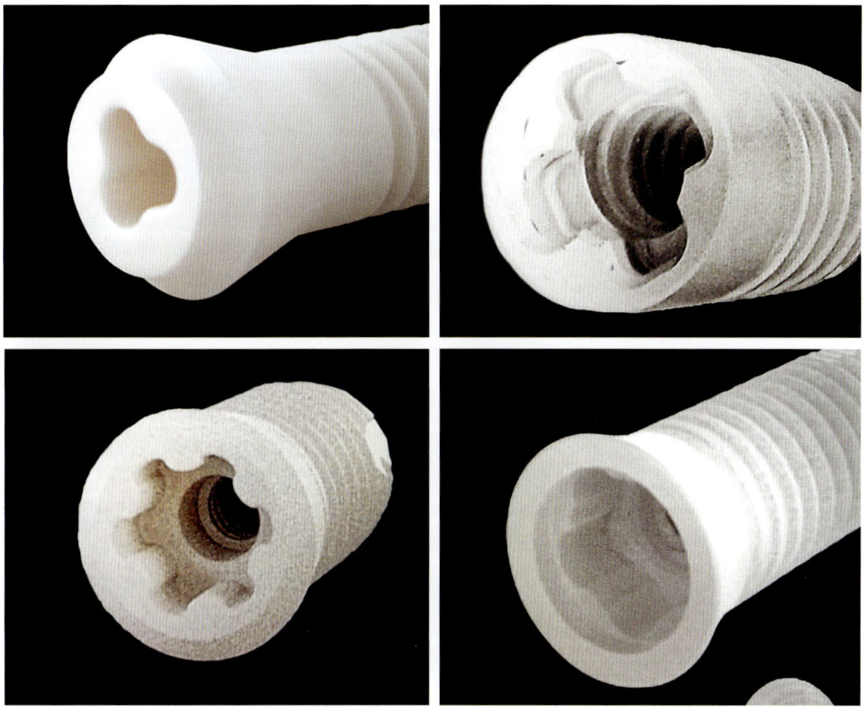

FIG 4-13 › Types of internal connections used in zirconia dental implants.

biologic response and osseointegration pattern.[39] Two main approaches have been suggested: microroughness optimization and/or the application of bioactive coatings.[40] A moderately rough surface topography is known to positively influence tissue healing,[41] and bioactive coatings such as hydroxyapatite (HA), silica, magnesium, and graphene are used for osteogenic stimulation.[42–46] Both approaches aim to increase surface wettability and energy.[47] The treatments performed on zirconia implant surfaces influence the adhesion, proliferation, and differentiation of osteoblasts, which facilitates osseointegration.[48] Studies report that modified zirconia implant surfaces show faster osseointegration than untreated ones, with good bone stability and histologic results showing no statistical differences between zirconia and titanium implants.[41–49] In addition, in vivo studies employing various animal models have shown that zirconia implants that have received surface treatment show a better pattern of osseointegration than untreated ones.[50,51]

Many physicochemical processes have been used to treat the surfaces of zirconia implants, including airborne-particle abrasion (ie, sandblasting), acid etching, selective infiltration etching (SIE), laser ablation, and UV surface treatment. Implants have been coated primarily with HA, bioglass, graphene, and peptides.

Airborne-particle abrasion

Airborne-particle abrasion is performed to obtain clean surfaces with ideal microroughness. This is fundamental to quality osseointegration, as evidenced by bone-to-implant contact (BIC) and removal torque, which indicate the amount of newly formed bone and the strength of union between the bone and implant.[52] Airborne-particle abrasion with 50- to 110-μm alumina (Al_2O_3) particles has been shown to increase the surface area for osteoblast fixation and thus accelerate the osseointegration process.[53] Other studies report that the degree of surface roughness obtained after blasting (which can vary from 1.3 to 4 μm) also plays a role in BIC.[54] Surface treatment of dental implants with airborne-particle abrasion accelerates the osseointegration process.[55,56] Gahlert et al[54] found significantly higher torque values for airborne particle–abraded zirconia implants (40.5 Ncm) than for zirconia implants with machined surfaces (25.9 Ncm). The implants were blasted with 0.2- to 0.5-μm alumina particles. Sennerby et al[57] reported a positive bone tissue response 6 weeks after the placement of airborne particle–abraded zirconia implants in rabbit bone. These implants showed a 4- to 5-fold increase in removal torque compared with machined zirconia implants. Other studies found that in airborne particle–abraded zirconia, the initial cell adhesion of osteoblasts was increased by up to 175% compared with machined zirconia.[55]

However, the forces generated during airborne-particle abrasion can induce phase transformation and microcrack formation, resulting in zirconia aging, a phenomenon known as *low-temperature degradation* (LTD).[58–60] In addition, airborne-particle abrasion can lead to a slight change in the elemental composition of the zirconia surface due to the unavoidable contamination with alumina.[61] These facts have led some authors to suggest the use of acid etching to remove the residues left after airborne-particle abrasion[62,63] and heat and etching to decrease the flexural strength of zirconia due to tetragonal to monoclinic phase transformation.[64,65]

Acid etching

Acid etching of zirconia surfaces can be carried out with hydrofluoric, acetic, citric, nitric, or sulfuric acid. Acid etching may be performed after airborne-particle abrasion to remove residue remaining on the zirconia surface. This combination of airborne-particle abrasion and acid etching became known in the dental field as *SLA treatment*. Airborne-particle abrasion of zirconia creates sharp-edged surfaces. Acid etching of the sandblasted surface rounds the edges and creates pits.[66] Studies have shown that altering surface topography via airborne-particle abrasion followed by acid etching can enhance the bioactive and osteoconductive properties of the surface, which can subsequently improve osteogenesis in clinical applications.[67,68]

According to Depprich et al,[69] the acid etching technique modifies not only the surface microtopography but also the submicron and nanometric topography of implant materials. Submicron and nanometric topographies influence cellular makeup and behavior, including orientation, motility, adhesion, and shape.

These topographic features play an important role in the initial stage of dental implant osseointegration.[70] Studies report that airborne particle–abraded zirconia implants that had their surfaces etched with 40% hydrofluoric acid (HF) for 1 hour reached an average roughness of about 1.3 µm (Ra). An increase in osteocalcin expression and cell adhesion was observed on these surfaces when compared with titanium surfaces and zirconia surfaces that were only machined (Ra of 0.54 and 0.59 µm, respectively). This confirms that higher roughness values correspond with areas most favorable for osteoblast adhesion.[66] Furthermore, a decrease in biofilm growth was observed on zirconia surfaces that were airborne-particle abraded and etched compared with titanium surfaces that were only airborne-particle abraded.[71] Representative examples of macro- and microsurface topographies are presented in Figs 4-14 and 4-15.

Although various acidic agents have been suggested in the literature for the surface treatment of implants, HF seems to be the best choice for osseointegration, resulting in higher values of implant removal torque.[63,73] Various volume concentrations (5% to 40%) and application times (1 to 2 hours) have been evaluated and resulted in different degrees of roughness on the zirconia surface. HF should be used at a maximum concentration of 5% to avoid any damage to the mechanical structure of zirconia.[74] Heat treatment after acid etching is also suggested in the literature, as it helps to smooth sharp edges caused by abrasion and acid etching for successful osseointegration.[75]

FIG 4-14 › *(a to c)* Macro- and microsurface topographies of a zirconia dental implant. (Courtesy of Prof A. Piattelli.)

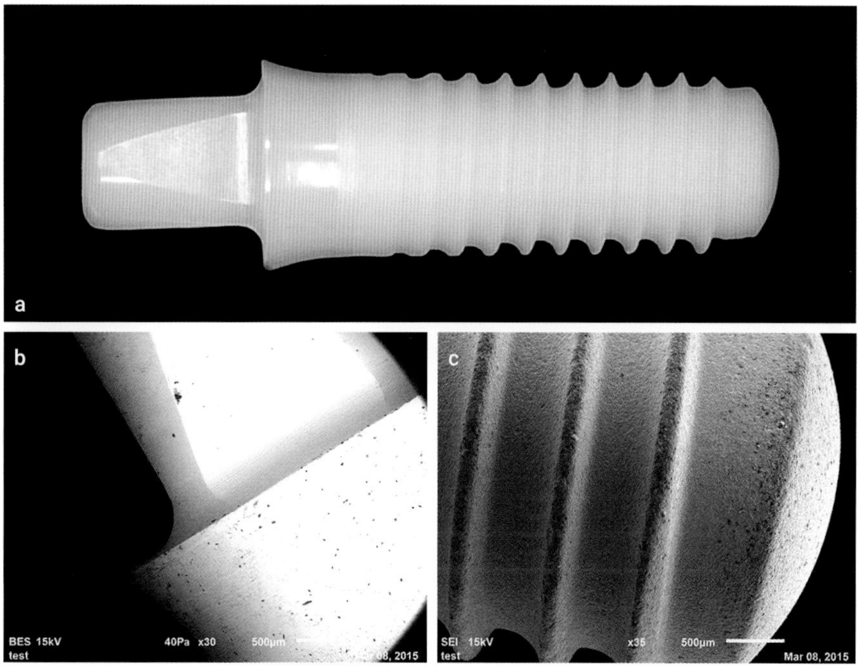

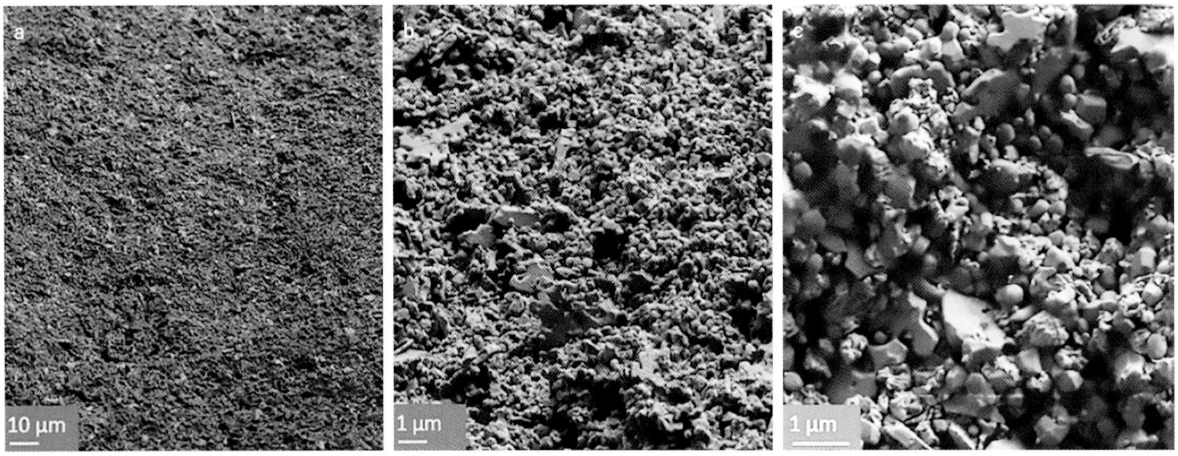

FIG 4-15 › Endosseous surface of a blasted and acid-etched zirconia-based implant at various SEM magnifications: *(a)* 500×, *(b)* 5,000×, and *(c)* 10,000×. (Reprinted with permission from Burkhardt et al.[72])

Laser surface treatment

Various types of lasers have been used to treat zirconia surfaces, including carbon dioxide (CO_2) lasers; erbium-doped yttrium aluminum garnet (Er:YAG) lasers; neodymium-doped yttrium aluminum garnet (Nd:YAG) lasers; erbium, chromium: yttrium-scandium-gallium-garnet (Er,Cr:YSGG) lasers; and femtosecond (FS) lasers.[76–79] Studies report that zirconia surfaces treated with CO_2 lasers showed an increase in the proliferation of osteogenic cells of 70% to 90% when compared with untreated surfaces, to the point of exhibiting osteoblast adherence. A progressive increase in cell proliferation was also observed when an Er,Cr:YSGG laser was used on zirconia surfaces.[80,81] Other studies have shown that adhesion, dissemination, proliferation, and differentiation of osteogenic cells can be improved with the use of lasers,[82–87] especially if an FS laser (100 fs, 795 nm, 10 nJ, 80 MHz) is employed.[88] In an in vivo study performed on dogs, the mean percentage of BIC of zirconia surfaces was about 48% after 3 months, which is statistically comparable to the BIC found with titanium surfaces.

UV light surface treatment

UV light surface treatment, also known as *photofunctionalization*,[89] is commonly used to remove contaminants from titanium implant surfaces, as well as to reactivate their biologic activity. UV treatment works by activating the potential for local hydrophilicity.[90,91] In recent years, UV light has been used to treat zirconia surfaces. Implants treated with UV light have shown improved bioactivity coupled with an increased hydrophilicity effect, allowing for initial interaction with proteins and cells, which is beneficial for the initial phases of osseointegration.[92–96] UV light is capable of inducing electron excitation, which increases the surface energy of zirconia. This is an important factor for improving the fixation, proliferation, and differentiation of osteoblasts. One study found that zirconia samples treated with UV light for 15 minutes showed a considerable increase in surface wettability,[54] which was confirmed again by another study, due to the change in surface contact angles from 56.4~69 degrees to 2.5~14.1 degrees.[97]

Calcium phosphate coatings

Coatings applied to zirconia surfaces have been proposed to increase bioactivity, improve antibacterial properties, and promote osteogenesis. Calcium phosphates are biologic apatites that stimulate bone repair and accelerate cell adhesion and proliferation.[98] In bone repair processes, HA and β-tricalcium phosphate (β-TCP) are the best-known calcium phosphates for promoting the bone tissue response due to their bioactivity and low solubility.[99]

HA and β-TCP present with chemical, structural, and biologic similarities to human bone, exhibiting a nontoxic and noninflammatory behavior in vivo. In view of such properties, these calcium phosphates have been widely used in implant coatings.[100–103] However, due to the stresses generated during the implantation process, these coatings can detach from the zirconia surface, resulting in compromised osseointegration.[104] Calcium phosphate particles may be deposited on the zirconia surface by different techniques, including plasma spraying,[105] dip coating,[104] electrochemical deposition,[106] spray coating,[107] and sol-gel,[108] which vary in deposition rates, costs, processing temperature, thickness control and homogeneity, porosity control, and surface quality.

Bioactive glass coatings

The bioactive properties of silica-based glasses make these materials favorable for coating dental implants because they promote the formation of HA when in contact with body fluids, which subsequently promotes osseointegration by stimulating the proliferation of osteoblasts.[109–111] The best-known bioactive glass is Bioglass 45S5 (Na_2O-CaO-SiO_2-P_2O_5).[111] The rapid formation of apatite in bone tissue suggests that osseointegration of dental implants may be favored by using bioactive glass coatings.[111–114] However, bioactive glasses may have insufficient mechanical properties due to their noncrystalline nature and brittleness. Due to different coefficients of thermal expansion (CTEs; 15.10^{-6} K^{-1} for bioactive glass and $10.8–12.5.10^{-6}$ K^{-1} for zirconia), cracks may be observed between the involved materials. Ideally, bioactive glass should have a slightly lower CTE than the substrate material.[111,112]

Graphene coatings

Graphene is one of the crystalline forms of carbon, as are diamond and graphite. Among its many applications in health care is as a coating for implant surfaces to improve the tribologic properties of implants and reduce wear.[115] Li et al[115] fabricated zirconia/graphene (ZrO_2/GNs) nanosheets with a thickness of 5 to 20 nm in 2014 using a plasma spray technique and investigated the microstructure and tribologic properties of this composite when applied to Ti-6Al-4V substrates. The nanosheets contributed to improved wear resistance and reduced the friction coefficient, which led to superior tribologic performance.[116] In 2022, composites made of yttria-stabilized zirconia and associated with graphene layers were fabricated and tested for resistance to degradation. The graphene-reinforced composite showed greater resistance to LTD than monolithic zirconia.[117] Another study reported a significant reduction in biofilm formation on graphene oxide–coated zirconia surfaces by means of an atmospheric pressure plasma generator.[118]

Conclusion

To date, the mass production of zirconia dental implants is based on established technologic processes such as blank machining and IM. Some manufacturers use postsintering HIP to reach full density and/or to eliminate machining flaws. AM has proven its potential for dental applications, especially for DLP, but at present, this technology looks more profitable for patient-specific devices, such as RAIs. While the reference material for ceramic dental implants is Y-TZP in conformity with ISO 13356 and ASTM F1873,[118,119] zirconia-based composite dental implants (eg, ATZ) are already in clinical use. Several other composites are being developed, but it is difficult to foresee their clinical applications. Ceramic implants have evolved from a one-piece design to a two-piece design, which offers more flexibility, and various manufacturers have this type of ceramic implant in their catalogs. Various surface treatments can be applied to promote the osseointegration of zirconia implants and make it comparable to that achieved with titanium implants. Airborne-particle abrasion and acid etching of the endosseous surfaces can be performed as part of the standard manufacturing process. Finally, other physical, chemical, and biologic surface processing methods are being investigated with promising results.

References

1. Kingery WD, Bowen HK, Uhlmann DR. Introduction to Ceramics, ed 2. Wiley, 1976.
2. Trunec M, Maca K. Advanced ceramic processes. In: Shen JZ, Kosmac T (eds). Advanced Ceramics for Dentistry. Butterworth-Heinemann, 2014:124–150.
3. Duret F [inventor]. Method for producing a dental prosthesis. French patent 2,536,654. 9 January 1987.
4. Mörmann WH, Brandestini M, Lutz F. The Cerec system: Computer-assisted preparation of direct ceramic inlays in one setting. Quintessenz 1987;38:457–470.
5. Hull CW. Apparatus for the production of three dimensional objects by stereolithography. US patent 4,575,330. 19 December 1989.
6. ISO/ASTM 52900:2021. Additive manufacturing–Part 3: Terms and definitions. International Organization for Standardization, 2021.
7. Lai J, Wang C, Wang M. 3D printing in biomedical engineering: Processes, materials, and applications. Appl Phys Rev 2021;8:021322.
8. Kumaresan S, Vaiyapuri S, Kang JH, et al. Perspective chapter: Additive manufactured zirconia-based bio-ceramics for biomedical applications. In: Shishkowsky IV (ed). Advanced Additive Manufacturing. In techOpen, 2022:1–36.
9. Methani MM, Cesar PF, Paula Miranda RB, S Morimoto, Özcan M, Revilla-León M. Additive manufacturing in dentistry: Current technologies, clinical applications, and limitations. Curr Oral Health Rep 2020;7:327–334.
10. Kim JC, Yeo ISL. Bone response to conventional titanium implants and new zirconia implants produced by additive manufacturing. Materials (Basel) 2021;14:4405.
11. Magnani G, Fabbri P, Leoni E, Salernitano E, Mazzanti F. New perspectives on zirconia composites as biomaterials. J Compos Sci 2021;5:244.
12. Jiang CP, Hentihu MFR, Cheng YC, Lei TY, Lin R, Chen Z. Development of 3D slurry printing technology with submersion—Light apparatus in dental application. Materials (Basel) 2021;14:7873.
13. Patil A, Davidson Jebaseelan D, Bomze D, Gopal V. Wear behaviour of lithography ceramic manufactured dental zirconia. BMC Oral Health 2023;23:276.
14. Yang SY, Koh YH, Kim HE. Digital light processing of zirconia suspensions containing photocurable monomer/camphor vehicle for dental applications. Materials (Basel) 2023;16:402.
15. Jung JM, Kim GN, Koh YH, Kim HE. Manufacturing and characterization of dental crowns made of 5-mol% yttria stabilized zirconia by digital light processing. Materials (Basel) 2023;16:1447.

16. Wang L, Yu H, Hao Z, Tang W, Dou R. Investigating the effect of solid loading on microstructure, mechanical properties, and translucency of highly translucent zirconia ceramics prepared via stereolithography-based additive manufacturing. J Mech Behav Biomed Mater 2023;144:105952.
17. Pirker W, Kocher A. Root analog zirconia implants: True anatomical design for molar replacement—A case report. Int J Periodontics Restorative Dent 2011;31:663–638.
18. Hodosh M, Povar M, Shklar G. The dental polymer implant concept. J Prosthet Dent 1969,22;371–380.
19. Driskell TD, O'Hara MJ, Sheets HD, Green GW Jr, Natiella JR, Armitage J. Development and application of ceramics and ceramic composites for implant dentistry. In: Hall CW, Hulbert SF, Levine SN, Young FA (eds). Bioceramics: Engineering in Medicine (Part 2). Interscience, 1972:345–361.
20. Pessanha-Andrade M, Sordi MB, Henriques B, Silva FS, Teughels W, Souza JCM. Custom-made root-analogue zirconia implants: A scoping review on mechanical and biological benefits. J Biomed Mater Res Part B 2018:106B:2888–2900.
21. Böse MWH, Hildebrand D, Beuer F, et al. Clinical outcomes of root-analogue implants restored with single crowns or fixed dental prostheses: A retrospective case series. J Clin Med 2020;23:2346.
22. Revilla-León M, Meyer MJ, Zandinejad A, Özcan M. Additive manufacturing technologies for processing zirconia in dental applications. Int J Comput Dent 2020;23:27–37.
23. Dantas T, Madeira S, Gasik M, Vaz P, Silva F. Customized root-analogue implants: A review on outcomes from clinical trials and case reports. Materials (Basel) 2021;14:2296.
24. Osman C, van der Veen AJ, Huiberts D, Wismeijer D, Alharbi N. 3D-printing zirconia implants: A dream or a reality? An in-vitro study evaluating the dimensional accuracy, surface topography and mechanical properties of printed zirconia implant and discs. J Mech Behav Biomed Mater 2017;75:521–528.
25. Cheng YC, Lin DH, Jiang CP, Lin YM. Dental implant customization using numerical optimization design and 3-dimensional printing fabrication of zirconia ceramic. Int J Numer Method Biomed Eng 2017;33:e2820.
26. Anssari Moin D, Hassan B, Wismeijer D. A novel approach for custom three-dimensional printing of a zirconia root analogue implant by digital light processing. Clin Oral Implants Res 2017;28:668–670.
27. Nakai H, Inokoshi M, Nozaki K, et al. Additively manufactured zirconia for dental applications. Materials (Basel) 2021;14:3694.
28. Rahaman M. Sintering of Ceramics. CRC Press, 2007.
29. German R. Sintering: From Empirical Observations to Scientific Principles. Butterworth-Heinemann, 2014.
30. Kang S. Sintering: Densification, Grain Growth and Microstructure. Butterworth-Heinemann, 2005.
31. Kuscer D, Shen JZ. Advanced direct forming processes for the future. In: Shen JZ, Kosmac T (eds). Advanced Ceramics for Dentistry. Butterworth-Heinemann, 2014:375–390.
32. Kosmač T, Oblak C, Jevnikar P, Funduk N, Marion L. The effect of surface grinding and sandblasting on flexural strength and reliability of Y-TZP zirconia ceramic. Dent Mater 1999;15:426–433.
33. Denry IL, Holloway JA. Microstructural and crystallographic surface changes after grinding zirconia-based dental ceramics. J Biomed Mater Res B Appl Biomater 2006;76:440–448.
34. Deng X, Zhang F, Liao Y, et al. Effect of grinding parameters on surface integrity and flexural strength of 3Y-TZP ceramic. J Eur Ceram Soc 2022;42:1635–1644.
35. Sandhaus S. Noveaux aspects de l'implantologie—Implant C.B.S. Julien Prelat, 1969.
36. Sandhaus S, Pasche K. Tenon radiculaire en zircone pour la realisation d'inlays-cores tout ceramique. Tribune Dentaire 1994;2:17–24.
37. Volz U. Zirkonoxid-Implantate mit zirkonoxid Kronen. Metallfreie rekonstruktion. Zahnarzt Impl 2003;19:176–180.
38. Dehestani M, Ilver L, Adolfsson E. Enhancing the bioactivity of zirconia and zirconia composites by surface modification. J Biomed Mater Res B Appl Biomater 2012;100:832–840.
39. Caravaca C, Shi L, Balvay S, et al. Direct silanization of zirconia for increased biointegration. Acta Biomater 2016;46:323–335.
40. Schünemann FH, Galárraga-Vinueza ME, Magini R, et al. Zirconia surface modifications for implant dentistry. Mater Sci Eng C Mater Biol Appl 2019;98:1294–1305.

41. Albrektsson T, Wennerberg A. Oral implant surfaces: Part 1—Review focusing on topographic and chemical properties of different surfaces and in vivo responses to them. Int J Prosthodont 2004;17:536–543.
42. Liu YT, Lee TM, Lui TS. Enhanced osteoblastic cell response on zirconia by bio-inspired surface modification. Colloids Surf B Biointerfaces 2013;106:37–45.
43. Pardum K, Treccani L, Volkmann E, et al. Magnesium-containing mixed coatings on zirconia for dental implants: Mechanical characterization and in vitro behavior. J Biomater Appl 2015;30:104–118.
44. Schienle S, Al-Ahmad A, Kohal RJ, et al. Microbial adhesion on novel yttria-stabilized tetragonal zirconia (Y-TZP) implant surfaces with nitrogen-doped hydrogenated amorphous carbon (a-C:H:N) coatings. Clin Oral Investig 2016;20:1719–1732.
45. Oh GJ, Yoon JH, Vu VT, et al. Surface characteristics of bioactive glass-infiltrated zirconia with different hydrofluoric acid etching conditions. J Nanosci Nanotechnol 2017;17:1645–1648.
46. Zhang C, Jiang Z, Zhao L. Mechanical properties and tribological behaviors of yttria-zirconia ceramics with additions of graphene oxide by hot-press sintering for dental implants. Surf Topogr Metrol Prop 2020;8:035010.
47. Noro A, Kaneko M, Murata I, Yoshinari M. Influence of surface topography and surface physicochemistry on wettability of zirconia (tetragonal zirconia polycrystal). J Biomed Mater Res B Appl Biomater 2013;101:355–363.
48. Altmann B, Rabel K, Kohal RJ, et al. Cellular transcriptional response to zirconia-based implant materials. Dent Mater 2017;33:241–255.
49. Rocchietta I, Fontana F, Addis A, Schupbach P, Simion M. Surface-modified zirconia implants: Tissue response in rabbits. Clin Oral Implants Res 2009;20:844–850.
50. Park YS, Chung SH, Shon WJ. Peri-implant bone formation and surface characteristics of rough surface zirconia implants manufactured by powder injection molding technique in rabbit tibiae. Clin Oral Implants Res 2013;24:586–591.
51. Gottlander M, Albrektsson T. Histomorphometric studies of hydroxyapatite-coated and uncoated CP titanium threaded implants in bone. Int J Oral Maxillofac Implants 1991;6:399–404.
52. Kosmac T, Oblak C, Jevnikar P, Funduk N, Marion L. The effect of surface grinding and sandblasting on flexural strength and reliability of Y-TZP zirconia ceramic. Dent Mater 1999;15:426–433.
53. Manzano G, Herrero R, Montero J. Comparison of clinical performance of zirconia implants and titanium implants in animal models: A systematic review. Int J Oral Maxillofacial Implants 2014;29:311–320.
54. Gahlert M, Gudehus T, Eichhorn S, Steinhauser E, Kniha H, Erhardt W. Biomechanical and histomorphometric comparison between zirconia implants with varying surface textures and a titanium implant in the maxilla of miniature pigs. Clin Oral Implants Res 2007;18:662–668.
55. Mihatovic I, Golubovic V, Becker J, Schwarz F. Bone tissue response to experimental zirconia implants. Clin Oral Investig 2017;21:523–532.
56. Barfeie A, Wilson J, Rees J. Implant surface characteristics and their effect on osseointegration. Br Dent J 2015;13:218.
57. Sennerby L, Dasmah A, Larsson B, Iverhed M. Bone tissue responses to surface-modified zirconia implants: A histomorphometric and removal torque study in the rabbit. Clin Implant Dent Relat Res 2005;7(suppl 1):S13–S20.
58. Al Qahtani WM, Schille C, Spintzyk S, et al. Effect of surface modification of zirconia on cell adhesion, metabolic activity and proliferation of human osteoblasts. Biomed Eng 2017;62: 75–87.
59. Fratucelli E, Candido LM, Pinelli LAP. Surface properties and flexural strength of a monolithic zirconia submitted to grinding and regenerative heat treatment. Int J Appl Ceramic Technol 2021;18:525–531.
60. Yang H, Xu YL, Hong G, Yu H. Effects of low-temperature degradation on the surface roughness of yttria-stabilized tetragonal zirconia polycrystal ceramics: A systematic review and meta-analysis. J Prosthet Dent 2021;125:222–230.
61. Blatt S, Pabst AM, Schiegnitz E, et al. Early cell response of osteogenic cells on differently modified implant surfaces: Sequences of cell proliferation, adherence and differentiation. J Craniomaxillofac Surg 2018;46:453–460.
62. Bächle M, Butz F, Hübner U, Bakalinis E, Kohal RJ. Behavior of CAL72 osteoblast-like cells cultured on zirconia ceramics with different surface topographies. Clin Oral Implants Res 2007;18:53–59.

63. Gahlert M, Röhling S, Wieland M, Eichhorn S, Küchenhoff H, Kniha H. A comparison study of the osseointegration of zirconia and titanium dental implants. A biomechanical evaluation in the maxilla of pigs. Clin Implant Dent Relat Res 2010;12:297–305.
64. Sriamporn T, Thamrongananskul N, Busabok C, Poolthong S, Uo M, Tagami J. Dental zirconia can be etched by hydrofluoric acid. Dent Mater J 2014;33:79–85.
65. Sato H, Yamada K, Pezzotti G, Nawa M, Ban S. Mechanical properties of dental zirconia ceramics changed with sandblasting and heat treatment. Dent Mater J 2008;27:408–414.
66. Bergemann C, Duske K, Nebe JB, et al. Microstructured zirconia surfaces modulate osteogenic marker genes in human primary osteoblasts. J Mater Sci Mater Med 2015;26:5350.
67. Karthigeyan S, Ravindran AJ, Bhat RTR, et al. Surface modification techniques for zirconia-based bioceramics: A review. J Pharm Bioallied Sci 2019;11(suppl 2):S131–S134.
68. Ito H, Sasaki H, Saito K, Honma S, Yajima Y, Yoshinari M. Response of osteoblast-like cells to zirconia with different surface topography. Dent Mater J 2013;32:122–129.
69. Depprich R, Zipprich H, Ommerborn M, et al. Osseointegration of zirconia implants compared with titanium: An in vivo study. Head Face Med 2008;4:30.
70. Meyer U, Büchter A, Wiesmann HP, Joos U, Jones DB. Basic reactions of osteoblasts on structured material surfaces. Eur Cell Mater 2005,9:39–49.
71. Flamant Q, Marro FG, Rovira JJR, et al. Hydrofluoric acid etching of dental zirconia. Part 1: Etching mechanism and surface characterization. J Eur Ceram 2016;36:121–124.
72. Burkhardt F, Harlass M, Adolfsson E, Vach K, Spies BC, Kohal RJ. A novel zirconia-based composite presents an aging resistant material for narrow-diameter ceramic implants. Materials (Basel) 2021;14:2151.
73. Xie H, Shen S, Qian M, Zhang F, Chen C, Tay FR. Effects of acid treatment on dental zirconia: An in vitro study. PloS One 2015;10:e0136263.
74. Wennerberg A, Albrektsson T. Effects of titanium surface topography on bone integration: A systematic review. Clin Oral Implants Res 2009;20:172–184.
75. Aboushelib MN, Salem NA, Taleb ALA, El Moniem NMA. Influence of surface nano-roughness on osseointegration of zirconia implants in rabbit femur heads using selective infiltration etching technique. J Oral Implantol 2013;39:583–590.
76. Delgado-Ruíz RA, Calvo-Guirado JL, Moreno P, et al. Femtosecond laser microstructuring of zirconia dental implants. J Biomed Mater Res B Appl Biomater 2011;96:91–100.
77. Paranhos MP, Burnett LH Jr, Magne P. Effect of Nd:YAG laser and CO2 laser treatment on the resin bond strength to zirconia ceramic. Quintessence Int 2011;42:79–89.
78. Aivazi M, Fathi M, Nejatidanesh F, et al. Effect of surface modification on viability of L929 cells on zirconia nanocomposite substrat. J Lasers Med Sci 2018;9:87–91.
79. Roitero E, Anglada M, Mücklich F, Jiménez-Piqué E. Mechanical reliability of dental grade zirconia after laser patterning. J Mech Behav Biomed Mater 2018;86:257–263.
80. Carvalho A, Grenho L, Fernandes MH, et al. Femtosecond laser microstructuring of alumina toughened zirconia for surface functionalization of dental implants. Ceram Int 2020;46: 1383–1389.
81. Kin H, Tugut F, Akin GE, Guney U, Mutaf B. Effect of Er:YAG laser application on the shear bond strength and microleakage between resin cements and Y-TZP ceramics. Lasers Med Sci 2012;27:333–338.
82. Hao L, Lawrence J, Chian KS. Osteoblast cell adhesion on a laser modified zirconia based bioceramic. J Mater Sci Mater Med 2005;16:719–726.
83. Hirota M, Hayakawa T, Ohkubo C, et al. Bone responses to zirconia implants with a thin carbonate-containing hydroxyapatite coating using a molecular precursor method. J Biomed Mater Res Part B Appl Biomater 2014;102:1277–1288.
84. Soares RD, Rodrigues JA, Cassoni A, et al. In vitro behavior of osteoblasts on zirconia after different intensities of erbium, chromium-doped: Yttrium, scandium, gallium, and garnet-laser irradiation. J Craniofac Surg 2016;27:784–788.
85. Vicente M, Gomes AL, Montero J, Rosel E, Seoane V, Albaladejo A. Influence of cyclic loading on the adhesive effectiveness of resin-zirconia interface after femtosecond laser irradiation and conventional surface treatments. Lasers Surg Med 2016;48:36–44.
86. Nassif W, Rifai M. Surface characterization and cell adhesion of different zirconia treatments: An in vitro study. J Contemp Dent Pract 2018;19:181–188.
87. Cunha W, Carvalho O, Henriques B, Silva FS, Özcan M, Souza JCM. Surface modification of zirconia dental implants by laser texturing. Lasers Med Sci 2022;37:77–93.

88. Calvo-Guirado JL, Aguilar-Salvatierra A, Delgado-Ruiz RA, et al. Histological and histomorphometric evaluation of zirconia dental implants modified by femtosecond laser versus titanium implants: An experimental study in fox hound dogs. Clin Implant Dent Relat Res 2013;17: 525–532.
89. Flanagan D. Photofunctionalization of dental implants. J Oral Implantol 2016;42:445–450.
90. Pyo SW, Park YB, Moon HS, Lee JH, Ogawa T. Photofunctionalization enhances bone-implant contact, dynamics of interfacial osteogenesis, marginal bone seal, and removal torque value of implants: A dog jawbone study. Implant Dent 2013;22:666–675.
91. Minamikawa H, Ikeda T, Att W, et al. Photofunctionalization increases the bioactivity and osteoconductivity of the titanium alloy Ti6Al4V. J Biomed Mater Res A 2014;102:3618–3630.
92. Tuna T, Wein M, Swain M, Fischer J, Att W. Influence of ultraviolet photofunctionalization on the surface characteristics of zirconia-based dental implant materials. Dent Mater 2015;31:14–24.
93. Yang Y, Zhou J, Liu X, Zheng M, Yang J, Tan J. Ultraviolet light-treated zirconia with different roughness affects function of human gingival fibroblastsin vitro: The potential surface modification developed from implant to abutment. J Biomed Mater Res B Appl Biomater 2015;103:116–124.
94. Brezavšček M, Fawzy A, Bächle M, Tuna T, Fischer J, Att W. The effect of UV treatment on the osteoconductive capacity of zirconia-based materials. Materials (Basel) 2016;24:958.
95. Henningsen A, Smeets R, Heuberger R, et al. Changes in surface characteristics of titanium and zirconia after surface treatment with ultraviolet light or non-thermal plasma. Eur J Oral Sci 2018;126:126–134.
96. Kobune K, Miura T, Sato T, Yotsuya M, Yoshinari M. Influence of plasma and ultraviolet treatment of zirconia on initial attachment of human oral keratinocytes: Expressions of laminin γ2 and integrin β4. Dent Mater J 2014;33:696–704.
97. Tuna T, Wein M, Altmann B, Steinberg T, Fischer J, Att W. Effect of ultraviolet photofunctionalization on the cell attractiveness of zirconia implant materials. Eur Cell Mater 2015;29:82–94.
98. Dorozhkin SV. Calcium orthophosphates in nature, biology and medicine. Materials (Basel) 2009;2:399–498.
99. Frame JW. Hydroxyapatite as a biomaterial for alveolar ridge augmentation. Int J Oral Maxillofac Surg 1987:16:642–655.
100. Sun L, Berndt CC, Gross KA, Kucuk A. Material fundamentals and clinical performance of plasma-sprayed hydroxyapatite coatings: A review. J Biomed Mater Res 2001;58:570–592.
101. Gómez-Morales J, Iafisco M, Delgado-López JM, Sarda S, Drouet C. Progress on the preparation of nanocrystalline apatites and surface characterization: Overview of fundamental and applied aspects. Prog Cryst Growth Charact Mater 2013;59:1–46.
102. Prakash C, Kansal HK, Pabla BS, Sanjeev P. Processing and characterization of novel biomimetic nanoporous bioceramic surface on β-Ti implant by powder mixed electric discharge machining. J Mater Engin Perform 2015;24:3622–3633.
103. Pardun K, Treccani L, Volkmann E, et al. Mixed zirconia calcium phosphate coatings for dental implants: Tailoring coating stability and bioactivity potential. Mater Sci Eng C Biol Appl 2015;48:337–346.
104. Ban S, Hasegawa J. Morphological regulation and crystal growth of hydrothermal-electrochemically deposited apatite. Biomaterials 2002;23:2965–2972.
105. Wolke JG, van Dijk K, Schaeken HG, de Groot K, Jansen JA. Study of the surface characteristics of magnetron-sputter calcium phosphate coatings. J Biomed Mater Res 1994;28: 1477–1484.
106. Kim J, Kang IG, Cheon KH, et al. Stable sol-gel hydroxyapatite coating on zirconia dental implant for improved osseointegration. J Mater Sci Mater Med 2021;32:81.
107. Catauro M, Bollino F, Papale F, Ciprioti SV. Investigation on bioactivity, biocompatibility, thermal behavior and antibacterial properties of calcium silicate glass coatings containing. J Non Cryst Solids 2015;422:16–22.
108. Rizwan M, Hamdi M, Basirun WJ. Bioglass R 45S5-based composites for bone tissue engineering and functional applications. J Biomed Mater Res A 2017;105:3197–3223.
109. Chen QZ, Thompson ID, Boccaccini AR. 45S5 Bioglass R-derived glass-ceramic scaffolds for bone tissue engineering. Biomaterials 2006;27:2414–2425.
110. Laranjeira MS, Carvalho A, Pelaez-Vargas A, et al. Modulation of human dermal microvascular endothelial cell and human gingival fibroblast behavior by micropatterned silica coating surfaces for zirconia dental implant applications. Sci Technol Adv Mater 2014;15:025001.

111. Kirsten A, Hausmann A, Weber M, Fischer J, Fischer H. Bioactive and thermally compatible glass coating on zirconia dental implants. J Dent Res 2015;94:297–303.
112. Skallevold HE, Rokaya D, Khurshid Z, Zafar MS. Bioactive glass applications in dentistry. Int J Mol Sci 2019;20:5960.
113. Fabris D, Fredel MC, Souza JCM, Silva FS, Henriques B. Biomechanical behavior of functionally graded S53P4 bioglass-zirconia dental implants: Experimental and finite element analyses. J Mech Behav Biomed Mater 2021;120:104565.
114. Cho BH, Ko WB. Preparation of graphene-ZrO2 nanocomposites by heat treatment and photocatalytic degradation of organic dyes. J Nanosci Nanotechnol 2013;13:7625–7630.
115. Li H, Xie Y, Li K, et al. Microstructure and wear behavior of graphene nanosheets-reinforced zirconia coating. Ceram Int 2014;40:12821–12829.
116. Rodríguez AM, González-Orellana C, García AAP, et al. Ageing-resistant zirconia/graphene-based nanostructures composites for use as biomaterials. J Eur Ceram Soc 2022;42;1784–1795.
117. Jang W, Kim HS, Alam K, Ji MK, Cho HS, Lim HP. Direct-deposited graphene oxide on dental implants for antimicrobial activities and osteogenesis. Int J Nanomed 2021;16:5745–5754.
118. ASTM-F1873. Standard specification for high-purity dense yttria tetragonal zirconium oxide polycrystal (Y-TZP) for surgical implant applications (withdrawn 2007). American Society for Testing and Materials, 1998.
119. ISO 13356:2015. Implants for surgery—Ceramic materials based on yttria-stabilized tetragonal zirconia (Y-TZP). International Organization for Standardization, 2015.

05

BIOLOGIC ASPECTS OF ZIRCONIA

Andrea Perna

The biocompatibility of a material is defined as its capacity "to perform with an appropriate host response in a specific application," according to the classic definition established during the 1986 Consensus Conference of the European Society for Biomaterials in Chester, England.[1] In the ensuing years, this definition evolved. According to Williams,[2] *biocompatibility* "refers to the ability of a biomaterial to perform its desired function with respect to a medical therapy, without eliciting any undesirable local or systemic effects in the recipient or beneficiary of that therapy, but generating the most appropriate beneficial cellular or tissue response in that specific situation, and optimizing the clinically relevant performance of that therapy." This new definition, although richer in detail, maintains the basic concept that *biocompatibility* refers to the biologic safety of a material joined with its functionality for the intended use.

Thus, to be considered biocompatible, materials used in the oral cavity must be *(1)* biologically safe, meaning that neither the biomaterial nor its degradation products cause inflammatory, allergic, autoimmune, toxic, mutagenic, or carcinogenic reactions, and *(2)* functionally safe, meaning they withstand the loads applied during clinical use throughout the expected lifetime of the product. Dental implants must also be able to integrate with the host bone.

Osseointegration is a term first used by Per-Ingvar Brånemark to indicate direct union between bone and an artificial implant, without the formation of connective tissue between the two surfaces.[3] Osseointegration is a time-dependent process that leads to the rigid fixation of alloplastic materials in the bone during functional loading.[4] Osseointegration of zirconia dental implants is discussed in detail in chapter 7. The present chapter deals mainly with the biologic safety of zirconia as reported in various studies testing its use as a biomaterial.

The first in vitro studies on the biologic safety of zirconia were carried out in the early 1990s,[5] with the results of the first in vivo studies reported 20 years earlier.[6] Since then a number of in vitro and in vivo studies have been carried out. Zirconia has been a standardized material for surgical implants since 1997, and its biologic safety is the foundation of its clinical use.[7,8] It is worthwhile to note that many studies have been carried out on experimental materials that are very different from those used in devices licensed for clinical use.

In Vitro Assays

In vitro assays have demonstrated that various zirconia powders and ceramics are not acutely toxic to cell lines including macrophages, lymphocytes, fibroblasts, and osteoblasts. However, powders (particularly nanometric powders) do stimulate higher cytotoxic reactions than ceramics, whatever the material. This is due to the high surface-to-mass ratio of powders and particulate in comparison with sintered ceramic bodies. Furthermore, whatever the mean diameter of a certain quantity of particulate is, a variable fraction of it will be nanometric in size. Nevertheless, there is general agreement about the biologic safety of both zirconia powders and ceramics.

A wide array of experimental parameters have been used for in vitro assays to assess the biologic safety of zirconia. Tested materials have varied both in physical form (powders or dense ceramics) and in chemical and physical characteristics (eg, reactive surface, chemical composition, purity, etc). Moreover, in vitro assays can be conducted using direct or indirect contact approaches. The chosen cell type—whether macrophages, lymphocytes, fibroblasts, or osteoblasts—may be from either stable cell lines or primary cell cultures, depending on the requirements of the experiment.

Testing conditions are also relevant for results. Tateishi et al[9] analyzed the results of a round robin test for the standardization of in vitro biocompatibility assays and observed significant differences between results obtained by different labs performing the same test with the same materials and cell lines.

LEUKOCYTE ASSAYS

Monocytes, lymphocytes, macrophages, and other cells of the immune system are a very important part of the hematologic elements contained in the connective tissue and constitute an effective tool for investigating the biologic safety of materials that are candidates for use in the human body.

Human lymphocytes harvested from healthy volunteers were used in the first in vitro tests on zirconia in 1991.[5] 3H-thimydine uptake tests were performed during phytohemagglutinin (PHA)–induced human lymphocyte proliferation. The cells were cultured in the presence of zirconia particulate. An inhibitory effect on the cells was observed and was dose-dependent at all material concentrations but lower for calcia partially stabilized zirconia (Ca-PSZ) than for titanium dioxide (rutile), which was used as a reference. Later, Greco et al[10] observed similar behavior in the mitogenesis of human lymphocytes during testing with alumina and zirconia powders.

Mebouta-Nkamgeu et al[11] observed a reduction in macrophage activity and potency of phagocytosis in the presence of zirconia powder. The cytotoxic effects were directly proportional to the concentration of powder and were enhanced when powder particle size exceeded 2 µm.

Catelas et al[12] observed apoptosis of murine 774 macrophages, which was dependent on the size and concentration of ceramic particles. This effect reached a plateau for particle concentrations above 150 particles/macrophage and a particle size of 1.3 µm. Ceramic particles were found to be less toxic than polyethylene particles, as previously reported by Purchio et al.[13]

In addition to evaluating the cytotoxicity of zirconia on immune cells, several authors have studied the production of inflammatory mediators by macrophage cell lines incubated with ceramics or metals. Sterner et al[14] investigated the tumor necrosis factor-α (TNF-α) response of macrophage-like human monocytes (THP-1) after exposure to several concentrations of alumina (Al_2O_3), zirconia (ZrO_2), and titanium (Ti) particles of various sizes. The greatest TNF-α response was observed with titanium particles, whereas zirconia exhibited no effects on the release of TNF-α.[14] Bu et al[15] found an increase in TNF-α as an inhibitor of the secretion of interferon-γ (IFN-γ) in human monocytes in the presence of zirconia powders. IFN-γ is a critical functional factor for osteoclast differentiation and subsequently for the osseointegration process.[15]

Obando-Pereda et al[16] observed that macrophages in culture with zirconium or titanium oxide particles expressed an increase in messenger ribonucleic acid (mRNA) levels for toll-like receptors (TLRs) 2, 3, 4, and 9 and their myeloid differentiation primary response 88 (MyD88); TIR-domain-containing adapter-inducing interferon-β (TRIF) and nuclear factor κ-light-chain-enhancer of activated B cells (NF-κB) adapters; and cytokines TNF-α, interleukin (IL)-1β, and IL-6. They also noted lower proinflammatory gene expression induced by zirconia particles in comparison with that induced by titanium particles.[16]

Some authors argue that the structural characteristics of the surface that interacts with the cell is more important than the chemical composition of the material. Wang et al[17] showned that hydrophilic surfaces tend to reduce the proinflammatory response by lowering the gene expression of TNF-α, IL-1, and IL-6 and promoting tissue resolution through the expression of cytokine IL-10. The topography and chemistry of the implant surface have a substantial impact on the behavior of macrophages.[17]

A summary of these leukocyte assays is provided in Table 5-1.

TABLE 5-1 › **Summary of leukocyte assays**

Study	Material	Physical form	Cell type	Test	Effect	Notes
Tateishi et al[9] (1992)	Ca-PSZ	Porous ceramic (30%) and powders	Human lymphocytes	Inhibition of cell mitogenesis after PHA induction	Dose-dependent cytotoxicity	
Greco et al[10] (1991)	Ca-PSZ	Powders	Human lymphocytes	Inhibition of cell mitogenesis after PHA induction	Dose-dependent cytotoxicity	Similar behavior of alumina and zirconia powder
Catelas et al[12] (1999)	ZrO_2	Powders	Human monocytes	Cell differentiation	Dose-dependent cytotoxicity (higher in alumina than in zirconia)	Enhanced cytotoxic effects when powder particle size > 2 µm
Purchio et al[13] (1995)	ZrO_2	Powders	Murine macrophages	Apoptosis	Dose-dependent cytotoxicity	No difference between ceramics and UHMWPE
Bu et al[15] (2017)	ZrO_2	Periprosthetic particles	THP-1 cells (human monocytic cell line)	TNF-α response using ELISA assay	ZrO_2 showed no effects on TNF-α release	
Obando-Pereda et al[16] (2014)	ZrO_2	Periprosthetic particles	THP-1 cells (human monocytic cell line)	Expression of IFN-γ and miR-29b detected by real-time RT-PCR or ELISA	TNF-α inhibited the secretion of IFN-γ in the presence of zirconia powders	IFN-γ is a critical functional factor for osseointegration
Wang et al[17] (2019)	ZrO_2	Periprosthetic particles	THP-1 cells (human monocytic cell line)	TLRs 2, 3, 4, and 9 by RT-PCR	Dose-dependent production	Zirconia-induced gene expression lower than that induced by titanium particles

ELISA = enzyme-linked immunosorbent assay; RT-PCR = reverse transcription polymerase chain reaction; UHMWPE = ultra-high molecular weight polyethylene.

FIBROBLAST ASSAYS

Bukat et al[18] reported the results of the first studies on zirconia cytotoxicity with fibroblasts. 3T3 fibroblasts were cultured on zirconia disks (30 vol% porosity). The adhesion and spreading of the fibroblasts on zirconia 12 hours from seeding was similar to that found on control surfaces (glass and plastic), a preliminary finding indicative of the lack of cytotoxicity of the ceramic.

Ito et al[19] investigated the cell reaction to zirconia particles generated by friction, observing cytotoxicity mainly by particles less than 0.22 nm in size. Similar results were reported much later by Kwon et al,[20] who used a culture of gingival fibroblasts. This dependence of the cytotoxic reactions on the surface-to-mass ratio of the material tested was also observed by Li et al,[21] who reported the results of cytotoxicity assays using human gingival fibroblast (HGF) colonies upon direct contact with human fibroblasts. Cell viability was assessed using mitochondrial function tests (MTT assay). Zirconia was much more toxic as a powder than in a sintered state. The difference is likely due to the higher surface-to-mass ratio of zirconia powders for sintering (zirconia precursors) in comparison with powders obtained by milling sintered ceramics.

Dion et al[22] used BALB/c 3T3 permanent cell lines and human umbilical venous endothelial cells (HUVECs) to evaluate the cytotoxicity of several ceramics, including zirconia. The results obtained from the cell viability and MTT assays showed the lack of cytotoxic effects of the tested ceramic powders on fibroblasts and endothelial cells. Harmand et al[23] used BALB 3T3 fibroblasts to demonstrate the absence of cytotoxicity with zirconia. They conducted agar overlay assays (indirect contact) as well as direct contact assays at 24 and 72 hours. Additionally, tests using cellular extracts were performed at 120 hours using four extraction vehicle concentrations: 100%, 50%, 10%, and 1%. Cytotoxicity was evaluated by viable cell count and MTT assay.

Uo et al[24] investigated the cytotoxicity of eight dental ceramics commonly used for restorations, including a zirconia ceramic (Denzir). HGFs were cultured with extraction solutions of the eight ceramic materials (1.25 cm^2/mL for 20 days at 37°C). The cytotoxicity was estimated by alamarBlue (Thermo Fisher Scientific) assay and DNA quantification, which showed the absence of significant cytotoxicity ($P > .05$) with the tested ceramic. Yamano et al[25] studied the cellular response of HGFs cultured on the surface of zirconia or titanium disks with either smooth or rough surfaces. The authors evaluated cell morphology via scanning electron microscopy (SEM), proliferation activity via MTT assay, and gene expression via polymerase chain reaction (PCR). The cells cultured on smooth zirconia proliferated significantly more quickly than on the other surfaces, but their spreading was the weakest. In comparison with titanium, gene expression of integrin α2 at 3 hours and integrin α5 and type 1 collagen at 48 hours were upregulated significantly on smooth zirconia.[25] The response of HGFs cultured on titanium and various zirconia surfaces was analyzed by Pae et al.[26] The titanium surfaces were machined, and the zirconia surfaces were smooth or grooved (100-μm depth). The cell proliferation activity was evaluated via MTT assay (24 hours and 48 hours), while the cell morphology was studied by SEM. The mean optical density values after 48 hours were greater for the titanium and grooved zirconia surfaces than for the smooth zirconia surfaces. SEM examination evidenced the attachment of HGFs to the grooves, with subsequent orientation of the cells along the grooves. Fibroblast-specific genetic expression evaluated by reverse transcription PCR was similar for the three groups.

Opposite results were reported by Fischer et al,[27] who investigated the influence of zirconia surface roughness on the adhesion of gingival fibroblasts, a key parameter for the formation of a mucosal seal around implant abutments. They seeded HGFs onto the zirconia surfaces after polishing with four grades of commercial polishing heads. After surface characterization (SEM, atomic force microscopy [AFM], and optical profilometry), cell proliferation was measured via a quantitative SEM technique and focal adhesion kinase (FAK), while phosphorylation status was measured by enzyme-linked immunosorbent assay (ELISA). Results showed an increase in proliferation on all polished surfaces compared with the control.

Table 5-2 summarizes the results of these studies.

TABLE 5-2 › Summary of fibroblast assays

Study	Material	Physical form	Cell type	Test	Effect	Notes
Bukat et al[18] (1992)	ZrO_2	Disks (30 vol% porosity)	3T3 fibroblasts	Direct contact SEM observation	Fibroblast adhesion and spreading	Cell monolayer on ceramic samples after 72 hours
Ito et al[19] (1993)	ZrO_2	Wear debris	Murine L929	Cell proliferation	More cytotoxicity in wear debris from zirconia than from titanium	Cytotoxicity dependent on specific surface
Kwon et al[20] (2014)	ZrO_2 with or without EMD	Disks	HGFs	Morphology (SEM), proliferation activity (MTT assay), and gene expression of the cells (PCR)	EMD affected the proliferation, attachment, and cell morphology of HGFs	

TABLE 5-2 *(cont)* › **Summary of fibroblast assays**

Study	Material	Physical form	Cell type	Test	Effect	Notes
Li et al[21] (1993)	ZrO_2	Powders and ceramic	HGFs	Direct contact MTT test	Powders more toxic than ceramic	50% reduction in CFE at a concentration of 50 µg/mL for zirconia
Dion et al[22] (1994)	ZrO_2	Powders	HUVECs, 3T3 fibroblasts	Indirect contact MTT test	No toxicity	
Harmand et al[23] (1995)	ZrO_2	Powders	3T3 fibroblasts	Agar overlay assays (indirect contact), MTT test	No toxicity	
Uo et al[24] (2003)	Y-PSZ	Powders	HGFs	Cytotoxicity by alamarBlue dye assay and DNA quantification	No toxicity	
Yamano et al[25] (2011)	ZrO_2	Ceramic disks with smooth or rough surfaces	HGFs	Morphology (SEM), proliferation activity (MTT assay), and gene expression of the cells (PCR)	Cells cultured on smooth zirconia proliferated significantly faster than cells on other surfaces	Upregulation of gene expression of integrin α2, integrin α5, and type 1 collagen on smooth zirconia
Pae et al[26] (2009)	ZrO_2	Smooth and grooved ceramic and titanium surfaces	HGFs	MTT assay, cell morphology (SEM)	Mean optical density was greater on grooved zirconia surfaces than smooth ones	
Fischer et al[27] (2017)	ZrO_2	CAD/CAM surfaces	HGFs	Proliferation via quantitative SEM technique and FAK, phosphorylation status measured by ELISA assay	Increase in proliferation on all polished surfaces in comparison with control	

CFE = cell-free gene expression; EMD = enamel matrix derivative; Y-PSZ = yttria partially stabilized zirconia.

OSTEOBLAST ASSAYS

Josset et al[28] evaluated the biocompatibility of zirconia and alumina ceramics using human osteoblast cell cultures in vitro and observed no cytostatic or cytotoxic effects. Cell proliferation kinetics and total protein synthesis in osteoblasts with zirconia or alumina were similar to those of control cells cultured on glass coverslips. Cell spreading on the surface of the two ceramics was similar. Immunochemistry assays evidenced extracellular matrices composed of collagen types 1 and 5, osteocalcin, osteonectin, bone sialoprotein, and cellular fibronectin.

Lohmann et al[29] analyzed the proliferation of MG63 osteoblastic cell lines in contact with alumina and zirconia particles. Transmission electron microscopy showed that MG63 cells phagocytosed alumina particles and exhibited ultrastructural changes consistent with cytotoxicity. Alumina particles decreased proliferation, alkaline phosphatase (ALP) activity, and tumor growth factor-β1 (TGF-β1) levels in MG63 cells, whereas zirconia particles increased proliferation and ALP-specific activity.

Hao et al[30] studied the effects of carbon dioxide (CO_2) laser irradiation on the adhesion of osteoblasts to zirconia surfaces using cultures of human fetal osteoblast cells (hFOBs). They found evidence of improved cell adhesion to the laser-treated samples, which was related to the change in the wettability of the irradiated surfaces.

The attachment of osteoblast-like cells (CAL72) on zirconia was investigated by Bächle et al.[31] The study was carried out on airborne particle–abraded and acid-etched zirconia and titanium to evaluate the influence of surface roughness and topography on cell behavior. No differences in cell proliferation and colonization of cells on the different substrates were detected at 12 days, regardless of the substrate conditions. Even rough untreated zirconia allowed cells to attach to the material.

Att et al[32] investigated the effects of the photochemical treatment of a zirconia surface with UV light on bone marrow–derived osteoblasts. Irradiation up to 48 hours increased the rates of attachment, spread, and proliferation of the cells, stimulating ALP and mineralization. These effects were due to transformation of the zirconia surface from hydrophobic to hydrophilic due to UV irradiation, which depending on the UV ray dose reduced the atomic percentage of surface carbon.

Aboushelib et al[33] investigated the influence of nanoporous zirconia and titanium surfaces on the attachment of human osteoblasts. By days 3 and 8 after seeding, they observed a significantly higher cell count on nanoporous zirconia and titanium surfaces compared with the polished samples. There were 25% more cells on the zirconia surfaces. Nanoporous zirconia specimens demonstrated similar ALP and intracellular protein content when compared with other tested groups.

Greater osteoblast cell activity of zirconia compared with titanium was observed by Song et al,[34] who evaluated the in vitro cellular behavior of MC3T3-E1 preosteoblast cells cultured on titanium and zirconia disks. They found that cell proliferation on titanium disks appeared to be significantly lower in comparison with that on zirconia disks ($P < .05$). Bubik et al[35] found similar cell behavior on zirconia and titanium but did not replicate these findings. They cultured hFOBs on disks made from commercially pure titanium and yttria-stabilized tetragonal zirconia polycrystal (Y-TZP) and observed changes in cell viability and lactate dehydrogenase (LDH) release after 1, 3, and 7 days. The mRNA expression of proliferative factors proliferation cell nuclear antigen (PCNA) and Ki67 and cellular adhesion (vinculin mRNA expression and immunofluorescence staining) were analyzed after 3 days in the culture. No significant difference was observed in commercially pure titanium and zirconia when compared with the control.

Herath et al[36] performed a study to assess the effects of zirconia surface characteristics on the attachment, proliferation, and differentiation of osteoblast-like cells. Zirconia ceramic surfaces supported cell attachment, proliferation, and differentiation regardless of their condition (sintered, abraded, polished, or porous), but the surfaces with grain boundary grooves or abraded grooves provided enhanced conditions for initial cell attachment. All cells retained the typical polygonal morphology of osteoblast-like cells, showing a preferential orientation along grooves on the surfaces. Moreover, overall cell proliferation and total DNA were higher on the polished surface than on the porous surface, as determined via alamarBlue assay.

Hadjicharalambous et al[37] compared in vitro adhesion, proliferation, and differentiation of mouse MC3T3-E preosteoblasts on three porous alumina and zirconia materials.[37] All three ceramics demonstrated strong cell attachment, but better cell spreading and growth was observed on zirconia-containing substrates. Moreover, cells expressed more ALP activity, increased collagen production, and increased calcium biomineralization on zirconia than on alumina.

The effect of a zirconia microgrooved surface on the behavior of hFOBs was investigated by Delgado-Ruíz et al.[38] They observed that an increase in surface area of zirconia due to microgrooving enhanced ALP and Alazarin red (ALZ), cell density size, and organization of hFOBs.

The behavior of human osteoblasts and HGFs in contact with zirconia and titanium implant surface materials after 14 days in culture was characterized by da Cruz et al.[39] Both osteoblasts and fibroblasts exhibited higher viability and proliferation compared with titanium. All groups showed an insignificant increase in ALP activity over time. Mineralization patterns demonstrated an increase in mineral content over time, which was higher in zirconia. Cell spreading was more evident on zirconia specimens than on titanium. The results suggest increased adhesion, viability, and proliferation of osteoblasts and gingival fibroblasts on zirconia surfaces compared with titanium.

The initial stem cell and preosteoblast cell adhesion and oxidative response on zirconia in comparison with titanium was investigated by Wei et al,[40] who studied human dental pulp stem cells (DPSCs) and murine preosteoblasts (MC3T3-E1) on zirconia and titanium surfaces. The morphologic features of both cell lines were comparable during cell adhesion processes, with continuous expansion of cell size and increasing cell viability on titanium and zirconia surfaces during the 24-hour culture time. Higher mean cell viability was observed on zirconia compared with titanium, with significantly higher DPSC viability at 12 hours after seeding (*P* < .05). In addition, both DPSCs and MC3T3-E1 cells on zirconia surfaces had higher mean reactive oxygen species levels after the 24-hour culture time compared with cells on titanium.

These osteoblast assays on zirconia are summarized in Table 5-3.

TABLE 5-3 › Summary of osteoblast assays

Study	Material	Physical form	Cell type	Test	Effect	Notes
Josset et al[28] (1999)	ZrO_2	Ceramic	Human osteoblast cells	Cytotoxicity by methylthiazole sulfate test, morphology via SEM	Cell proliferation kinetics and total protein synthesis similar to control cells	
Lohmann et al[29] (2002)	ZrO_2	Powders	MG63 osteoblastic cells	SEM	Increased zirconia particle proliferation and ALP activity	Decrease in cell proliferation and cytotoxic effect with alumina
Hao et al[30] (2005)	Y-PSZ	Ceramics, with or without CO_2 laser irradiation	hFOBs	Cell adhesion (SEM)	Improved adhesion of cells on the laser-treated samples compared with the untreated samples	
Bächle et al[31] (2007)	Y-PSZ	Airborne particle–abraded and acid-etched surfaces	Osteoblast-like cells (CAL72)	Cell proliferation versus surface topography (SEM)	No differences in cell proliferation and colonization on different substrates	Roughened Y-TZP enhanced proliferation of CAL72
Att et al[32] (2009)	ZrO_2	UV-treated machined zirconia disks	Murine bone marrow–derived osteoblasts	Cell adhesion and proliferation (SEM)	UV irradiation increased the rate of cell attachment, spreading, and proliferation; ALP; and mineralization	Effects depended on UV ray dose
Aboushelib et al[33] (2013)	ZrO_2	Nanoporous versus polished zirconia surfaces	Human osteoblasts	Cell morphology (SEM) and proliferation (cell count)	Porous surfaces enhanced cell growth and attachment compared with polished surfaces	

TABLE 5-3 *(cont)* › **Summary of osteoblast assays**

Study	Material	Physical form	Cell type	Test	Effect	Notes
Song et al[34] (2014)	ZrO_2	Ceramic disks	Murine preosteoblasts (MC3T3-E1)	Cell morphology and proliferation (SEM, X-ray spectrometer, and X-ray diffraction), protein expression (RT-PCR)	Proliferation on titanium disks significantly lower than on zirconia disks	Interconnecting pores of the zirconia scaffolds showed enhanced proliferation and cell differentiation
Bubik et al[35] (2017)	Y-TZP	Ceramic disks	hFOBs	Cell viability, proliferation, and adhesion	No difference between commercially pure titanium and Y-TZP	
Herath et al[36] (2015)	ZrO_2	Ceramics	Osteoblast-like cells	Cell proliferation	Zirconia ceramics supported cell attachment, proliferation, and differentiation	Greater proliferation and total DNA on polished surfaces
Hadjicharalambous et al[37] (2015)	ZrO_2	Porous zirconia versus alumina	Mouse preosteoblasts (MC3T3-E1)	Cell adhesion, proliferation, and differentiation	Better cell spreading and growth observed on zirconia substrates	Enhanced collagen production and calcium biomineralization on zirconia
Delgado-Ruíz et al[38] (2016)	ZrO_2	Zirconia implants with microgrooved surfaces	hFOBs	Cell morphology and density (SEM)	Higher ALP and ALZ, greater cell density, and larger cell size due to microgrooving	
Da Cruz et al[39] (2019)	Y-TZP	Implant surfaces, disks	Human osteoblasts	Cell viability and proliferation (resazurin assay), cell morphology and adhesion (SEM)	Improved cell viability and proliferation greater with PEEK and Y-TZP compared with titanium, cell spreading higher with PEEK and Y-TZP specimens	Mineralization patterns more apparent in the Y-TZP group
Wei et al[40] (2019)	ZrO_2	Surfaces	Murine preosteoblast cells (MC3T3-E1), DPSCs	Cell viability and morphology (tetrazolium-based colorimetric assay, SEM, and ELISA assay)	Higher mean cell viability observed with zirconia compared to titanium within a 24-hour culture period	Cells had higher mean reactive oxygen species levels on zirconia surfaces than titanium ones

PEEK = polyetheretherketone; RT-PCR = reverse transcription polymerase chain reaction; Y-PSZ = yttria partially stabilized zirconia.

In Vivo Tests

In vitro tests are fundamental for evaluating material biocompatibility, but complex physiologic phenomena related to organs and other systems in the body mean that evidence gained via in vitro testing must also be supported by tests in vivo.

The first in vivo study on the biologic safety of zirconia was performed by Helmer and Driskell,[6] who implanted zirconia samples in monkey femurs and observed apparent bone growth around the material with no adverse reactions. Connective tissue was present at the interface of the bone and ceramic, and over time it gradually transformed into bone in direct contact with the ceramic.[6] Hulbert et al[41] examined the soft tissue response to three different ceramics, including calcia-stabilized zirconia, by implanting disks with porosity in the range of 45 to 150 μm into the muscles and connective tissue of rabbits for up to 9 months without finding any adverse reactions. The samples were encapsulated by fibrous tissue, and fibrous layers were thinner around samples with larger pores.[41]

Some early studies were performed to investigate the use of zirconia as a coating on metallic implants. In 1973, Bortz and Onesto[42] reported the results of a wide research program aimed at developing several different products, including artificial trachea, vascular prostheses, and contraceptive devices, obtained by flame spraying zirconia on supports made of AISI 316 stainless steel or copper. Implants placed in the trachea of dogs and rabbits failed due to fibrous tissues invading the implant lumen, whereas implants placed in the vena cava of dogs showed the absence of clotting 6 weeks postoperatively. Tests on contraceptive devices showed a fibrous reaction to implants. Overall, the inflammatory reaction observed in these experimental implants was less than those observed with cobalt-chromium alloys.[42] Further research on tissue reactions to zirconia coatings was performed by Cranin et al,[43] who implanted zirconia-coated endosteal implants in beagles, and Monticelli et al,[44] who described the clinical use of zirconia-coated endoprosthesis stems. Studies on zirconia coatings to promote direct apposition of bone to metallic implants are still in progress.[45,46]

The first study to investigate the suitability of zirconia for dental devices was performed by Nagai et al,[47] who implanted zirconia pins in the subfacial tissues and mandibular bones of Wistar rats for up to 56 days. By 28 days, the zirconia ceramic pins implanted in the subfacial tissues were completely encapsulated by dense fibrous tissues, as observed previously by Hulbert et al.[41] By 28 days after placement, zirconia pins inserted in the mandibular bones were surrounded by new trabecular bone, which was replaced with mature bone tissue by 56 days postoperatively. Garvie et al[48] implanted magnesia partially stabilized zirconia (Mg-PSZ) in the paraspinal muscles of rabbits for 6 months and observed no adverse soft tissue response to the implants, confirming the results of this seminal work. Furthermore, by the end of the studied implantation period in vivo, the surface phase content, surface roughness, and strength of the implants remained unchanged. Similar findings were reported by Christel et al,[49] Satoh and Niwa,[50] and Ichikawa et al.[51] The study by Satoh and Niwa[50] involved implanting zirconia screws in the femoral condyle of rabbits. The histology of retrieved block specimens after 12 and 18 months from implant placement evidenced new bone surrounding the screws and the apposition of trabecular bone against the surface of the zirconia.[50]

Greco et al[52] implanted sintered zirconia samples in the tibial metaphysis of New Zealand White rabbits. In the follow-ups that lasted for up to 12 months, no pathologic processes related to local or systemic toxicity due to the alloplastic implants were observed. Evidence of reparative osteogenesis was found around the implants, with trabecular and lamellar bone in direct contact with the ceramic surfaces. In a few cases fibrous interposition was observed.[52]

Hayashi et al[53] implanted zirconia, alumina, and 316L stainless steel screws in the medial and lateral femoral condyles of dogs. The follow-up of the implants lasted up to 96 weeks from insertion. The bone-to-implant contact (BIC) index was similar for the three materials at the end of the follow-up (81% to 86%). However, the implants were placed in unloaded sites, and the difference in stiffness did not play any role in implant macrostrains and interfacial stresses, which may be significant for bone apposition in loaded sites.

Miani et al[54] placed submerged zirconia cylinder implants into the distal root site of beagles immediately after tooth extraction. The follow-up period lasted 60 or 120 days. Osteotropic fluorochromes were injected into the animals at 21, 14, and 7 days before the end of the follow-up time. Clinical examination at the end of the follow-up time did not reveal inflammatory or degenerative processes due to the presence of the material. Radiography indicated bone with a regular and uniform texture surrounding the implants that appeared to be in direct contact with the zirconia surface. The direct apposition of newly formed bone, confirmed in the histologic sections, evidenced the osseointegrative capacity of zirconia implants.

In a study by Akagawa et al,[55] zirconia screw implants placed in the right premolar sites of four beagle dogs were inserted by tapping and divided into two groups: loaded or unloaded. The premolars had been removed 3 months before implant placement. A noble metal superstructure connected loaded implants. Histology demonstrated direct bone apposition without interposed fibrous tissue at the bone-zirconia interface. Healthier gingiva was observed around implants in the nonloaded group, along with reduced marginal bone loss, compared with implants in the loaded group.

These studies, along with the one performed later by Dubruille et al,[56] paved the way for the clinical use of zirconia as a dental implant. The osseointegration of zirconia implants is widely acknowledged today and described in several reviews.[57–59]

A summary of these in vivo biocompatibility studies on zirconia is provided in Table 5-4.

TABLE 5-4 › **Summary of in vivo tests on zirconia**

Study	Material	Physical form	Animal model	Implant site	Tissue response	Notes
Helmer and Driskell[6] (1978)	ZrO_2 (6% Y_2O_3)	Pellets	Monkeys	Femur	No adverse response	Apparent bone ingrowth
Hulbert et al[41] (1972)	Ca-PSZ	Dense and porous tubes	Rabbits	Paraspinal muscles	No toxicity or immunogenic reactions	Bone ingrowth depending on pore size
Bortz and Onesto[42] (1973)	ZrO_2	Coated tubes	Rabbits, dogs	Trachea	Fibrous growth in lumen	
Cranin et al[43] (1975)	ZrO_2	Coating	Dogs	Mandibular bone		
Chung et al[45] (2013)	ZrO_2	Coating	Rabbits	Tibia	Greater BIC and higher removal torque values with zirconia-coated implants	Removal torque depended on surface roughness
Hamad et al[46] (2018)	ZrO_2	Coating	Rabbits	Tibia	High removal torques in zirconia-coated implants	Zirconia coating enhanced osseointegration
Nagai et al[47] (1982)	ZrO_2	Pins	Rats	Abdominal subfascial tissue, mandibular bone	Fibrous encapsulation in soft tissue, growth of bony trabeculae in mandibular bone	
Garvie et al[48] (1984)	Mg-PSZ	Bars	Rabbits	Paraspinal muscle	No adverse response	
Christel et al[49] (1989)	Y-PSZ	Cylinders	Rats	Paraspinal muscle	No significant differences between Y-PSZ and alumina	
Satoh and Niwa[50] (1992)	ZrO_2	Screws	Rabbits	Femoral condyle	New bone surrounding the screws	Trabecular bone apposition on zirconia surfaces

TABLE 5-4 *(cont)* › **Summary of in vivo tests on zirconia**

Study	Material	Physical form	Animal model	Implant site	Tissue response	Notes
Ichikawa et al[51] (1992)	Y-TZP	Cylinders	Rats	Dorsal subcutis	Fibrous tissue growth around the sample	
Greco et al[52] (1993)	Ca-PSZ	Cylinders	Rabbits	Tibia	No toxic effects, new bone formation	
Hayashi et al[53] (1992)	ZrO_2	Cylinders	Dogs	Distal femoral epiphysis	Fibrous membrane, no adverse response	
Miani et al[54] (1993)	Y-TZP	Cylinders	Dogs	Mandibular bone	No inflammatory or degenerative processes	Uniform texture of the bone surrounding the implants
Akagawa et al[55] (1993)	Y-TZP	Cylinders	Dogs	Mandibular bone	Direct bone apposition on zirconia without interposing fibrous tissue	No fibrous tissue observed
Dubruille et al[56] (1999)	ZrO_2	Cylinders	Dogs	Mandibular bone	No significant statistical difference between the three implant types	

Y-PSZ = yttria partially stabilized zirconia.

Carcinogenicity and Genotoxicity Studies

It is known that high-purity dense zirconia qualified for implantable devices does not induce carcinogenicity or mutagenicity. These effects are related to nanopowders and are related more to the physical form than to material chemistry. Nanopowders have a surface-to-mass ratio of several square meters per gram, with a much more reactive surface than sintered ceramics.

Early studies on the biologic safety of zirconia addressed the issues of carcinogenicity and mutagenicity. Hulbert et al,[41] who implanted zirconia samples in rabbits, reported the absence of both carcinogenicity and immunologic effects. The absence of carcinogenic and teratogenic effects was also reported by Satoh and Niwa[50] after Ames tests on Chinese hamster cells cultured in the presence of zirconia.

Covacci et al[60] investigated the mutagenic and oncogenic effects of zirconia ceramics obtained by sintering high-purity powder to assess its suitability for medical devices. Assays were made using mouse embryo–derived fibroblast C3H/10T½ cultures. Ceramics made from a low-purity zirconia powder were tested for comparison, and fibroblasts irradiated by a linear accelerator were used as a positive control.

The results obtained showed that the high-purity zirconia did not elicit either a mutagenic or transforming effect on cells, whereas impure zirconia resulted in the formation of clones similar to those resulting from x-ray treatment of cells.

Absence of mutagenicity and carcinogenicity of zirconia ceramic was also observed by Josset et al,[28] who cultured human osteoblasts on sintered zirconia disks for up to 30 days to detect any changes in DNA synthesis and cell proliferation. The evaluation was carried out via DNA image cytometry and the quantification of nucleolar organization regions (NORs). The results showed that in comparison with control cells, neither material altered the number of homologous sets of chromosomes present in a cell or the cell growth rate. These results were in accordance with the absence of any inducing effect on DNA synthesis or proliferation.

On the other hand, Atalay et al[61] reported DNA damage and apoptosis when performing in vitro investigation of the genotoxic and apoptotic effects of 20-nm zirconia nanopowders on an L929 mouse fibroblast cell line. Three different concentrations of 20-nm zirconia nanoparticles (50 µg/mL, 100 µg/mL, and 150 µg/mL) were used. Single-cell gel electrophoresis (ie, *comet assay*) and flow cytometry demonstrated that the nanopowders induced DNA damage at all tested concentrations.

Table 5-5 summarizes these studies.

TABLE 5-5 › Summary of carcinogenicity and genotoxicity studies on zirconia

Study	Material	Physical form	Model	Implant site/type of assay	Effect
Hulbert et al[41] (1972)	Ca-PSZ	Porous and nonporous tubes	Rabbits	Paraspinal muscle	No carcinogenic or immunogenic reactions
Satoh and Niwa[50] (1992)	ZrO_2	Powder	Chinese hamster cells	Ames tests	No carcinogenic or teratogenic effects
Covacci et al[60] (1999)	Y-TZP	Ceramic disks	Murine embryo–derived fibroblasts (C3H/10T½)	Mutation and transformation frequency	High-purity zirconia did not elicit a mutagenic or transforming effect on cells
Josset et al[28] (1999)	Y-TZP	Ceramic disks	Human osteoblasts	DNA synthesis	No DNA alterations
Atalay et al[61] (2018)	ZrO_2	Nanoparticles (20 nm) at different concentrations (50 µg/mL, 100 µg/mL, and 150 µg/mL)	L929 mouse fibroblasts	Genotoxic and apoptotic effects in in vitro conditions by comet assay and flow cytometry methods	Zirconia nanoparticles induced DNA damage and apoptosis at all concentrations

Conclusion

Extensive analyses have been performed showing zirconia's superior abilities compared with materials like titanium and alumina. These include zirconia's ability to promote cell proliferation, partly by modulating gene expression. The configuration of the reaction surface plays a pivotal role and highlights the need to develop materials that maximize both cell proliferation and adhesion to enhance osseointegration. Zirconia's combination of biocompatibility, absence of carcinogenicity and toxicity, and mechanical strength make it an excellent candidate for prosthetic implant coatings. Its mechanical and biologic properties render it particularly suitable for dental implants. Although aging can negatively impact zirconia's mechanical properties, this does not appear to compromise clinical outcomes in dentistry. Future research should focus on optimizing the biomedical applications of zirconia, particularly in areas such as ceramic bonding, anchoring techniques, and strategies to mitigate material aging.

References

1. Williams DF. Definitions in Biomaterials. Elsevier, 1987.
2. Williams DF. On the mechanisms of biocompatibility. Biomaterials 2008;29:2941–2953.
3. Carlsson L, Röstlund T, Albrektsson B, Albrektsson T, Brånemark PI. Osseointegration of titanium implants. Acta Orthop Scand 1986;57:285–289.
4. Zarb CA, Albrektsson T. Nature of implant attachments. In: Brånemark PI, Zarb C, Albrektsson T (eds). Tissue-Integrated Prostheses Osseointegration in Clinical Dentistry. Quintessence, 1985:88–98.
5. Greco F, Piantelli S, Maccauro G, Arena M, Piconi C. Valutazione della biocompatibilità in vitro dell'ossido di titanio e dell'ossido di zirconio. Biomateriali 1991;5:119.
6. Helmer JD, Driskell TD. Research on bioceramics. In: Hulbert SF, Young FA (eds). Use of Ceramics as Surgical Implants. Gordon and Breach, 1978:123–126.
7. ISO 13356:2015 Implants for surgery—Ceramic materials based on yttria-stabilized tetragonal zirconia (Y-TZP). International Organization for Standardization, 1997.
8. ASTM F-1873 Standard specification for high-purity dense yttria tetragonal zirconium oxide polycrystal (Y-TZP) for surgical implant applications. American Society for Testing and Materials, 1998.
9. Tateishi T, Ushida T, Aoki H, et al. Round-robin test for standardization of biocompatibility test procedure by cell culture method. In: Doherty PJ, Williams RL, Williams DF, Lee AJC (eds). Biomaterial-Tissue Interfaces. Vol 10: Advances in Biomaterials. Elsevier, 1992:89–97.
10. Greco F, Specchia N, Maccauro G, Arena M, Piconi C. Risultati preliminari delle prove di biocompatibilità in vivo di compatti ceramici a base di zirconia. Biomateriali 1991;1:47.
11. Mebouta-Nkamgeu E, Adnet JJ, Bernard J, et al. In vitro effects of zirconia and alumina particles on human blood monocyte derived macrophages: X-ray microanalysis and flow cytometric studies. J Biomed Mater Res 2000;52:587–594.
12. Catelas I, Petit A, Zukor DJ, Marchand R, Yahia L, Huk OL. Induction of macrophage apoptosis by ceramic and polyethylene particles in vitro. Biomaterials 1999;20:625–630.
13. Purchio RA, Zavaglia CAC, Consolaro A. Zirconia biocompatibility for femoral hip prosthesis. In: Ravaglioli A (ed). Bioceramics. Faenza, 1995:313–318.
14. Sterner T, Schutze N, Saxler G, Jakob F, Rader CP. Effects of clinically relevant alumina ceramic, zirconia ceramic and titanium particles of different sizes and concentrations on TNF-α release in a human macrophage cell line. Biomed Tech 2004;49:340–344.
15. Bu YM, Zheng DZ, Wang L, Liu J. Abrasive endoprosthetic wear particles inhibit IFN-γ secretion in human monocytes via upregulating TNF-α-induced miR-29b. Inflammation 2017;40:166–173.
16. Obando-Pereda GA, Fischer L, Stach-Machado DR. Titanium and zirconia particle-induced pro-inflammatory gene expression in cultured macrophages and osteolysis, inflammatory hyperalgesia and edema in vivo. Life Sci 2014;97:96–106.
17. Wang Y, Zhang Y, Sculean A, Bosshardt DD, Miron RJ. Macrophage behavior and interplay with gingival fibroblasts cultured on six commercially available titanium, zirconium, and titanium-zirconium dental implants. Clin Oral Investig 2019;23:3219–3227.

18. Bukat A, Fassina P, Greco F, Piantelli S, Piconi C, Zaghini N. GSP made Ca-PSZ for biomedical applications. In: Hulbert JE, Hulbert SF (eds). Bioceramics 3. Rose-Hulman Institute of Technology, 1992:355–366.
19. Ito A, Tateishi T, Niwa S, Tange S. In vitro evaluation of the cytocompatibility of wear particles generated by UHMWPE zirconia friction. Clin Mater 1993;12:203–209.
20. Kwon YD, Choi HJ, Lee H, Lee JW, Weber HP, Pae A. Cellular viability and genetic expression of human gingival fibroblasts to zirconia with enamel matrix derivative (Emdogain S). J Adv Prosthodont 2014;6:406–414.
21. Li J, Liu Y, Hermansson L, Söremark R. Evaluation of biocompatibility of various ceramic powders with human fibroblasts in vitro. Clin Mater 1993;12:197–201.
22. Dion I, Bordenave L, Lefebvre F, et al. Physico-chemistry and cytotoxicity of ceramics: Part 1: Characterization of ceramic powders. J Mater Sci Mater Med 1994;5:18–24.
23. Harmand MF, Naji A, Lorini G, Priem TH, Piconi C. Cytotoxicity study of ceramic powders for plasma spray coating. Proceedings of the 12th ESB Conference on Biomaterials, Porto, Portugal, 1995.
24. Uo M, Sjögren G, Sundh A, Watari F, Bergman M, Lerner U. Cytotoxicity and bonding property of dental ceramics. Dent Mater 2003;19:487–492.
25. Yamano S, Ma AK, Shanti RM, Kim SW, Wada K, Sukotjo C. The influence of different implant materials on human gingival fibroblast morphology, proliferation, and gene expression. Int J Oral Maxillofac Implants 2011;26:1247–1255.
26. Pae A, Lee H, Kim H-S, Kwon YD, Woo YH. Attachment and growth behaviour of human gingival fibroblasts on titanium and zirconia ceramic surfaces Biomed Mater 2009;4:025005.
27. Fischer NG, Wong J, Baruth A, Cerutis RD. Effect of clinically relevant CAD/CAM zirconia polishing on gingival fibroblast proliferation and focal adhesions. Materials (Basel) 2017;10:1358.
28. Josset Y, Oum'Hamed Z, Zarrinpour A, Lorenzato M, Adnet JJ, Laurent-Maquin D. In vitro reactions of human osteoblasts in culture with zirconia and alumina ceramics. J Biomed Mater Res 1999;47:481–493.
29. Lohmann CH, Dean DD, Köster G, et al. Ceramic and PMMA particles differentially affect osteoblast phenotype. Biomaterials 2002;23:1855–1863.
30. Hao L, Lawrence J, Chian KS. Osteoblast cell adhesion on a laser modified zirconia based bioceramic. J Mater Sci Mater Med 2005;16:719–726.
31. Bächle M, Butz F, Hübner U, Bakalinis E, Kohal RJ. Behavior of CAL72 osteoblast-like cells cultured on zirconia ceramics with different surface topographies. Clin Oral Implants Res 2007;18:53–59.
32. Att W, Takeuchi M, Suzuki T, Kubo K, Anpo M, Ogawa T. Enhanced osteoblast function on ultraviolet light-treated zirconia. Biomaterials 2009;30:1273–1280.
33. Aboushelib MN, Osman E, Jansen I, Everts V, Feilzer AJ. Influence of a nanoporous zirconia implant surface on cell viability of human osteoblasts. J Prosthodont 2013;22:190–195
34. Song YG, Cho IH. Characteristics and osteogenic effect of zirconia porous scaffold coated with β-TCP/HA. J Adv Prosthodont 2014;6:285–294.
35. Bubik S, Payer M, Arnetzl G, et al. Attachment and growth of human osteoblasts on different biomaterial surfaces. Int J Comput Dent 2017;20:229–243.
36. Herath HM, Di Silvio L, Evans JR. Osteoblast response to zirconia surfaces with different topographies. Mater Sci Eng C Mater Biol Appl 2015;57:363–370.
37. Hadjicharalambous C, Buyakov A, Buyakova S, Kulkov S, Chatzinikolaidou M. Porous alumina, zirconia and alumina/zirconia for bone repair: Fabrication, mechanical and in vitro biological response. Biomed Mater 2015;10:025012.
38. Delgado-Ruíz RA, Gomez Moreno G, Aguilar-Salvatierra A, Markovic A, Mate-Sánchez JE, Calvo-Guirado JL. Human fetal osteoblast behavior on zirconia dental implants and zirconia disks with microstructured surfaces. An experimental in vitro study. Clin Oral Implants Res 2016;27:e144–e153.
39. da Cruz MB, Marques JF, Peñarrieta-Juanito GM, et al. Hard and soft tissue cell behavior on polyetheretherketone, zirconia, and titanium implant materials. Int J Oral Maxillofac Implants 2019;34:39–46.
40. Wei C, Gong T, Pow EHN, Botelho MG. Adhesive and oxidative response of stem cell and pre-osteoblasts on titanium and zirconia surfaces in vitro. J Investig Clin Dent 2019;10:e12407.
41. Hulbert SF, Morrison SJ, Klawitter JJ. Tissue reaction to three ceramics of porous and non porous structure. J Biomed Mater Res 1972;6:347–374.
42. Bortz SA, Onesto EJ. Flame sprayed bioceramics. Cer Bull 1973;52:898

43. Cranin AN, Schnitman PA, Rabkin SM, Onesto EJ. Alumina and zirconia coated vitallium oral endosteal implants in beagles. J Biomed Mater Res 1975;9:257–262.
44. Monticelli G, Santori F, Sandrolini-Cortesi S. First consideration on the use of ZrO2 in hip prosthesis stem coating. Artificial Organs 1981;5:185.
45. Chung SH, Kim HK, Shon WJ, Park YS. Peri-implant bone formations around (Ti, Zr)O(2)-coated zirconia implants with different surface roughness. J Clin Periodontol 2013;40: 404–411.
46. Hamad TI, Fatalla AA, Waheed AS, Azzawi ZGM, Cao YG, Song K. Biomechanical evaluation of nanozirconia coatings on Ti-6Al-7Nb implant screws in rabbit tibias. Curr Med Sci 2018;38:530–537.
47. Nagai N, Takeshita N, Hayashi J. Biological reaction of zirconia ceramic as a new implant material in the dental field. Jpn J Oral Biol 1982;24:759–762.
48. Garvie RC, Urbani C, Kennedy D, McNeuer JC. Biocompatibility of magnesia partially stabilized zirconia (Mg-PSZ) ceramics. J Mater Sci 1984;10:3224–3228.
49. Christel P, Meunier A, Heller M, Torre JP, Cales B, Peille CN. Mechanical properties and short term in vivo evaluation of yittrium-oxide-partially-stabilized zirconia. J Biomed Mater Res 1989;23:45–61.
50. Satoh Y, Niwa S. Tissue/biomaterial interface characteristics of zirconia ceramics. In: Hulbert JE, Hulbert SF (eds). Bioceramics 3. Rose-Hulman Institute of Technology, 1992:101–108.
51. Ichikawa Y, Akagawa Y, Nikai H, Tsuru H. Tissue compatibility and stability of a new zirconia ceramic in vivo. J Prosthet Dent 1992;68:322–326.
52. Greco F, Piantelli S, Maccauro G, Arena M, Piconi C. Risposta biologica ai materiali ceramici: Risultati delle prove in vitro ed in vivo. Minerva Ortop Traumatol 1993;44:913–918.
53. Hayashi K, Matsuguchi N, Uenoyama K, Sugioka Y. Re-evaluation of the biocompatibility of bioinert ceramics in vivo. Biomaterials 1992;13:195–200.
54. Miani C, Piconi C, Piselli D, Ponti M. Experimental in vivo studies on zirconia in oral implantology. Italian Osseoint J 1993;3:23–34.
55. Akagawa Y, Ichikawa Y, Nikai H, Tsuru H. Interface histology of unloaded and early loaded partially stabilized zirconia endosseous implant in initial bone healing. J Prosthet Dent 1993;69:599–604.
56. Dubruille JH, Viguier E, Le Naour G, Dubruille MT, Auriol M, Le Charpentier Y. Evaluation of combinations of titanium, zirconia, and alumina implants with two bone fillers in the dog. Int J Oral Maxillofac Implants 1999;14:271–277.
57. Pieralli S, Kohal RJ, Jung RE, Vach K, Spies BC. Clinical outcomes of zirconia dental implants: A systematic review. J Dent Res 2017;96:38–46.
58. Roehling S, Schlegel KA, Woelfler H, Gahlert M. Zirconia compared to titanium dental implants in preclinical studies—A systematic review and meta-analysis. Clin Oral Implants Res 2019;30:365–395.
59. Lorusso F, Noumbissi S, Francesco I, Rapone B, Khater AGA, Scarano A. Scientific trends in clinical research on zirconia dental implants: A bibliometric review. Materials 2020;4:5534.
60. Covacci V, Bruzzese N, Maccauro G, et al. In vitro evaluation of the mutagenic and carcinogenic power of high purity zirconia ceramic. Biomaterials 1999;20:371–376.
61. Atalay H, Çelik A, Ayaz F. Investigation of genotoxic and apoptotic effects of zirconium oxide nanoparticles (20 nm) on L929 mouse fibroblast cell line. Chem Biol Interact 2018;296:98–104.

06

BIOMECHANICS OF DENTAL IMPLANTS

Loredana Cerroni

The biomechanical properties of dental implants are very important because dental restorations must support high mechanical loads under masticatory function, and biomechanical stresses can influence tissue behavior at the implant interface.[1] Titanium implants or titanium or zirconia alloy implants are selected on the basis of physical and mechanical properties, including the material's tensile, fracture, and fatigue strengths; ductility; toughness; and structural modulus of elasticity. Titanium implants are still the most common choice for oral rehabilitation because of their inherent biocompatibility and favorable mechanical properties. Many variables can influence the biomechanical properties of an implant-supported prosthesis, including the implant connection system, insertion torques, and abutment screw material, and a variety of complications associated with dental implants and prothesis superstructures have been identified and broadly classified as biologic, technical, or esthetic. Mechanical complications affect the structural integrity of the implant, abutment, and prosthetic superstructure.[2] This chapter describes relevant biomechanical principles and reviews literature comparing the results found with titanium and zirconia implants.

Implant Stability

Implant stability is the capacity of an implant to withstand loads in axial and lateral directions, as well as in rotation. Implant stability is achieved via bone-to-implant contact (BIC). Primary stability occurs just after implant placement and is biomechanical in nature, related mostly to the quality of bone at the implant site. The surgical protocol used to prepare the implant site also plays a role in primary stability. Site preparation and insertion torque influence the strength, rigidity, and capacity of the implant to resist micromovements before tissue healing. The achievement of BIC is also directly related to crestal bone loss, which could lead to the formation of a pocket—usually in the coronal region of the implant. The first radiologic sign of dental implant failure is the development of angular bone loss around the neck of the implant.[3,4] Implant design, surgical protocol, and bone and implant friction phenomena all play an important role in primary implant stability.[5,6]

Implant Design

Three major macroscopic features characterize the design of endosseous implants: *(1)* thread design, *(2)* a solid body press-fit design (cylindrical, conical), and *(3)* a porous-coated surface.[7] Implants should be selected with consideration for achieving primary implant stability. Bone has the capacity to grow into the irregularities of implants to establish interlocking biomechanical bonding. Later, implant stability decreases a few weeks after placement because the amount of bone resorption at the bone-implant interface is greater than the apposition of new bone.[8] Because the shape of implant threads and thread pitch determine the surface area available for trabecular bone interaction, they are important design parameters.[7]

Finite element analysis (FEA) is optimal for evaluating the biomechanics and complex clinical behavior of dental implants, in particular for thread analyses. Kong et al[9] concluded that thread pitch plays a great role in protecting dental implants placed under axial loading. Thread pitches exceeding 0.8 mm were found to provide good biomechanical properties for type 2 bone according to the Lekholm and Zarb classification.[9]

Implants must also have sufficient strength to transmit appropriate forces to bone and resist failure upon repeated loading.[1,10] Dental implants are exposed to various mechanical stresses from swallowing, mastication, and parafunctions (eg, grinding, clenching), which result in applications of force to the restorative crown leading to simultaneous mechanical movement and potential deformation of the restoration structure. Depending on the degree of osseointegration and mucosal integration, this mechanical force can be correctly transferred to the bone and mucosa.[11] Implant longevity is influenced not only by the intensity and duration of forces but also by their direction. Bone is an anisotropic tissue, and during mastication, various forces affect its viscoelastic properties. Bone reacts to strain by increasing in stiffness.

Optimum biomechanical and functional behavior of the bone-implant interface can be achieved by proper design of the implant surface, with the aim of avoiding cortical and trabecular bone loss.[12] An implant is "overloaded" when the functional loading exerted on it exceeds a given stress level and leads to possible complications, such as peri-implant bone resorption. The stress level leading to overload depends on various factors, including bone remodeling properties, healing time (osseointegration), and the direction and nature (shear or compression) of the applied stress. Good primary implant stability and low initial stresses are key factors for long-term implant stability.[13]

Osseointegration

Secondary implant stability is a prerequisite for implant loading and long-term clinical success. Secondary stability of the implant is achieved via osseointegration, which is the direct structural and functional connection between living bone and the loaded implant surface without the interposition of connective tissue. The overall stability of an implant decreases during the first weeks after implantation but increases again as osseointegration occurs. The mechanism underlying fibrous tissue development is excessive micromotion, and fibrous tissue formation is largely independent of the implant biomaterial but strongly dependent on biomechanics. Local interfacial strains may also affect the molecular and cellular interactions with the implant surface that regulate the biologic response.[6]

Roughening the implant surface is one option for reducing mobility at the bone-implant interface, as the resulting increased surface friction increases the resistance of the implant to shear forces.[14] A stronger biomechanical bond can be obtained with rough implant surfaces, and surface roughness can influence the degree of osseointegration. For example, the size and distribution of peaks and valleys on an implant surface can significantly influence the overall intimacy and mechanical interlocking of the bone and implant. Surface treatments increase the surface area of the implant adjacent to bone and allow for improved implant resistance to tensile strength and torsion.[15,16]

Topographic variation can be achieved by coating machined titanium implants with titanium plasma spray (TPS) or by performing airborne-particle abrasion with titanium or soluble/resorbable materials with or without acid etching anodizing (alumina oxide and H_2SO_4/HCl18).[10] Etching alone removes the marks from the machining technique but seldom provides significantly increased roughness on a micrometer scale.[17] These procedures influence the implant microtopography profile that drives initial interactions with the organic deposits (primarily fibrin) from blood and tissue fluids and the local healing characteristics of bone.[18]

The ideal surface roughness of dental implants is in the range of 1 to 10 μm. This level of roughness is likely to maximize the interlocking between mineralized bone and the surface of the implant. A close implant-bone interaction is beneficial for improving the capacity of the restoration to withstand high levels of loading.[19] Abraded titanium implants with a roughness of 1.5 μm induce a better bone response than machined implants, as evidenced by removal torque values.[20]

Dental Implant Complications

The most common types of failure associated with dental implants are loss of preload, screw loosening, and implant and abutment fracture.[21,22] Resonance frequency analysis (RFA), percussion frequency analysis (Periotest), and insertion torque measurements have been recommended for assessing implant stability. RFA and percussion frequency analysis are used to assess the bone-implant interface and may be used for monitoring implants over time. Percussion frequency analysis is sensitive to extrinsic variables such as implant positioning, abutment length, and implant location within the jaw.[23] Insertion torque measurements are used to assess conditions at the time of implant placement and can be used to predict implant survival and estimate healing time before loading.[24,25]

Usually endosseous implants and abutments are joined to one another with a screw. The loosening of this screw is a major mechanical complication and can occur due to inadequate insertion torque, plastic deformation of the screw, settling effect of the surface, movement occurring during mastication, or loss of preload. (Preload is the compressive force generated across a joint when a screw is tightened and is responsible for keeping the joint closed.) Tightening is aimed to obtain optimum preload, which will maximize the life of the screw and protect it from loosening and fatigue. Insertion torque creates tension between the mating threads and the head of the abutment screw, which determines the elongation.[22] The elastic recovery of the screw maintains the abutment-prothesis system by creating a clamping force. There is a linear relationship between insertion torque and screw preload.[2,26]

Greater preload values result in greater force required to loosen the screw. The application of an adequate torque value is crucial for clinical success. Low insertion torque values can result in mechanical failure of the implant-abutment assembly after cyclic loading.[26] Higher torque values provide greater screw resistance, but if they exceed the yield strength of the screw, they may lead to plastic deformation and loss of the screw's mechanical properties.[2] The relationship between applied torque and preload depends on several factors, including screw geometry, material properties, and surface texture; the degree of lubrication; rate of tightening; and integrity of the joint.

The implant-abutment connection provides a means to apply torque to screw the body of the implant into bone and provide a stage-two connection for the abutment. The joint design influences the fracture strength of the implant-abutment connection. Internal and external connection designs are available. The external hexagon connection was the first connection system adopted by Brånemark, with diameter, height, and insertion torque being modified over time. The external hexagon connection offers little contact between the restoration and the hexagonal part of the implant head, allows for a degree of rotation between the platform and the internal hexagon of the restoration, and creates high tension in the screw connection. Under high occlusal loads, there is a greater risk of abutment micromovement, instability of the joint, and subsequent abutment screw loosening.[27,28] Internal hexagon connections exhibit improved mechanical resistance, higher removal torque values (indicating higher preload), and less screw loosening. Connections that have exhibited superior resistance to fracture strength include internal conical, long internal, and slot implant-abutment interface connections.[29] Conical connections are a particular kind of internal connection in which the abutment is secured to the implant using the mechanical properties of a machine taper.[28] Internal conical connections of various degrees can exhibit deformation, but only the 8-degree connection has been found to fracture at the head of the screw.[30] A platform-switching model has been found to decrease stress transfer at the marginal bone level but results in more stress at the level of the abutment or abutment screw.

Carvalho et al[31] used FEA to investigate the effects of various abutment materials and platform connections on stress distribution in anterior single-implant–supported restorations. Nine experimental groups were modeled from the combination of three platform connections (external hexagon, internal hexagon, and Morse tapered) and three abutment materials (titanium, zirconia, and hybrid). The platform connection influenced the stress on the abutments more than the abutment material did.[31]

Biomechanical Properties of Zirconia Implants

Titanium is the most common material used for dental implants due to its excellent biocompatibility and mechanical properties, but although the crown that abuts the titanium implant may be esthetically optimal, in cases of thin peri-implant mucosa and soft tissue recessions, the gray color of the titanium implant shows through the thin peri-implant mucosa, thus impairing the esthetic results.[32,33] Furthermore, titanium particles have been reported to cause degenerative changes in peri-implant tissue, where they are phagocytosed by macrophages and neutrophils activated as part of the biologic response.[34] Therefore ceramic implants made of yttria-stabilized zirconia (YSZ) or alumina-toughened zirconia (ATZ) are a great alternative for patients who are allergic to titanium. Ceramic implants resist acid corrosion, prevent the formation of bacterial plaque, and favor creeping attachment.[35,36] Zirconia implants used to replace missing teeth have proved to address patient needs with a lasting positive effect.[37]

Yttria-stabilized tetragonal zirconia (Y-TZP) exhibits high flexural strength, favorable hardness, high fracture toughness, and a Weibull parameter of 10 to 12.9. Thus, zirconia is considered a feasible alternative to titanium dental implants.[38–40] In addition to having excellent cosmetic results, zirconia implants were found to allow for good osseointegration and satisfactory soft tissue responses.[41,42]

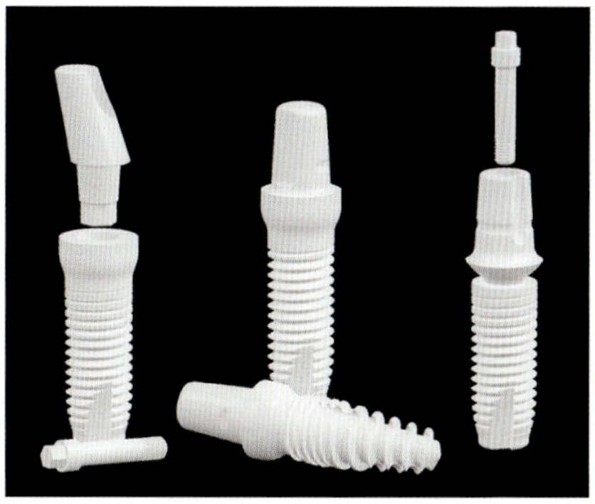

FIG 6-1 › One- and two-piece Z-Systems implants with a laser-modified surface.

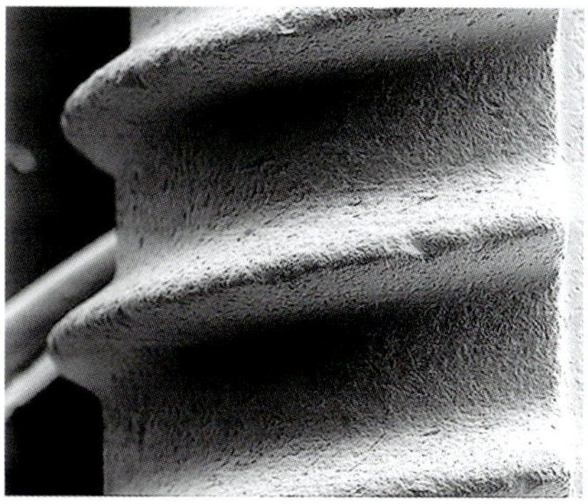

FIG 6-2 › Airborne particle–abraded surface of a whiteSKY implant. The microstructure is in the 500-µm range for rapid bone adaptation.

Three different thread-form configurations in zirconia implants were evaluated in a study by Caglar et al[32]: V-shaped threads (Z-Systems implants), buttress-shaped threads (Ziterion implants), and combined square- and V-shaped threads (whiteSKY implants, Bredent Medical). 3D FEA showed that von Mises, compressive, and tensile stresses in the cortical bone under oblique and horizontal loading conditions were lower with whiteSKY implants than with the other implants because whiteSKY implants have no threading in the neck region. The highest stresses occurred in the cortical bone around Z-Systems implants. These implant systems have since been improved and are currently on the market (Figs 6-1 and 6-2).

In another study, zirconia implants showed less resistance to failure than titanium implants, though the difference between the titanium and zirconia implants was minimal because one is more rigid and the other more tenacious.[36] For restoring single-tooth gaps and replacing up to three adjacent missing teeth, zirconia implants can be considered a treatment option with outcomes comparable to those of titanium implants.[43]

ZIRCONIA IMPLANT DESIGN

Fuh et al[44] compared the biomechanical effects of various zirconia and titanium implants with different thread designs and interfacial conditions (bonding and contact with different frictional coefficients) on bone stress in conditions of both conventional delayed loading and immediate loading. Increased frictional coefficients did not reduce bone stresses around the implants; however, sliding was reduced, which might improve primary implant stability and thereby facilitate osseointegration. Promising 5-year clinical outcomes were found for one-piece zirconia implants with no difference between different diameters and lengths.[45]

BONE-TO-IMPLANT CONTACT

Machined zirconia implants have shown BIC percentages similar to those of titanium implants in most studies in animal models without functional loading and at different observation periods.[46] Kohal et al[47] reported a higher percentage of osseointegration for unloaded zirconia implants; they also found direct BIC of approximately 82% for unloaded zirconia implants and 70% for loaded zirconia implants.

The first zirconia implant (Sigma 1) was developed by Sandhaus in 1984. It was constructed with an internal hexagonal abutment connection. The Sigma implants were inserted in the mandibles of dogs 6 months after filling surgical defects with coralline-derived calcium carbonate (Biocoral, Inoteb). The osseointegration of Sigma implants has been compared with implants made of alumina and experimental grade 1 titanium. The BIC was higher than that of titanium implants after 10 months.[48] A study investigating BIC% around one-piece zirconia and titanium implants placed in the jaws and femurs of domestic sheep showed superior BIC% values for zirconia compared with titanium implants after 12 weeks of healing in the sheep mandibles. Implants were placed using a single-stage transgingival protocol and were nonsubmerged.[49]

A higher failure rate of one-piece zirconia implants was demonstrated in some clinical studies.[50,51] Overloading and implant design were the main reasons for zirconia implant fracture. In one study, implants with reduced diameters (3.25 mm) showed lower survival (58.5%) compared with implants with a diameter of 4.0 mm (88.9%) and 5.0 mm (78.6%).[52]

Because titanium implants with roughened surfaces have been found to be more acceptable than machined zirconia, research has considered various approaches to produce microroughened zirconia implants with reliable fracture toughness and fatigue strength.[53] It was demonstrated that commercially available first-generation zirconia implants with an abraded surface topography showed a survival probability of 82.4% up to and after 3 years of functional loading.[54] The more roughened surface of abraded and acid-etched zirconia implants increased bone integration and primary implant stability compared with machined zirconia.[55,56]

Oliva et al[57] reported the first clinical evaluation of 100 one-piece CeraRoot zirconia implants with two different levels of surface roughness after 1 year of follow-up. The overall success rate was 98%. With a total of 831 implants with the same roughened surfaces followed for up to 5 years (an average of 3.40 ± 0.21 years), the overall implant success rate was 95%. The success rate of the acid-etched surface group was significantly better than that of the other two.[58] Failures were clustered in the first year after loading. Figures 6-3 and 6-4 show SEM images of the CeraRoot 34 thread and implant body.

Comparable rates of bone apposition in sintered zirconia, laser-modified zirconia, airborne particle–abraded zirconia, and acid-etched titanium implants have been observed at 6 and 12 weeks of healing in a rabbit model.[59] In a study by Payer et al,[60] radiographic bone levels, the condition of the peri-implant mucosa, and

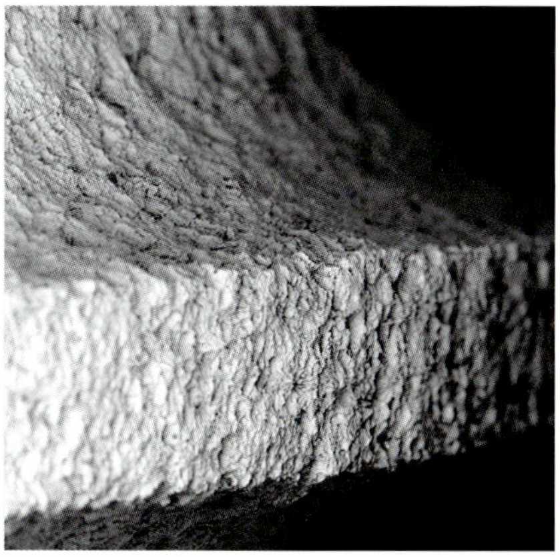

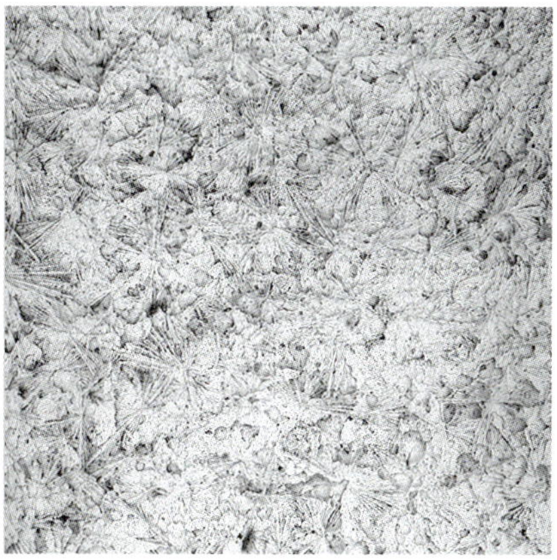

FIGS 6-3 AND 6-4 › SEM images of the CeraRoot 34 implant thread.

implant survival for up to 24 months were recorded, and there was no significant difference in success rates between two-piece zirconia implants and two-piece titanium implants. The bonded zirconia implant–abutment connection appeared to be sufficient for the clinical application throughout the observed period.

In 36-month follow-up studies on the success and survival of one-piece zirconia implants, survival rates ranged between 97.5% and 98.5%, which are almost identical with those of titanium implants.[61] Significant bone apposition has been found around Straumann Pure Ceramic implants between 1 and 3 years after occlusal loading.[62] On the contrary, the survival rates of ZiUnite implants (Nobel Biocare) are inferior to those reported for immediately loaded one-piece titanium and zirconia implants of similar shape. Bone remodeling analysis has revealed high frequencies of bone loss > 2 mm.[63] In another study, the clinical outcomes of 16 two-piece zirconia implants in comparison with 15 titanium implants 80 months after delivery of all-ceramic (lithium disilicate) single-tooth restorations were not significantly different.[34] It has been shown that zirconia implant survival rates have increased significantly between 2004 and 2017 and that the fracture incidence of zirconia dental implants has been significantly reduced from 3.4% to 0.2%.[49–64]

Gahlert et al[65] reported the first clinical and radiographic data on 36 monotype YSZ implants (Straumann Pure Ceramic implants) with airborne particle–abraded, large grit, acid-etched surfaces (Fig 6-5). Implant survival and success rates were 97.5% and 97.2%, respectively, after a mean follow-up of 58.7 months. There was a mean peri-implant marginal bone level loss of 0.99 mm (± 0.59) (Fig 6-6).

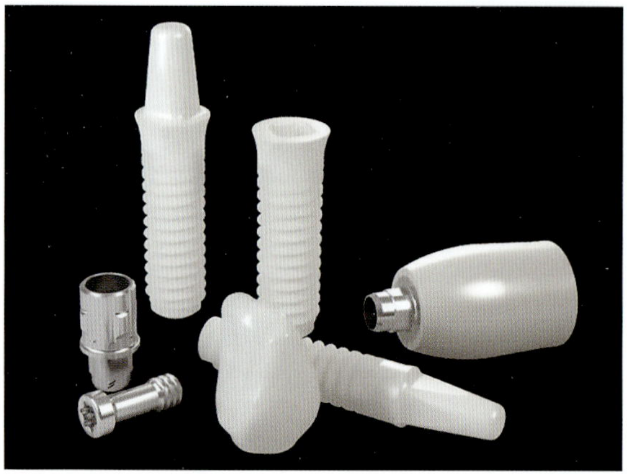

FIG 6-5 › The Straumann Pure Ceramic Implant System.

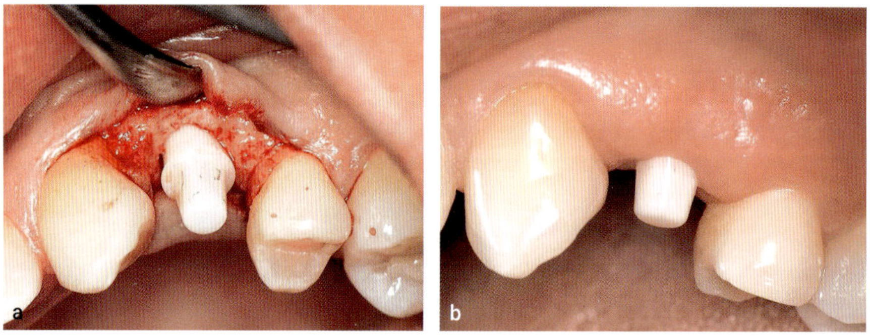

FIG 6-6 › *(a)* One-piece Straumann Pure Ceramic Implant in situ. *(b)* Healed implant site before prosthetic restoration. (Reprinted with permission from Gahlert et al.[65])

REMOVAL TORQUE TESTING

Ceramic implant failure can be due to physical, chemical, or mechanical factors. Removal torque testing in a rabbit model showed that moderately roughened zirconia implants are four to five times more resistant than machined zirconia implants after 6 weeks of healing.[66] Gahlert et al[67] evaluated the removal torque values of machined zirconia implants, airborne particle–abraded zirconia implants, and SLA titanium implants. The machined zirconia implants showed statistically significant lower removal torque values than the other two implant types, and the SLA titanium implants showed significantly higher removal torque values than the abraded zirconia surface at 8 and 12 weeks. Roughening zirconia implants has a beneficial effect on interfacial shear strength,[67] though the tissue response to altered surface topography need not necessarily reflect the change of the surface alone. When the surface topography is changed, the surface chemistry or physics may also change simultaneously.[46] These factors seem to play important roles in the osseointegration of modified zirconia implants.

Manufacturing errors introduced during zirconia implant fabrication and subsequent surface treatment may compromise implant strength. Common material defects include pores and microcracks on a submillimeter scale.[56,68] Kohal et al[69] reported that yttria partially stabilized zirconia (Y-PSZ) implants showed stress distribution similar to that of commercially pure titanium implants in the anterior maxilla.[33] Surface modifications on zirconia implants may have a positive effect on BIC. However, water diffusion can alter the stability of the tetragonal phase due to the humid atmosphere. Furthermore, grinding or airborne-particle abrasion of the zirconia surface may cause tetragonal to monoclinic phase transformation, which can increase the material's susceptibility to aging and reduce material toughness.[38] Studies have shown that high cyclic contact loading during mastication can initiate crack nucleation and propagation via subcritical crack growth.[50]

IMPLANT FRACTURE

Failure analysis of fractured dental zirconia implants has revealed that many fractured implants were located in the anterior of the maxilla and mandible and fractured due to mechanical overloading. Kohal et al[70] evaluated the fracture strength of titanium implants with metal-ceramic crowns, Empress I crowns, and Procera (alumina-based; Nobel Biocare) crowns before and after exposure to an artificial mouth. In the unloaded group, fracture strength was not statistically different. After a chewing load of 1.2 million cycles, fracture strength values for metal-ceramic and Procera crowns were significantly higher than for the loaded Empress I crowns. Zirconia implants restored with Procera crowns possibly fulfill the biomechanical requirements for anterior teeth. All the investigated all-ceramic crowns, as well as the implants, met the minimum requirements for clinical use, as the lowest fracture strength value was 290 N.

Silva et al[71] examined the effects of full-crown preparation and found that the fracture strength of zirconia implants with and without preparation was similar (1,111.7 N versus 1,023.3 N). On the contrary, Andreiotelli and Kohal[72] showed that when one-piece zirconia implants (Sigma) were prepared, fracture occurred at 539 to 607 N after a simulation of 5 years of clinical service, whereas fracture occurred at 725 to 850 N when not prepared. However, the mean fracture strength of zirconia implants was clinically acceptable.

Zirconia implants are sold as one- and two-piece implants. The last one-piece implants were recently introduced because implementing the connection between the zirconia implant and the abutment screw was technically complicated.[73] Early studies on zirconia implants were limited to one-piece implants. Thoma et al[74] aimed to test whether marginal bone level alterations with loaded zirconia implants are similar to marginal bone level alterations with grade 4 titanium one-piece dental implants. Zirconia implants were more prone to fracture than titanium implants both before and after loading with implant-supported crowns.[74] The failures occurred during the period between the healing phase and 6 months after loading. The implant neck seemed to be the point of weakness, and the fracture rate seemed to depend on bruxism and implant design, in particular the narrow diameter. These implants with reduced diameters (3.25 mm) cannot be recommended for further clinical use.[75]

Ferraz et al[76] investigated stress distribution in zirconia and titanium implants and their biomechanical responses in alveolar sockets of the anterior region of the maxilla through 3D FEA. The tested implants were Straumann Zirconia Pure Ceramic Implant Monotype, Zirconia Pure Ceramic ZLA, and Roxolid Titanium Bone-Level SLA. CI RD Straumann PUREbase and Straumann RC Variobase abutments were attached to the Pure ZLA and Titanium Bone-Level implants, respectively. IPS e.max press ceramic crowns (Ivoclar Vivadent) were installed over all the implants. Under oblique forces, stress distribution was more concentrated in the ZLA implants and in the abutments of the Roxolid SLA implants. Zirconia Pure Ceramic Implant Monotype presented the lowest levels of stress.

In a 3D FEA study, Choi et al[77] applied two loading conditions to emulate the occlusal loading that may occur in the oral cavity during mastication. An inclined force (175 N) was applied at an inclination of 30 degrees relative to the axis of the implant, and a vertical force (175 N) was applied relative to the axis of the implant. The stress transmission of the abutment, abutment screw, and implant were evaluated using von Mises stresses on the titanium and zirconia systems. The zirconia model exhibited higher von Mises stresses in the abutments than the titanium model but at a level lower than the fracture strength of the material.[77]

IMPLANT-ABUTMENT CONNECTION

Early failure rates of zirconia implant systems developed and tested so far have generally been higher than those of titanium implants.[78] There are several limitations to the use of one-piece zirconia implants. For example, the surgical placement of the implant may not always meet the prosthodontic requirements. Depending on the angle at which the implant is placed, secondary corrections of the shape by grinding may be necessary; this must be avoided when possible because it severely affects the fracture strength of zirconia.[72,79] Moreover, single-piece implants are immediately exposed to forces from the tongue or as a result of mastication.[80] In contrast, in two-piece zirconia implants, the unfavorable implant angle and position can be compensated for by the abutment, and two-stage implant surgery is also possible.[77] Abutment fracture was described in a clinical study on two-piece zirconia implants. The line of fracture was located at the base of the implant-abutment connection.[81] The authors investigated the effect of the tightening torque of the abutment screw on the stability of the implant-abutment connection in a two-piece zirconia implant system using FEA. When a torque of 35 Ncm was applied, the two-piece zirconia system showed a maximum stress value near 660 MPa (75% of the yield strength of the Ti-6Al-4V alloy), which is the optimal preload recommended for abutment screws. An internal hexagonal implant connection was used in this study.[77]

Spies et al[82] compared the fracture resistance of two differently connected two-piece implant systems with one-piece ATZ implants. In the group of two-piece implants, one subgroup had its abutment fixed into the implant by a titanium screw while the other had its ATZ abutment bonded into the implant. After dynamic loading, the one-piece implants showed an increase in fracture resistance, whereas both two-piece implants showed a decrease. Debonding was noted only for the group with abutments cemented into the implants. The authors concluded that these implant systems had sufficient fracture resistance values to withstand physiologic bite forces in vivo.

Preis et al[73] investigated the influence of different implant-abutment connections on the long-term in vitro performance and fracture resistance of two-piece zirconia implant systems for anterior application under simulation of loading and aging. The abutments were cemented or screwed with a carbon fiber–reinforced polymer screw to an ATZ implant. In another group, the abutments were screwed with titanium screws on Y-TZP implants. Only the bonded abutment system was free of mechanical failures. In the screwed abutment system group, all specimens presented abutment fractures combined with either partial fracture of the implants or fractures of the screws.[73] Joos et al[83] compared the behavior of incisor- and molar-shaped monolithic screw-retained zirconia crowns with two-piece titanium implants in an in vitro chewing simulation including artificial aging. The connection of the screw-retained zirconia crowns showed similar survival rates in both implant systems.[83] In in vitro studies where implant stability and fracture resistance were tested according to ISO 14801,[84] zirconia implant systems have shown good resistance to masticatory forces.[64,85,86]

Table 6-1 reviews some of the studies that have been performed to evaluate the results found with various zirconia and titanium implants.

TABLE 6-1 › Clinical studies on zirconia implants with follow-ups of at least 2 years

	Implant type and number	Prosthetic reconstruction	Follow-up	Clinical parameters	Survival/ success rate	Mean MBL	Notes
Blaschke and Volz[41] (2006)	66 Z-Systems implants	Single-crown reconstruction after 4–6 months	2 y	PI, BOP, PD, CAL	98%/NR	NR	No implant failed after the prosthesis was fitted.
Oliva et al[58] (2010)	831 CeraRoot implants	3M Lava All-Ceramic single-crown reconstructions after 4–11 months	3 y	BOP	95%/NR	NR	Zirconia dental implants with roughened surfaces might be a viable alternative for tooth replacement.
Borgonovo et al[39] (2013)	35 whiteSKY implants (28 at follow-up)	3M Lava All-Ceramic zirconia SCs or partial dentures after 6 months	4 y	BOP, PD, PI	100%/ 100%	1.63 mm	Zirconia showed good marginal bone preservation.
Gahlert et al[52] (2013)	170 Z-Look3 implants	87 SCs, 25 with FDPs and 7 with RHDs after 3 months	3 y	PI, PD, BOP	82.4%/ NR	NR	30 implants were lost due to lack of osseointegration or fracture. The survival rate was lower for anterior implants and for implants in the maxilla.
Payer et al[80] (2013)	20 whiteSKY implants	Immediate CAD/CAM provisional restorations (after 4–6 months, all-ceramic Ivoclar Vivadent e.max CAD block crowns)	2 y	BOP, PD, PI, Periotest, PES	95%/95%	1.29 mm	The main focus of the pilot study was to evaluate the applicability of an immediate adhesive CAD/CAM restoration of Y-TZP implants without a microgap and without using removable protection devices.
Cionca et al[81] (2015)	76 Zeramex XT Implants (CeramTec)	Zirconia abutments and ceramic SCs after 6 months	2 y	PD, BOP, PI	86%/NR	NR	Failures were due to aseptic loosening.

BOP = bleeding on probing; CAL = clinical attachment level; FDP = fixed dental prosthesis; MBL = marginal bone loss; NR = not reported; PD = probing depth; PES = pink esthetic score; PI = plaque index; RHD = removable hybrid denture; SC = single crown.

TABLE 6-1 *(cont)* **Clinical studies on zirconia implants with follow-ups of at least 2 years**

	Implant type and number	Prosthetic reconstruction	Follow-up	Clinical parameters	Survival/ success rate	Mean MBL	Notes
Grassi et al[42] (2015)	32 whiteSKY implants	Provisional SCs or partial dentures immediately after surgery, definitive ceramic crowns with a zirconia base after 3–4 months	5 y	PD, PI, REC	96.8%/ NR	1.23 mm	Radiographic and clinical evaluations after 5 years showed satisfactory amounts of MBL and acceptable soft tissue health.
Payer et al[60] (2015)	16 Ziterion Varioz implants	Straight or angulated prefabricated standard ceramic abutments (Ziterion zirconia abutments) and all-ceramic lithium disilicate SCs (e.max CAD blocks) after 4–6 months	2 y	BI, PI, Periotest, PES	93.3%/ 93.3%	1.48 mm	Rubber dam placement at crestal levels is a prerequisite for proper adhesive fixation of the zirconia abutment to the zirconia implant.
	15 Ziterion Variot two-piece implants				100%/ 100%	1.43 mm	
Spies et al[37] (2015)	53 Ziraldent FR1 ATZ implants (Metoxit)	Provisional restorations for 6 weeks in the mandible or 14 weeks in the maxilla, final prosthetic reconstructions of all-ceramic SCs (IPS e.max CAD LT, Ivoclar Vivadent) and three-unit partial dentures (IPS e.max ZirCAD and IPS e.max ZirPress LT, Ivoclar Vivadent)	3 y	PD, CAL, BI, PROM	94.2%/ 95.9% grade I success; 100% grade II success*	0.79 mm	The survival rate of the ceramic implant system seems comparable to reported survival rates of titanium implants when immediately restored.

BOP = bleeding on probing; CAL = clinical attachment level; MBL = marginal bone loss; NR = not reported; PD = probing depth; PES = pink esthetic score; PI = plaque index; PROM = patient-reported outcome measures; REC = gingival recession; SC = single crown.
*Grade II success was assigned to implants showing no further pathology but a bone loss/resorption ≤ 3 mm.

TABLE 6-1 *(cont)* › **Clinical studies on zirconia implants with follow-ups of at least 2 years**

	Implant type and number	Prosthetic reconstruction	Follow-up	Clinical parameters	Survival/ success rate	Mean MBL	Notes
Roehling et al[53] (2016)	161 Z-Look3 implants (3.25 mm, 4.0 mm, and 5.0 mm)	112 SCs, 31 FDPs, 4 RHDs after 3 months	7 y	GI, PI, BI	77.3%/ 77.6%	0.97 mm	Fractures were associated with decreasing implant diameter (3.25 mm) and with bruxism. Fractures during the loading period were observed in 11 implants with single-tooth reconstructions and 7 implants with FDPs. All implant fractures occurred at the abraded part (threads) of the coronal part of the implant body.
Kniha et al[62] (2018)	117 Straumann Pure Ceramic Implants (105 at follow-up)	NR	3 y	PD	100%/ 95.4%	+0.54 mm	Zirconia implants presented with little bone loss up to 1 year, but significant bone apposition was observed up to 3 years. A significant association was found between the papilla deficit and the height of the contact point.
Kohal et al[63] (2018)	65 ZiUnite implants	Final crowns of Nobel Biocare NobelProcera zirconia with Nobel Biocare NobelRondo as veneering material after 2–4 months	3 y	PI, BOP, PD	90.8%/ 95.9% grade I success; 100% grade II success*	1.45 mm	35% of implants lost at least 2 mm of bone, and 22% of implants lost more than 3 mm.
Lorenz et al[35] (2019)	83 Z-Look3 implants	NR	7 y	BOP, PI, PD, REC, PES	100%/ NR	1.20 ± 0.76 mm	No major complications such as implant or screw fractures occurred, and no signs of an acute or advanced peri-implant infection were observed.

BOP = bleeding on probing; FDP = fixed dental prosthesis; GI = gingival index; MBL = marginal bone loss; NR = not reported; PD = probing depth; PES = pink esthetic score; PI = plaque index; REC = gingival recession; RHD = removable hybrid denture; SC = single crown.
*Grade II success was assigned to implants showing no further pathology but a bone loss ≤ 3 mm.

TABLE 6-1 *(cont)* **Clinical studies on zirconia implants with follow-ups of at least 2 years**

	Implant type and number	Prosthetic reconstruction	Follow-up	Clinical parameters	Survival/ success rate	Mean MBL	Notes
Kohal et al[88] (2020)	53 Metoxit ATZ implants	27 SCs were fabricated out of IPS e.max CAD LT and 13 three-unit FPDs were fabricated out of IPS e.max ZirCAD veneered with IPS e.max ZirPress LT	5 y	PI, CAL, PD, REC, PROM	94.3%/ 91.7%	0.81 ± 0.77 mm	Significantly higher MBL was associated with implants supporting FDPs compared to SCs, especially before delivery of the definitive reconstructions.
Koller et al[34] (2020)	16 Ziterion Varioz implants	Straight or angulated prefabricated standard ceramic Ziterion abutments and all-ceramic lithium disilicate SCs (e.max CAD blocks) after 4–6 months	7 y	BOP, PI, Periotest, PES	85.7%/ NR	1.38 mm	Two zirconia implants were lost after crown delivery, and one titanium implant was removed at follow-up due to peri-implantitis. There was no fracture of implants and no fracture or debonding of abutments.
	15 Ziterion Variot two-piece implants				93.3%/ NR	1.17 mm	
Gahlert et al[65] (2022)	44 Straumann Pure Ceramic Implants (36 at follow-up)	Provisional prosthesis placed at 3 months, final prosthesis (lithium disilicate glass-ceramic or zirconia ceramic crowns) placed at 6–7 months	5 y	PI, BOP	97.7%/ 97.2%	0.99 ± 0.59 mm	The clinical and radiographic evaluation showed no signs of peri-implantitis.
Kraus et al[85] (2022)	44 OsseoSpeed Astra Tech two-piece dental implants (Dentsply Sirona)	One-piece customized CAD/CAM zirconia abutments (Atlantis, Dentsply Sirona) for all patients, 22 screw-retained and 22 cemented all-ceramic SCs	5 y	PD, BOP, PI	95.5%/ 81.2%	NR	Cemented restorations showed a significantly higher complication rate (73.7%, split evenly between biologic and technical complications) compared with screw-retained restorations (22.7%, only technical complications).

BOP = bleeding on probing; CAL = clinical attachment level; FDP = fixed dental prosthesis; GI = gingival index; MBL = marginal bone loss; NR = not reported; PD = probing depth; PES = pink esthetic score; PI = plaque index; REC = gingival recession; PROM = patient-reported outcome measures; SC = single crown.

Conclusion

Although zirconia implants are still viewed with suspicion by dentists, data obtained from the literature and the 2021 Statement of the European Society of Ceramic Implantology (ESCI)[64] can be used to support their biomechanical soundness and use, even though titanium implants are predictable and have been on the market for many years:

- Esthetics: Zirconia implants are a good alternative to titanium implants when patients prefer an all-ceramic rehabilitation.
- Biocompatibility: The biocompatibility of zirconia implants has been thoroughly investigated, with the main lymphocyte, fibroblast, chondrocyte, osteoblast, and macrophage responses reported. The behavior of zirconia materials has been found to be similar to that of pure titanium with respect to osteoblast histology, gene expression, and morphology.[33]
- In vitro studies have shown that zirconia implants with microroughened surfaces show osseointegration similar to that of titanium implants.
- An overall survival rate of zirconia implants of 94% has been reported after 5 years of functional loading[87] (see Table 6-1).

Although one-piece zirconia implants may not be as prosthetically versatile as desired, there are two-piece zirconia implants available, though there is little published clinical data comparing them to one-piece implants (see chapter 8 for more information).

References

1. Li J, Jansen JA, Walboomers XF, van den Beucken JJ. Mechanical aspects of dental implants and osseointegration: A narrative review. J Mech Behav Biomed Mater 2020;103:103574.
2. Alzahrani KM. Implant bio-mechanics for successful implant therapy: A systematic review. J Int Soc Prev Community Dent 2020;10:700–714.
3. Lindquist LW, Rockler B, Carlsson GE. Bone resorption around fixtures in edentulous patients treated with mandibular fixed tissue-integrated prostheses. J Prosthet Dent 1988;59:59–63.
4. Lin D, Li Q, Li W, Swain M. Dental implant induced bone remodeling and associated algorithms. J Mech Behav Biomed Mater 2009;2:410–432.
5. Meredith N. Assessment of implant stability as a prognostic determinant. Int J Prosthodont 1998;11:491–501.
6. Haïat G, Wang HL, Brunski J. Effects of biomechanical properties of the bone-implant interface on dental implant stability: From in silico approaches to the patient's mouth. Annu Rev Biomed Eng 2014;16:187–213.
7. Gaviria L, Salcido JP, Guda T, Ong JL. Current trends in dental implants. J Korean Assoc Oral Maxillofac Surg 2014;40:50–60.
8. Albrektsson T. Hard tissue implant interface. Aust Dent J 2008;53(suppl 1):S34–S38.
9. Kong L, Zhao Y, Hu K, et al. Selection of the implant thread pitch for optimal biomechanical properties: A three-dimensional finite element analysis. Adv Eng Software 2009;40:474–478.
10. Cooper LF. A role for surface topography in creating and maintaining bone at titanium endosseous implants. J Prosthet Dent 2000;84:522–534.
11. Gasik M, Lambert F, Bacevic M. Biomechanical properties of bone and mucosa for design and application of dental implants. Materials (Basel) 2021;14:2845.
12. Stanford CM. Biomechanical and functional behavior of implants. Adv Dent Res 1999;13:88–92.
13. Mathieu V, Vayron R, Richard G, et al. Biomechanical determinants of the stability of dental implants: Influence of the bone-implant interface properties. J Biomech 2014;47:3–13.
14. Sykaras N, Iacopino AM, Marker VA, Triplett RG, Woody RD. Implant materials, designs, and surface topographies: Their effect on osseointegration. A literature review. Int J Oral Maxillofac Implants 2000;15:675–690.
15. Steigenga JT, al-Shammari KF, Nociti FH, Misch CE, Wang HL. Dental implant design and its relationship to long-term implant success. Implant Dent 2003;12:306–317.

16. Cervino G, Meto A, Fiorillo L, et al. Surface treatment of the dental implant with hyaluronic acid: An overview of recent data. Int J Environ Res Public Health 2021;18:4670.
17. Albrektsson T, Wennerberg A. On osseointegration in relation to implant surfaces. Clin Implant Dent Relat Res 2019;21(suppl 1):4–7.
18. Lemons JE. Biomaterials, biomechanics, tissue healing, and immediate-function dental implants. J Oral Implantol 2004;30:318–324.
19. Le Guéhennec L, Soueidan A, Layrolle P, Amouriq Y. Surface treatments of titanium dental implants for rapid osseointegration. Dent Mater 2007;23:844–854.
20. Wennerberg A, Albrektsson T. Effects of titanium surface topography on bone integration: A systematic review. Clin Oral Implants Res 2009;20(suppl 4):172–184.
21. Winkler S, Ring K, Ring JD, Boberick KG. Implant screw mechanics and the settling effect: Overview. J Oral Implantol 2003;29:242–245.
22. Nithyapriya S, Ramesh AS, Kirubakaran A, Mani J, Raghunathan J. Systematic analysis of factors that cause loss of preload in dental implants. J Indian Prosthodont Soc 2018;18:189–195.
23. Baltayan S, Pi-Anfruns J, Aghaloo T, Moy PK. The predictive value of resonance frequency analysis measurements in the surgical placement and loading of endosseous implants. J Oral Maxillofac Surg 2016;74:1145–1152.
24. Hobkirk JA, Wiskott HW; Working Group 1. Biomechanical aspects of oral implants. Consensus report of Working Group 1. Clin Oral Implants Res 2006;17(suppl 2):52–54.
25. Elias CN, Rocha FA, Nascimento AL, Coelho PG. Influence of implant shape, surface morphology, surgical technique and bone quality on the primary stability of dental implants. J Mech Behav Biomed Mater 2012;16:169–180.
26. Xia D, Lin H, Yuan S, Bai W, Zheng G. Dynamic fatigue performance of implant-abutment assemblies with different tightening torque values. Biomed Mater Eng 2014;24:2143–149.
27. Binon P. The external hexagonal interface and screw joint stability: A primer on threaded fasteners in implants dentistry. Quintessence Dent Technol 2000;23:91–105.
28. Vinhas AS, Aroso C, Salazar F, López-Jarana P, Ríos-Santos JV, Herrero-Climent M. Review of the mechanical behavior of different implant-abutment connections. Int J Environ Res Public Health 2020;17:8685.
29. Steinebrunner L, Wolfart S, Ludwig K, Kern M. Implant abutment interface design affects fatigue and fracture strength of implants. Clin Oral Implants Res 2008;19:1276–1284.
30. Norton MR. In vitro evaluation of the strength of the conical implant-to-abutment joint in two commercially available implant systems. J Prosthet Dent 2000;83:567-571.
31. Carvalho MA, Sotto-Maior BS, Del Bel Cury AA, Pessanha Henriques GE. Effect of platform connection and abutment material on stress distribution in single anterior implant-supported restorations: A nonlinear 3-dimensional finite element analysis. J Prosthet Dent 2014;112:1096–1102.
32. Caglar A, Bal BT, Aydin C, Yilmaz H, Ozkan S. Evaluation of stresses occurring on three different zirconia dental implants: Three-dimensional finite element analysis. Int J Oral Maxillofac Implants 2010;25:95–103.
33. Cerroni L. Ceramics for dentistry: Commercial devices and their clinical analysis. In: Palmero P, Cambier F, De Barra E (eds). Advances in Ceramic Biomaterials: Materials, Devices and Challenges. Woodhead Publishing, 2017:181–248.
34. Koller M, Steyer E, Theisen K, Stagnell S, Jakse N, Payer M. Two-piece zirconia versus titanium implants after 80 months: Clinical outcomes from a prospective randomized pilot trial. Clin Oral Implants Res 2020;31:388–396.
35. Lorenz J, Giulini N, Hölscher W, Schwiertz A, Schwarz F, Sader R. Prospective controlled clinical study investigating long-term clinical parameters, patient satisfaction, and microbial contamination of zirconia implants. Clin Implant Dent Relat Res 2019;21:263–271.
36. Martinez-Mondragon M, Urriolagoitia-Sosa G, Romero-Ángeles B, et al. Numerical analysis of zirconium and titanium implants under the effect of critical masticatory load. Materials (Basel) 2022;15:7843.
37. Spies BC, Balmer M, Patzelt SB, Vach K, Kohal RJ. Clinical and patient-reported outcomes of a zirconia oral implant: Three-year results of a prospective cohort investigation. J Dent Res 2015;94:1385–1391.
38. Piconi C, Maccauro G. Zirconia as a ceramic biomaterial. Biomaterials 1999;20:1–25.
39. Borgonovo AE, Censi R, Vavassori V, et al. Evaluation of the success criteria for zirconia dental implants: A four-year clinical and radiological study. Int J Dent 2013;2013:463073
40. Depprich R, Naujoks C, Ommerborn M, Schwarz F, Kübler NR, Handschel J. Current findings regarding zirconia implants. Clin Implant Dent Relat Res 2014;16:124–137.
41. Blaschke C, Volz U. Soft and hard tissue response to zirconium dioxide dental implants—A clinical study in man. Neuro Endocrinol Lett 2006;27(suppl 1):69–72 [erratum 2007;28:iii].

42. Grassi FR, Capogreco M, Consonni D, Bilardi G, Buti J, Kalemaj Z. Immediate occlusal loading of one-piece zirconia implants: Five-year radiographic and clinical evaluation. Int J Oral Maxillofac Implants 2015;30:671–680.
43. Pieralli S, Kohal RJ, Jung RE, Vach K, Spies BC. Clinical outcomes of zirconia dental implants: A systematic review. J Dent Res 2017;96:38–46.
44. Fuh LJ, Hsu JT, Huang HL, Chen MY, Shen YW. Biomechanical investigation of thread designs and interface conditions of zirconia and titanium dental implants with bone: Three-dimensional numeric analysis. Int J Oral Maxillofac Implants 2013;28:e64–e71.
45. Gul A, Papia E, Naimi-Akbar A, Ruud A, Vult von Steyern P. Zirconia dental implants; the relationship between design and clinical outcome: A systematic review. J Dent 2024;143:104903.
46. Hafezeqoran A, Koodaryan R. Effect of zirconia dental implant surfaces on bone integration: A systematic review and meta-analysis. Biomed Res Int 2017;2017:9246721.
47. Kohal RJ, Weng D, Bächle M, Strub JR. Loaded custom-made zirconia and titanium implants show similar osseointegration: An animal experiment. J Periodontol 2004;75:1262–1268.
48. Piconi C. La zirconia negli impianti dentali. In: Piconi C, Rimondini L, Cerroni L (eds). La zirconia in odontoiatria. Elsevier, 2008:136–156.
49. Siddiqi A, Khan AS, Zafar S. Thirty years of translational research in zirconia dental implants: A systematic review of the literature. J Oral Implantol 2017;43:314–325.
50. Roehling S, Schlegel KA, Woelfler H, Gahlert M. Performance and outcome of zirconia dental implants in clinical studies: A meta-analysis. Clin Oral Implants Res 2018;29(suppl 16):135–153.
51. Morton D, Gallucci G, Lin WS, et al. Group 2 ITI Consensus Report: Prosthodontics and implant dentistry. Clin Oral Implants Res 2018;29(suppl 16):215–223.
52. Gahlert M, Burtscher D, Pfundstein G, Grunert I, Kniha H, Roehling S. Dental zirconia implants up to three years in function: A retrospective clinical study and evaluation of prosthetic restorations and failures. Int J Oral Maxillofac Implants 2013;28:896–904.
53. Roehling S, Woelfler H, Hicklin S, Kniha H, Gahlert M. A retrospective clinical study with regard to survival and success rates of zirconia implants up to and after 7 years of loading. Clin Implant Dent Relat Res 2016;18:545–558.
54. Roehling S, Schlegel KA, Woelfler H, Gahlert M. Zirconia compared to titanium dental implants in preclinical studies—A systematic review and meta-analysis. Clin Oral Implants Res 2019;30:365–395.
55. Gahlert M, Gudehus T, Eichhorn S, Steinhauser E, Kniha H, Erhardt W. Biomechanical and histomorphometric comparison between zirconia implants with varying surface textures and a titanium implant in the maxilla of miniature pigs. Clin Oral Implants Res 2007;18:662–668.
56. Gahlert M, Roehling S, Sprecher CM, Kniha H, Milz S, Bormann K. In vivo performance of zirconia and titanium implants: A histomorphometric study in mini pig maxillae. Clin Oral Implants Res 2012;23:281–286.
57. Oliva J, Oliva X, Oliva JD. One-year follow-up of first consecutive 100 zirconia dental implants in humans: A comparison of 2 different rough surfaces. Int J Oral Maxillofac Implants 2007;22:430–435.
58. Oliva J, Oliva X, Oliva JD. Five-year success rate of 831 consecutively placed zirconia dental implants in humans: A comparison of three different rough surfaces. Int J Oral Maxillofac Implants 2010;25:336–344.
59. Hoffmann O, Angelov N, Zafiropoulos GG, Andreana S. Osseointegration of zirconia implants with different surface characteristics: An evaluation in rabbits. Int J Oral Maxillofac Implants 2012;27:352–358.
60. Payer M, Heschl A, Koller M, Arnetzl G, Lorenzoni M, Jakse N. All-ceramic restoration of zirconia two-piece implants—A randomized controlled clinical trial. Clin Oral Implants Res 2015;26:371–376.
61. Balmer M, Spies BC, Kohal RJ, Hämmerle CH, Vach K, Jung RE. Zirconia implants restored with single crowns or fixed dental prostheses: 5-year results of a prospective cohort investigation. Clin Oral Implants Res 2020;31:452–462.
62. Kniha K, Schlegel KA, Kniha H, Modabber A, Hölzle F, Kniha K. Evaluation of peri-implant bone levels and soft tissue dimensions around zirconia implants—A three-year follow-up study. Int J Oral Maxillofac Surg 2018;47:492–498.
63. Kohal RJ, Spies BC, Bauer A, Butz F. One-piece zirconia oral implants for single-tooth replacement: Three-year results from a long-term prospective cohort study. J Clin Periodontol 2018;45:114–124.
64. Scientific Advisory Board and Board of Directors of the European Society for Ceramic Implantology. The clinical application of two-piece zirconia implants. European Society for Ceramic Implantology, 2021. https://esci-online.com/wp-content/uploads/2021/10/ESCI-Statement-2-piece-zirconia-implants-final-engl.pdf. Accessed 30 May 2024.

65. Gahlert M, Kniha H, Laval S, Gellrich NC, Bormann KH. Prospective clinical multicenter study evaluating the 5-year performance of zirconia implants in single-tooth gaps. Int J Oral Maxillofac Implants 2022;37:804–811.
66. Sennerby L, Dasmah A, Larsson B, Iverhed M. Bone tissue responses to surface-modified zirconia implants: A histomorphometric and removal torque study in the rabbit. Clin Implant Dent Relat Res 2005;7(suppl 1):S13–S20.
67. Gahlert M, Röhling S, Wieland M, Eichhorn S, Küchenhoff H, Kniha H. A comparison study of the osseointegration of zirconia and titanium dental implants. A biomechanical evaluation in the maxilla of pigs. Clin Implant Dent Relat Res 2010;12:297–305.
68. Osman RB, Swain MV. A critical review of dental implant materials with an emphasis on titanium versus zirconia. Materials (Basel) 2015;8:932–958.
69. Kohal RJ, Papavasiliou G, Kamposiora P, Tripodakis A, Strub JR. Three-dimensional computerized stress analysis of commercially pure titanium and yttrium-partially stabilized zirconia implants. Int J Prosthodont 2002;15:189–194.
70. Kohal RJ, Klaus G, Strub JR. Zirconia-implant-supported all-ceramic crowns withstand long-term load: A pilot investigation. Clin Oral Implants Res 2006;17:565–571.
71. Silva NR, Coelho PG, Fernandes CA, Navarro JM, Dias RA, Thompson VP. Reliability of one-piece ceramic implant. J Biomed Mater Res B Appl Biomater 2009;88:419–426.
72. Andreiotelli M, Kohal RJ. Fracture strength of zirconia implants after artificial aging. Clin Implant Dent Relat Res 2009;11:158–166.
73. Preis V, Kammermeier A, Handel G, Rosentritt M. In vitro performance of two-piece zirconia implant systems for anterior application. Dent Mater 2016;32:765–774.
74. Thoma DS, Benic GI, Muñoz F, et al. Marginal bone-level alterations of loaded zirconia and titanium dental implants: An experimental study in the dog mandible. Clin Oral Implants Res 2016;27:412–420.
75. Gahlert M, Burtscher D, Grunert I, Kniha H, Steinhauser E. Failure analysis of fractured dental zirconia implants. Clin Oral Implants Res 2012;23:287–293.
76. Ferraz CC, Barros RM, Ferraz FC, Mundstock ÁA, Maior BS. Analysis of stress distribution in ceramic and titanium implants in alveolar sockets of the anterior region of the maxilla. J Clin Exp Dent 2019;11:e850–e857.
77. Choi H, Hong MH. Finite element analysis of the effect of tightening torque on the connection stability of a two-piece zirconia implant. Adv Materials Sci Eng 2022;2022:1456475.
78. Cionca N, Hashim D, Mombelli A. Zirconia dental implants: Where are we now, and where are we heading? Periodontol 2000 2017;73:241–258.
79. Kohal RJ, Knauf M, Larsson B, Sahlin H, Butz F. One-piece zirconia oral implants: One-year results from a prospective cohort study. 1. Single tooth replacement. J Clin Periodontol 2012;39:590–597.
80. Payer M, Arnetzl V, Kirmeier R, Koller M, Arnetzl G, Jakse N. Immediate provisional restoration of single-piece zirconia implants: A prospective case series—Results after 24 months of clinical function. Clin Oral Implants Res 2013;24:569–575.
81. Cionca N, Müller N, Mombelli A. Two-piece zirconia implants supporting all-ceramic crowns: A prospective clinical study. Clin Oral Implants Res 2015;26:413–418.
82. Spies BC, Nold J, Vach K, Kohal RJ. Two-piece zirconia oral implants withstand masticatory loads: An investigation in the artificial mouth. J Mech Behav Biomed Mater 2016;53:1–10.
83. Joos M, Sailer I, Filippi A, Mukaddam K, Rosentritt M, Kühl S. Stability of screw-retention in two-piece zirconia implants: An in vitro study. Clin Oral Implants Res 2020;31:607–614.
84. ISO 14801:2016 Dentistry–Implants–Dynamic loading test for endosseous dental implants, ed 3. International Organization for Standardization, 2016.
85. Kraus RD, Espuelas C, Hämmerle CHF, Jung RE, Sailer I, Thoma DS. Five-year randomized controlled clinical study comparing cemented and screw-retained zirconia-based implant-supported single crowns. Clin Oral Implants Res 2022;33:537–547.
86. Bethke A, Pieralli S, Kohal RJ, et al. Fracture resistance of zirconia oral implants in vitro: A systematic review and meta-analysis. Materials (Basel) 2020;13:562.
87. Spitznagel FA, Balmer M, Wiedemeier DB, Jung RE, Gierthmuehlen PC. Clinical outcomes of all-ceramic single crowns and fixed dental prostheses supported by ceramic implants: A systematic review and meta-analyses. Clin Oral Implants Res 2022;33:1–20.
88. Kohal RJ, Spies BC, Vach K, Balmer M, Pieralli S. A prospective clinical cohort investigation on zirconia implants: 5-year results. J Clin Med 2020;9:2585.

07

HARD AND SOFT TISSUE RESPONSES TO ZIRCONIA IMPLANTS

Stefan Roehling and Michael Gahlert

Replacing missing teeth with implants has become a routine dental procedure and relies on the biologic stabilization of the implant in bone tissue (ie, osseointegration). Besides implant material, implant design, bone quality, surgical technique, and loading protocol, the implant surface itself is one of the most critical factors for achieving successful and long-lasting osseointegration.[1] For titanium implants, the evolution of machined surfaces to microrough surface topographies was the key factor for successful establishment as part of daily clinical practice.

It has been scientifically shown that roughening titanium implant surfaces to a certain degree leads to accelerated and improved osseointegration.[2] A similar evolution has been observed with zirconia implants. The first generation of zirconia implants had rather smooth surfaces and thus lower clinical survival rates than titanium implants.[3] High fracture rates were also reported.[3,4] In the last two decades, however, practical experiences with handling zirconia as an implant material and optimized manufacturing processes have allowed for the development of microrough surface topographies for zirconia implants that significantly improve osseointegration.[5] Scientific investigations have shown that the newest generation of zirconia implants with microrough surfaces demonstrate a capacity for osseointegration similar to that of titanium implants.[6–10] The evolution of industrial processes and subsequent quality control has also resulted in improved biomechanical properties of zirconia implants, resulting in a clinical fracture rate of only 0.2%.[11]

Based on optimized implant designs and surface topographies, achieving successful osseointegration is no longer the most challenging task for clinicians, even in compromised situations. Instead, esthetic outcomes, especially in the anterior region, have become more important today. A natural appearance of the crown (white esthetics) and soft tissues (pink esthetics) with healthy and irritation-free peri-implant soft tissue conditions is very important. The soft tissue margin and interdental peri-implant papilla formation, along with healthy and regular vertical peri-implant soft tissue dimensions represented by the biologic width, are very important. In addition, gingival tissues around implants serve a barrier function like that of dentogingival tissues around teeth, helping to prevent bacterial peri-implant diseases.[12] Thus, peri-implant soft tissue integration represented by epithelial and connective tissue is as important as osseointegration.[13]

This chapter presents the current scientific results from studies investigating hard and soft tissue integration around zirconia implants.

Hard Tissue Integration

The evidence-based investigation of the hard tissue integration of zirconia began in the early 1990s. Results from experimental studies showed that zirconia had excellent osteoconductive properties and could integrate directly with osseous host tissue.[14,15] However, because implants with a smooth surface topography were investigated in these early studies, a fibrous layer of connective tissue was also found between the implant surfaces and surrounding bone tissue for single implants.[15,16] Since the beginning of the 2000s, experimental studies have thus focused on developing zirconia implants with microrough surface topography.

In 2004, the first experimental study investigating loaded zirconia and titanium implants was published.[17] After extraction of the anterior teeth and 5 months of healing, 12 custom-made zirconia and titanium implants were inserted into the maxillae of 6 monkeys. The titanium implants were airborne-particle abraded and acid etched, whereas the zirconia implants were only airborne-particle abraded to create a microrough surface. After 3 months of unloaded healing, the implants were functionally loaded with crowns. After 5 months of loading, the authors reported similar soft and hard tissue integration for both types of implants.[17]

To date, many different procedures have been reported for creating microrough topographies on zirconia implant surfaces, including additive methods (coating) and subtractive methods (airborne-particle abrasion, acid etching, airborne-particle abrasion combined with acid and lye etching, and laser treatment).[5] Unlike with titanium, the production method itself (eg, injection molding [IM] using a microrough mold or sintering procedures using rough pore formers) can be used to create microsurface topographies on zirconia implants.[5] Experimental studies have shown that increasing the surface roughness of zirconia implants directly correlates with an improved capacity for osseointegration.[5,16,18]

Now microrough zirconia implant surfaces can be produced with topographies similar to microrough titanium implants via moderately rough airborne-particle abrasion with large grits and acid etching (SLA) (Fig 7-1). Initially, this specific zirconia implant surface topography was created via a low-pressure IM technique using a mold with a microrough topography followed by an etching procedure with hot hydrofluoric acid.[6–9] Later the manufacturing and surface treatment procedures were further developed so that currently this microrough surface topography can be produced on zirconia implants using a specially designed mild airborne-particle abrasion procedure followed by an etching procedure with hydrofluoric acid (zirconia large-grit airborne-particle abrasion and acid etching [ZLA]) (Fig 7-2). The airborne particle–abraded and acid-etched surfaces of zirconia implants have a similar topography as titanium implants with SLA surfaces (see Fig 7-1). However, with regard to quantitative surface analysis, the microrough zirconia implant surface shows a reduced mean Sa value (Sa = 0.70 μm) compared with titanium (Sa = 1.15 μm).[2]

ZLA surfaces have been investigated extensively and compared directly with titanium SLA implants in several experimental studies, with both unloaded and loaded implants being evaluated.[6–10] Qualitative histologic analyses have shown

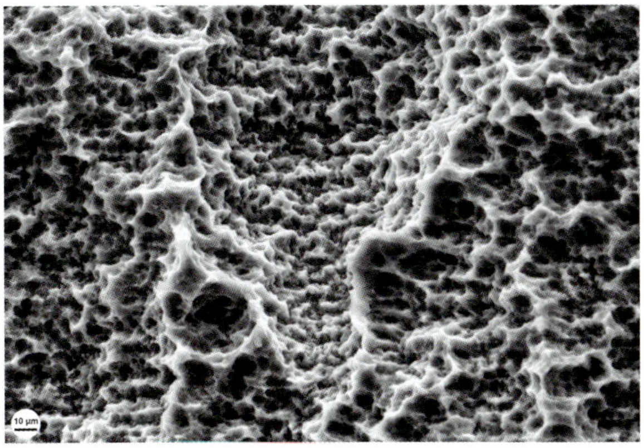

FIG 7-1 › Electron micrograph of an airborne particle–abraded and acid-etched (SLA) titanium surface. Calculations were performed with the use of a Gaussian filter with a cutoff wavelength of 30 µm. (Information provided by Straumann Group.)

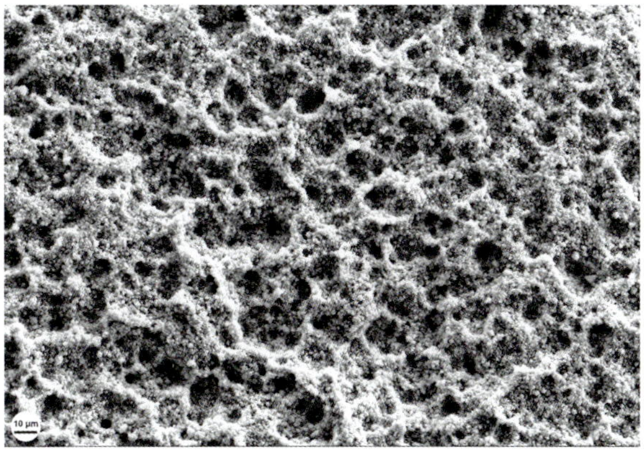

FIG 7-2 › Electron micrograph of an airborne particle–abraded and acid-etched zirconia surface (ZLA). This surface topography is similar to zirconia implants produced via low-pressure IM followed by acid etching.[6–9] Calculations were performed with the use of a Gaussian filter with a cutoff wavelength of 30 µm. (Information provided by Straumann Group.)

FIG 7-3 › Undecalcified, ground, and polished methyl methacrylate section stained with toluidine blue showing direct contact between the bone *(blue)* and implant surfaces *(gray)*. Complete and intimate osseointegration can be seen for the zirconia *(a)* and titanium *(b)* implants.

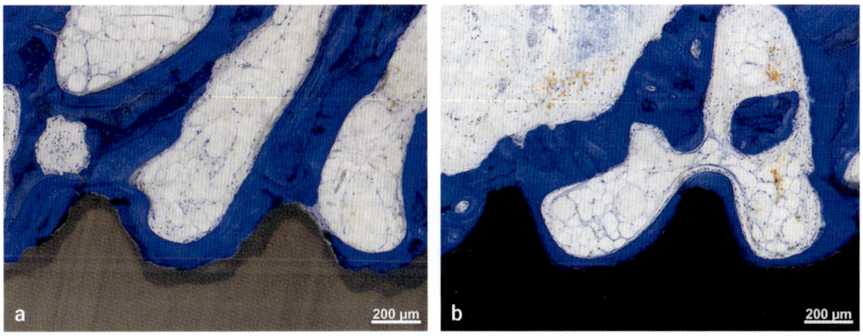

that after 4, 8, and 12 weeks of unloaded healing, peri-implant bone tissue can be found in direct contact with implant surfaces and active osseointegration can be observed for both materials (Fig 7-3). Quantitative histomorphometric analyses have revealed no significant differences between titanium and zirconia regarding bone-to-implant contact (BIC) and bone density.[7,8] Moreover, results from biomechanical removal torque testing after 4, 8, and 12 weeks of unloaded healing were similar for zirconia and titanium.[6,9] In addition, in a study by Jenner et al,[10] loaded two-piece zirconia ZLA and titanium SLA implants were investigated in five dogs. After extraction of the mandibular premolars and molars, 60 implants (30 zirconia implants and 30 titanium implants) were alternately placed bilaterally in healed sites. After 6 weeks of unloaded transmucosal healing,

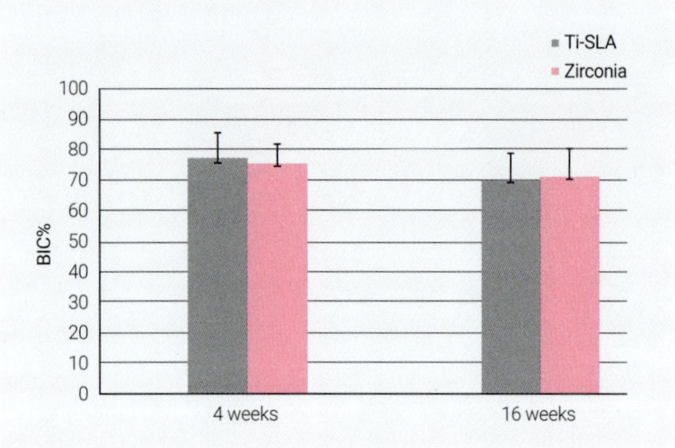

FIG 7-4 › BIC of SLA and ZLA surfaces.

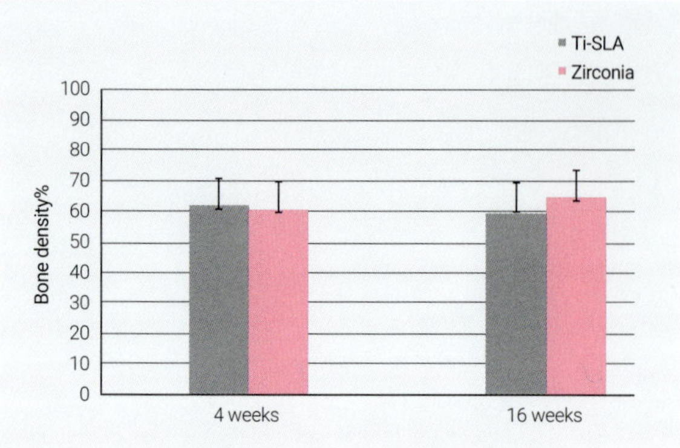

FIG 7-5 › Bone density of SLA and ZLA surfaces.

full-ceramic single-tooth restorations were cemented in place. After 4 and 16 weeks of functional loading, histomorphometric evaluation of BIC and bone density revealed no statistically significant differences between the zirconia and titanium implants[10] (Figs 7-4 and 7-5).The results of the latter studies clearly indicate that there are no qualitative and quantitative differences between the osseointegrative capacity of the investigated ZLA and titanium SLA implants in unloaded and loaded conditions.[6–10]

The osseointegration of zirconia and titanium implant surfaces has also been evaluated in a meta-analysis of preclinical studies. A total of 37 studies were included for data extraction. Bone tissue, BIC, bone density, and removal torques were evaluated. The authors concluded that titanium and zirconia implants demonstrate a similar capacity for hard tissue integration.[5]

Predictable osseointegration is not only a key factor for good clinical performance but is also important with respect to augmentation procedures. Many clinical situations require simultaneous bone augmentation and implant placement. Accordingly, a microrough zirconia implant surface that allows for osseointegration in healed sites should also be suitable for guided bone regeneration (GBR) procedures. An experimental study in seven dogs investigated the GBR of peri-implant bone defects associated with titanium and zirconia implants. After extraction of the maxillary premolars and molars in each dog, four standardized semi-saddle bone defects were created and three zirconia implants and one titanium implant were placed. After a healing period of 3 months, histomorphometric analyses were performed. The authors concluded that zirconia and titanium implants did not perform differently regarding osseous regeneration.[19]

Soft Tissue Integration

MATERIAL-RELATED FACTORS

The cuff of peri-implant junctional epithelial tissue provides biologic protection and seals against subgingival bacterial infections. The connective tissue also prevents uncontrolled downward growth of the epithelium toward the crestal bone.[12,13] Consequently, bacterial adhesion, clinical signs of inflammation or inflammatory cells in the peri-implant soft tissue, and peri-implant blood circulation are relevant factors when considering soft tissue integration.

In one experimental study on different types of machined and microrough zirconia and titanium implant surfaces, significantly reduced biofilm formation was reported with zirconia.[20] Moreover, a significantly reduced volume of leukocytes infiltrating the peri-implant epithelium has been shown around zirconia healing abutments compared with titanium ones after 2 months.[21] Similar results were confirmed in a clinical study with measurements taken after 6 months of unloaded healing. The authors reported a "higher rate of inflammation-associated processes" in the peri-implant soft tissues around titanium healing abutments compared with zirconia ones. These results were related to an increased amount of bacteria around titanium.[22] Moreover, the authors of a clinical study investigating the soft tissue around titanium and zirconia implant abutments in 10 patients using 2D laser speckle imaging and thermography found significantly improved microcirculation in peri-implant soft tissues for zirconia abutments compared with titanium ones, as well as an assumed advantage with regard to the maintenance of the immune function of the peri-implant soft tissue.[23] It must be noted that the latter studies investigated titanium and zirconia abutments, healing abutments, or experimental disks, and the relevance of these results to zirconia implants is not clear. However, from a material point of view, zirconia might have some biologic advantages over titanium with regard to soft tissue integration.

QUALITATIVE AND QUANTITATIVE FACTORS

Qualitatively, typical epithelial and gingival structures are found around implants, as with natural teeth. The epithelial tissue consists of a keratinized oral epithelium, a nonkeratinized sulcular epithelium at the top of the papilla, and a junctional epithelium in direct contact with the implant surface. Below the junctional epithelium, gingival connective tissue separates the bone from the epithelium. The sum of the vertical dimensions of the sulcular epithelium—sulcus depth, junctional epithelium, and connective tissue contact (CTC)—represents the biologic width (BW).[13]

Experimental studies have shown similar soft tissue integration for zirconia and titanium implants. Qualitatively, typical epithelial structures like keratinized oral epithelium, nonkeratinized sulcular epithelium, and a thin layer of junctional epithelium in direct contact with the implant surface can be observed (Fig 7-6). However, a keratinized sulcular epithelium around unloaded tissue-level zirconia implants after 8 weeks of follow-up has also been reported.[24] Beneath the epithelial tissue, a connective tissue zone separates the bone from the junctional epithelium.[17,24–26] In the connective tissue zone, collagen fibers are mainly aligned

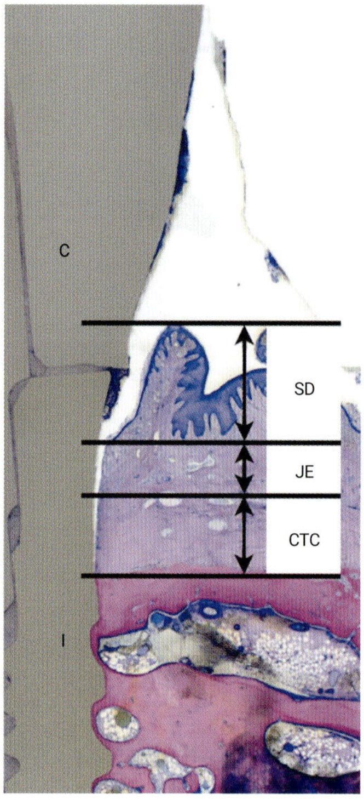

FIG 7-6 › BW dimensions around a two-piece zirconia dental implant. SD = sulcus depth; JE = junctional epithelium; CTC = connective tissue contact; I = zirconia implant; C = zirconia crown. (Undecalcified, ground, and polished methyl methacrylate section stained with Giemsa–eosin.)

parallel with the implant surface.[26] A similar fiber orientation has been observed in the connective tissue around titanium implants with a transmucosal zirconia implant shoulder.[27] One study in pigs even reported a significantly increased collagen organization in the connective tissue zone around unloaded zirconia implants compared with titanium implants.[24]

Only a few experimental studies provide detailed information regarding quantitative soft tissue integration around zirconia implants. When zirconia implants were directly compared to titanium implants, no significant differences were reported with regard to the dimensions of the epithelial tissue—sulcular and junctional epithelium, epithelial tissue length (ETL), CTC, and BW. For zirconia, mean values of 1.41 to 3.57 mm, 0.49 to 1.62 mm, and 2.71 to 5.05 mm have been reported for ETL, CTC, and BW dimensions, respectively. The corresponding values for titanium are 1.28 to 2.9 mm, 1.23 to 2.4 mm, and 2.78 to 5.2 mm, respectively.[17,24–26,28,29] Only one study in pigs records a significantly shorter sulcular and a longer junctional epithelium for zirconia (0.76 mm ± 0.25 and 1.24 mm ± 0.54, respectively) compared to titanium (1.4 mm ± 0.56 and 0.8 mm ± 0.45, respectively) after 8 weeks of unloaded healing. In addition to that, the authors reported a significantly improved collagen organization on zirconia compared with titanium and concluded that there was "more mature and pronounced soft tissue integration for this ceramic implant than for a standard titanium implant."[24]

In dogs, submerged versus nonsubmerged implant healing did not have any significant effect on soft tissue integration and the BW proportions associated with unloaded monotype tissue-level zirconia and titanium implants after 4 months of healing. However, the position of the microgap seemed to be relevant, as the submerged implants that required 0.5 to 1 mm deeper placement of the implant shoulder tended to have an insignificantly lower mucosal height compared with nonsubmerged implants.[25] Moreover, unloaded or immediate loading of nonsubmerged monotype tissue-level zirconia and two-piece titanium implants did not have any significant effect on the total BW proportions after 3 months of healing. However, detailed information on sulcular depth, junctional epithelium, and CTC dimensions was not provided.[29]

Similar results were shown when different zirconia implant materials (yttria-stabilized zirconia [YSZ] implants and partially stabilized zirconia [PSZ]/alumina nanocomposite implants) were investigated after 12 weeks of immediate loading in dogs. Interestingly, increased epithelial tissue length was associated with decreased CTC.[26] When different implant designs were evaluated after 24 weeks of loading in a dog model, no significant differences were found with regard to epithelial tissue contact and BW dimensions between monotype and two-piece tissue-level zirconia implants. However, the individual implant design had an effect on peri-implant mucosal height.[28]

Quantitative soft tissue integration has also been evaluated in a systematic review. Altogether six experimental preclinical studies were considered for data extraction and meta-analysis of BW proportions, resulting in estimated mean values of 3.5 mm (CI: 2.9–4.2) and 3.2 mm (CI: 2.7–3.7) for titanium and zirconia, respectively. The statistical analysis showed that implant material and follow-up time did not have any significant effect on the reported BW dimensions. In addition, unloaded and conventionally loaded protocols resulted in similar BW values. However, significantly increased BW dimensions were noted with immediately loaded implants compared with conventionally loaded implants. The authors concluded that zirconia and titanium implants demonstrate a similar soft tissue integration capacity, though faster maturation processes of epithelial and connective tissues around zirconia implants were assumed.[5]

CLINICAL FACTORS

Only limited clinical data is available for the objective assessment of soft tissue integration of fully ceramic/zirconia implants with regard to papilla formation capacity and pink esthetics. When applying the papilla index according to Jemt,[30] a statistically significant increase in peri-implant papilla formation over time has been reported. At crown cementation, only 17% of the papillae revealed indices of 2 and 3, whereas 3 years after implant placement, this distribution significantly increased up to 56%.[31] Non-irritated and healthy papilla formation were also evaluated in clinical studies using the pink esthetic score (PES) according to Furhauser et al.[32] Continuously increasing PES scores between crown cementation and the 24-month follow-up period were reported for one- and two-piece tissue-level zirconia implants.[33,34] Significantly increased PES values were observed for two-piece zirconia implants restored with zirconia abutments and ceramic crowns (PES range: 6.9–11.2) compared with titanium implants restored with titanium abutments and ceramic crowns (PES range: 2.4–10.8) after 2 years of follow-up.[33]

The distance between the alveolar crest of the neighboring tooth and the lowest point of the contact area of the crown appears to be an important factor for interdental papilla formation for one-piece zirconia implants.[35,36] A retrospective clinical study showed that when this distance was ≤ 5 mm, the papilla was present in 100% of all cases. When the distance increased up to 10 mm, the papilla was still present in 67% of the cases.[35] Moreover, immediate and delayed implant placement protocols resulted in similar papilla growth formation around one-piece tissue-level zirconia implants 12 months after crown cementation. There were no visible defects of the peri-implant papilla observed with 81.3% and 86.5% of immediate and delayed placement implants, respectively. However, nonvisible papilla deficits were correlated with distances of 7 to 8 mm or less.[36]

In another clinical study, researchers assessed the esthetic aspects of adjacent zirconia and titanium implants in the anterior maxilla between 3 and 12 months after crown insertion. A total of 40 patients and 109 adjacent implants (47 titanium implants and 62 zirconia implants) were included, and the authors reported that the papillae were fully present (with a Jemt score of 3) in around 39.1% of adjacent zirconia implants and only 17.4% of adjacent titanium implants. The papilla deficit was significantly higher (1.64 mm with a standard deviation of 1.35 mm) around titanium implants than zirconia implants (0.92 mm with a standard deviation of 0.94 mm) ($P < .01$). Esthetic parameters such as the interdental contact area did not differ significantly between titanium and zirconia implants.[37]

Conclusion

In experimental studies comparing ceramic implants with titanium implants, material characteristics do not have any significant effects on peri-implant soft and hard tissue integration. Direct osseointegration around zirconia and titanium implant surfaces has been observed, with similar quantitative results reported when microrough surfaces were investigated under loaded and unloaded conditions. Likewise, similar qualitative and quantitative soft tissue integration parameters have been reported for one- and two-piece tissue-level zirconia implants and two-piece tissue-level titanium implants. Thus, with regard to the morphogenesis of peri-implant soft and hard tissues, similar physiologic processes might be supposed for both materials. However, faster maturation processes of epithelial and connective tissues around zirconia implants have been noted.

Zirconia implant design and the position of the microgap influence the height of the peri-implant mucosa, with a clinically significant increase in papilla height formation over time. For titanium and zirconia implants, the distance between the alveolar crest at the neighboring tooth and the lowest point of the contact area of the crown are considered important factors for peri-implant papilla formation.

References

1. Albrektsson T, Brånemark PI, Hansson HA, Lindstrom J. Osseointegrated titanium implants. Requirements for ensuring a long-lasting, direct bone-to-implant anchorage in man. Acta Orthop Scand 1981;52:155–170.
2. Roehling S, Meng B, Cochran D. Sandblasted and acid etched implant surfaces with or without high surface free energy—Experimental and clinical background. In: Wennerberg A, Albrektsson T, Jimbo R (eds). Implant Surfaces and their Biological and Clinical Impact. Springer, 2015:93–136.
3. Roehling S, Woelfler H, Hicklin S, Kniha H, Gahlert M. A retrospective clinical study with regard to survival and success rates of zirconia implants up to and after 7 years of loading. Clin Implant Dent Relat Res 2016;18:545–558.
4. Gahlert M, Burtscher D, Grunert I, et al. Failure analysis of fractured dental zirconia implants. Clin Oral Implants Res 2012;23:287–293.
5. Roehling S, Schlegel KA, Woelfler H, Gahlert M. Zirconia compared to titanium dental implants in preclinical studies—A systematic review and meta-analysis. Clin Oral Implants Res 2019;30:365–395.
6. Bormann KH, Gellrich NC, Kniha H, Dard M, Wieland M, Gahlert M. Biomechanical evaluation of a microstructured zirconia implant by a removal torque comparison with a standard Ti-SLA implant. Clin Oral Implants Res 2012;23:1210–1216.
7. Gahlert M, Roehling S, Sprecher CM, Kniha H, Milz S, Bormann K. In vivo performance of zirconia and titanium implants: A histomorphometric study in mini pig maxillae. Clin Oral Implants Res 2012;23:281–286.
8. Gahlert M, Roehling S, Wieland M, Sprecher CM, Kniha H, Milz S. Osseointegration of zirconia and titanium dental implants: A histological and histomorphometrical study in the maxilla of pigs. Clin Oral Implants Res 2009;20:1247–1253.
9. Gahlert M, Rohling S, Wieland M, Eichhorn S, Kuchenhoff H, Kniha H. A comparison study of the osseointegration of zirconia and titanium dental implants. A biomechanical evaluation in the maxilla of pigs. Clin Implant Dent Relat Res 2010;12:297–305.
10. Janner SFM, Gahlert M, Bosshardt DD, et al. Bone response to functionally loaded, two-piece zirconia implants: A preclinical histometric study. Clin Oral Implants Res 2018;29:277–289.
11. Roehling S, Schlegel KA, Woelfler H, Gahlert M. Performance and outcome of zirconia dental implants in clinical studies: A meta-analysis. Clin Oral Implants Res 2018;29(suppl 16):135–153.
12. Berglundh T, Lindhe J, Ericsson I, Marinello CP, Liljenberg B, Thomsen P. The soft tissue barrier at implants and teeth. Clin Oral Implants Res 1991;2:81–90.
13. Cochran DL, Hermann JS, Schenk RK, Higginbottom FL, Buser D. Biologic width around titanium implants. A histometric analysis of the implanto-gingival junction around unloaded and loaded nonsubmerged implants in the canine mandible. J Periodontol 1997;68:186–198.
14. Akagawa Y, Ichikawa Y, Nikai H, Tsuru H. Interface histology of unloaded and early loaded partially stabilized zirconia endosseous implant in initial bone healing. J Prosthet Dent 1993;69:599–604.
15. Chang YS, Oka M, Nakamura T, Gu HO. Bone remodeling around implanted ceramics. J Biomed Mater Res 1996;30:117–124.
16. Sennerby L, Dasmah A, Larsson B, Iverhed M. Bone tissue responses to surface-modified zirconia implants: A histomorphometric and removal torque study in the rabbit. Clin Implant Dent Relat Res 2005;7(suppl 1):S13–S20.
17. Kohal RJ, Weng D, Bachle M, Strub JR. Loaded custom-made zirconia and titanium implants show similar osseointegration: An animal experiment. J Periodontol 2004;75:1262–1268.
18. Gahlert M, Gudehus T, Eichhorn S, Steinhauser E, Kniha H, Erhardt W. Biomechanical and histomorphometric comparison between zirconia implants with varying surface textures and a titanium implant in the maxilla of miniature pigs. Clin Oral Implants Res 2007;18:662–668.
19. Benic GI, Thoma DS, Sanz-Martin I, et al. Guided bone regeneration at zirconia and titanium dental implants: A pilot histological investigation. Clin Oral Implants Res 2017;28:1592–1599.
20. Roehling S, Astasov-Frauenhoffer M, Hauser-Gerspach I, et al. In vitro biofilm formation on titanium and zirconia implant surfaces. J Periodontol 2017;88:298–307.
21. Welander M, Abrahamsson I, Berglundh T. The mucosal barrier at implant abutments of different materials. Clin Oral Implants Res 2008;19:635–641.
22. Degidi M, Artese L, Scarano A, Perrotti V, Gehrke P, Piattelli A. Inflammatory infiltrate, microvessel density, nitric oxide synthase expression, vascular endothelial growth factor expression, and proliferative activity in peri-implant soft tissues around titanium and zirconium oxide healing caps. J Periodontol 2006;77:73–80.

23. Kajiwara N, Masaki C, Mukaibo T, Kondo Y, Nakamoto T, Hosokawa R. Soft tissue biological response to zirconia and metal implant abutments compared with natural tooth: Microcirculation monitoring as a novel bioindicator. Implant Dent 2015;24:37–41.
24. Linares A, Grize L, Munoz F, et al. Histological assessment of hard and soft tissues surrounding a novel ceramic implant: A pilot study in the minipig. J Clin Periodontol 2016;43:538–546.
25. Koch FP, Weng D, Kramer S, Wagner W. Soft tissue healing at one-piece zirconia implants compared to titanium and PEEK implants of identical design: A histomorphometric study in the dog. Int J Periodontics Restorative Dent 2013;33:669–677.
26. Igarashi K, Nakahara K, Haga-Tsujimura M, Kobayashi E, Watanabe F. Hard and soft tissue responses to three different implant materials in a dog model. Dent Mater J 2015;34:692–701.
27. Tete S, Mastrangelo F, Bianchi A, Zizzari V, Scarano A. Collagen fiber orientation around machined titanium and zirconia dental implant necks: An animal study. Int J Oral Maxillofac Implants 2009;24:52–58.
28. Thoma DS, Benic GI, Munoz F, et al. Histological analysis of loaded zirconia and titanium dental implants: An experimental study in the dog mandible. J Clin Periodontol 2015;42:967–975.
29. Delgado-Ruiz RA, Calvo-Guirado JL, Abboud M, et al. Histologic and histomorphometric behavior of microgrooved zirconia dental implants with immediate loading. Clin Implant Dent Relat Res 2014;16:856–872.
30. Jemt T. Regeneration of gingival papillae after single-implant treatment. Int J Periodontics Restorative Dent 1997;17:326–333.
31. Spies BC, Balmer M, Patzelt SB, Vach K, Kohal RJ. Clinical and patient-reported outcomes of a zirconia oral implant: Three-year results of a prospective cohort investigation. J Dent Res 2015;94:1385–1391.
32. Furhauser R, Florescu D, Benesch T, Haas R, Mailath G, Watzek G. Evaluation of soft tissue around single-tooth implant crowns: The pink esthetic score. Clin Oral Implants Res 2005;16:639–644.
33. Payer M, Heschl A, Koller M, Arnetzl G, Lorenzoni M, Jakse N. All-ceramic restoration of zirconia two-piece implants—A randomized controlled clinical trial. Clin Oral Implants Res 2015;26:371–376.
34. Payer M, Arnetzl V, Kirmeier R, Koller M, Arnetzl G, Jakse N. Immediate provisional restoration of single-piece zirconia implants: A prospective case series—Results after 24 months of clinical function. Clin Oral Implants Res 2013;24:569–575.
35. Kniha K, Gahlert M, Hicklin S, Bragger U, Kniha H, Milz S. Evaluation of hard and soft tissue dimensions around zirconium oxide implant-supported crowns: A 1-year retrospective study. J Periodontol 2016;87:511–518.
36. Kniha K, Kniha H, Mohlhenrich SC, Milz S, Holzle F, Modabber A. Papilla and alveolar crest levels in immediate versus delayed single-tooth zirconia implants. Int J Oral Maxillofac Surg 2017;46:1039–1044.
37. Kniha K, Bock A, Peters F, et al. Aesthetic aspects of adjacent maxillary single-crown implants—Influence of zirconia and titanium as implant materials. Int J Oral Maxillofac Surg 2020;49:1489–1496.

08

ONE- AND TWO-PIECE ZIRCONIA IMPLANT DESIGNS

Michael Payer

The ideal type of implant-abutment connection for ceramic implant systems has not yet been determined. The majority of zirconia implants are still manufactured as one-piece systems, and one-piece ceramic implants fabricated from yttria-stabilized tetragonal zirconia polycrystal (Y-TZP) were the first to fulfill requirements for clinical applications. However, in an ongoing scientific debate, justified doubts about one-piece implants have been raised based on the high fracture rates of ceramic implants made of mono- or polycrystalline aluminum oxide and evaluated in early clinical trials and experimental investigations.[1,2] In a recent systematic review and meta-analysis conducted by Bethke et al[3] on in vitro studies, the authors found that one-piece implants are generally more fracture resistant than two-piece implants, even though some of the included studies showed very promising results for two-piece zirconia implants. Within the group of one-piece implants, those fabricated from alumina-toughened zirconia (ATZ) seemed to be more fracture resistant than implants made from Y-TZP. This chapter reviews the available literature on one- and two-piece designs for zirconia implants.

One-Piece Zirconia Implants

When using one-piece zirconia implants (Fig 8-1) for clinical applications, strict prosthetically driven ("backward") planning is highly recommended, as both the implant and abutment positions are determined during surgery. Modifications to the abutment angle in one-piece zirconia implants is contraindicated because intraoral grinding may induce superficial phase transformation, resulting in early material aging and a higher risk of fracture.[2,4] Unfortunately, angled abutments to facilitate restorative requirements are so far not available for one-piece implant systems, which limits their prosthetic versatility and can lead to compromised implant positioning. This is a potential drawback of one-piece zirconia implants, especially in the esthetic zone.[5] In addition, only limited data is available on the use of zirconia implants in patients requiring augmentation procedures to compensate for hard and soft tissue deficits.[6]

Another fact to consider when using one-piece implants is that loading forces on the supramucosal part of the implant abutment will result immediately after implant placement due to masticatory activity and tongue movements.[7] To compensate for immediate loading of one-piece implants, manufacturers have recommended using protective splints during the healing period. However, even if a patient is provided with a removable splint that fits perfectly, it remains unclear whether a single-piece implant will be allowed to heal in a stress-free environment, especially because patient compliance is required. Nonremovable provisional bridging devices between adjacent teeth could guarantee load-free healing, though there are limitations with respect to free-end situations and compromised oral hygiene.

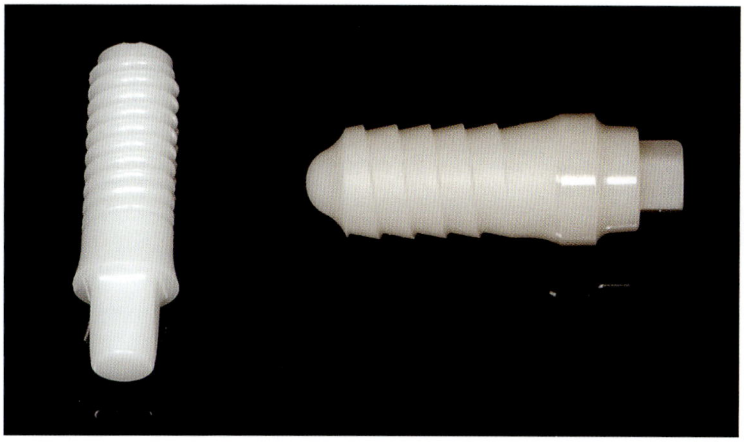

FIG 8-1 › Different designs of one-piece zirconia implants.

One-piece implants are usually constructed with a submucosally submerged prosthetic platform, and a provisional device or a soft tissue–forming device should be applied after insertion. Otherwise, the mucosa will have to be detached traumatically prior to impression taking for fabrication of the provisional or permanent restoration.[5] Immediate provisionalization and conditioning of the peri-implant soft tissues is therefore recommended for one-piece zirconia implants, even though data on immediate provisionals and loading of these implants is limited.[8] In any case, exposure to immediate loading seems to be inevitable for one-piece implants and generally occurs regardless of the type of provisional restoration used.[9]

So far, cementation and adhesive techniques are the only options available for securing restorations to one-piece implants. However, the lack of an implant-abutment interface (microgap) in one-piece implants may be appealing and advantageous from a biologic point of view because it avoids creating a niche for the retention of microbiota and plaque accumulation in comparison with conventional two-piece systems. For example, Hermann et al[10] studied the biologic width (BW) around one- and two-piece implant systems in a dog model and found that the presence of a microgap and its location with respect to the alveolar crest had a significant impact on the amount of peri-implant bone loss. In nonsubmerged one-piece implant systems without a microgap placed at the crest, it was found that the BW was similar to that of natural teeth and that there was a more stable coronal position of the gingival margin when compared with a two-piece system with a microgap at the crest.[10]

In another clinical study on 26 patients, Hartman and Cochran[11] found a physiologic distance between the bone and the implant-crown interface around one-piece implants that is established early and maintained over time. These results demonstrate that the magnitude of initial bone remodeling around one-piece dental implants depends on the apicocoronal position of the implant border. The distance from the crown-implant interface to the point of bone-to-implant contact (BIC) was found to be consistent with a BW like that found around natural dentition.[11]

In another animal trial in five laboratory-bred male American hounds, Hermann et al[12] found that crestal bone changes around two-piece nonsubmerged titanium implants are significantly influenced by movement between the implants and abutments and not necessarily by the size of the microgap. They observed significant crestal bone loss in two-piece implant systems in combination with possible movements between the implant components even with the smallest-sized microgaps of less than 10 μm.[12] Although the animal studies of Hartman and Cochran[11] and Hermann et al[12] were conducted with titanium implants, the nature of their findings appears to be related to basic physiologic and biologic phenomena occurring around both implants and natural teeth, so one may expect validity irrespective of the type of implant material being used, including for one-piece zirconia implants.

Another issue frequently discussed in the context of one-piece zirconia implants is reduced plaque affinity in comparison with titanium, and subsequently a reduced incidence of peri-implant infection. In a preclinical study using a dog model, Roehling et al[13] observed a significantly reduced occurrence of ligature-induced inflammation and bone loss around implants with airborne particle–abraded and acid-etched zirconia (ZLA) surfaces in comparison with titanium implants with airborne particle–abraded and acid-etched (SLA) surfaces.[13] These results, in combination with the findings on the effect of microgaps found in two-piece implants systems, could represent a plausible microbiologic-based argument for the use of one-piece zirconia implants.

This hypothesis is further supported by results from an experimental investigation by Clever et al[14] that aimed to assess clinical and microbiologic parameters around zirconia and titanium implants compared with those around natural teeth during experimental plaque accumulation. Clinical parameters such as the gingival index, plaque index, bleeding on probing, and pocket probing depth were assessed. In addition, microbiologic samples were analyzed for total bacterial cell counts, as well as *Tannerella forsythia* and *Prevotella intermedia* counts. A statistically significant difference over time was observed between groups in terms of gingival index, plaque index, and bleeding on probing. The lowest mean total number of bacterial cells was measured around natural teeth, followed by zirconia implants, with the highest values measured around titanium implants. Compared with the soft tissues around zirconia implants and natural teeth, the soft tissues around titanium implants developed stronger inflammatory responses to experimental plaque accumulation in terms of the total number of bacterial cells and *T forsythia* and *P intermedia* counts.[14] However, clear clinical evidence from experimental and preclinical trials proving the superiority of zirconia implants is still lacking.

Another substantial problem with one-piece zirconia implants is the challenge of proper vertical implant positioning and fixation.[11] Implants are frequently inserted further submucosally to reduce the risk of the restoration margins peeking through the soft tissue, especially in anterior regions. With one-piece implants, however, this may lead to an increased risk of excessive luting cement left in the submucosal areas, as there is no option for screw-retained restorations. Excess cement on the implant or in the surrounding soft tissues has been associated with peri-implant disease.[15] Unfortunately, cement remnants are not always visible on radiographs[16] but only upon clinical examination after removal of the restoration. By that time, local infection and substantial tissue damage may have already occurred.[17] On the other hand, cementation has become popular for prosthesis fixation because it is relatively simple and eliminates time-consuming technical adjustments to correct problems such as prosthetic screw loosening. Passivity of fit, improved esthetics, the ease of examining occlusion, and economic benefits are other clear advantages of cementation techniques over screw-retained prostheses.[18]

In a systematic review, Wittneben et al[19] found no statistically significant difference between cement- and screw-retained restorations regarding survival and failure rates. Overall, however, screw-retained prostheses exhibited fewer technical and biologic complications. The authors also found no statistically significant differences between the failure rates of the different restoration types nor between ceramic titanium and gold abutment materials. Thus, the failure rates of cement-retained restorations do not seem to be influenced by the type of abutment material but rather by the cement itself.[19] Proposed techniques to avoid leaving behind excess cement include palatal venting and precementation using custom analogs.[20]

CLINICAL STUDIES

Pieralli et al[21] conducted a systematic review limited to randomized controlled trials and prospective clinical trials reporting survival rates and marginal bone loss to evaluate the success of one- and two-piece zirconia implants restored with single crowns or three-unit fixed partial dentures.[21] Furthermore, at least 15 patients per study were required as a supplementary criterion of inclusion in the review. In accordance with these inclusion criteria, nine studies totaling 326 patients restored with 398 implants were included. Of the included zirconia implants (made from Y-TZP and ATZ), 97% (382) were one-piece implants not currently available commercially and followed for 19.7 months (only 16 implants varied from this design[22]). Survival analysis revealed an estimated 1-year survival rate for zirconia implants of 95.6%. Limited to the short-term prognosis of this estimate, it was concluded that this survival rate is comparable to that of titanium implants supporting similar single crowns and fixed dental prostheses.[21]

In another systematic review and meta-analysis by Roehling et al,[23] electronic and manual searches were performed to identify clinical studies investigating zirconia dental implants with a mean follow-up of at least 12 months. Primary outcomes were implant survival and peri-implant marginal bone loss. Secondary outcomes included technical and biologic complications, as well as esthetic outcomes. Meta-analyses were performed to estimate implant survival and marginal bone loss. According to the inclusion criteria, 18 studies were included for data extraction. One-piece (14 studies) and two-piece (4 studies) zirconia implants were investigated. Commercially available (510 implants in 398 patients) and noncommercially available zirconia implants (618 implants and 343 patients) were evaluated. Of the 18 clinical studies that were included in the analysis, only 3 were prospective randomized clinical trials comparing titanium (n = 71) with zirconia (n = 89) or immediately (n = 20) and conventionally (n = 20) loaded zirconia implants. Fifteen publications reported observational studies. Of those, 11 were prospective and 4 were retrospective. Since 2004, the survival rates of commercially available implants significantly improved compared with noncommercially available implants. Regarding commercially available one-piece zirconia implants, the meta-analysis by Roehling et al found 1- and 2-year mean survival

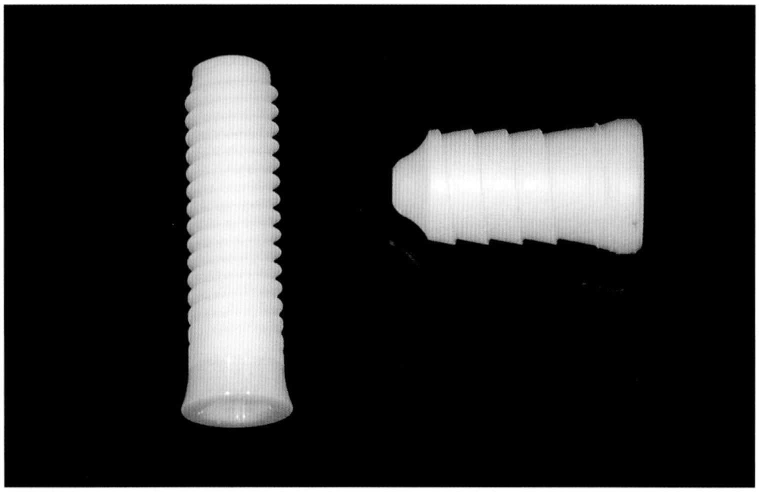

FIG 8-2 › Different designs of two-piece zirconia implants.

rates and peri-implant marginal bone loss after 1 year that were similar to those reported for titanium implants.[23]

Thus, both reviews concluded from the available short- and medium-term data that one-piece zirconia implants may be considered a reliable treatment option that should continue to be evaluated in additional follow-ups. Obviously, zirconia implants in one-piece designs provide sufficient stability for clinical application and a low risk profile for technical complications and failures attributable to material limitations. However, due to their aforementioned limitations, ongoing research with experimental and clinical trials is being performed to identify reliable two-piece connection options for ceramic implants (Fig 8-2).

Two-Piece Zirconia Implants

Due to the material properties of ceramics, screw connections for zirconia two-piece implants using all-ceramic components could not be made at first. Thus, the first generations of two-piece zirconia implant systems connected implants and abutments via adhesive fixation techniques. However, using adhesive abutment fixation with two-piece zirconia implants in daily clinical practice requires consideration of several factors. First, the data regarding the performance of subgingival adhesive abutment fixation on crestal bone levels is available only for medium-term applications.[6] Furthermore, in some cases, especially in the posterior mandible, proper adhesive abutment fixation could require rubber dam use, which may be challenging.[22] In addition, thorough removal and cleaning of excess adhesive material must be performed after abutment installation to avoid biologic complications with prosthetic superstructures. Adhesive techniques conveniently eliminate microgaps[12] but still have a rather experimental character and present complexities in clinical application, though they have proved capable of withstanding loading forces in experimental and clinical trials.[6]

In recent years, progress has been made, and new designs and materials have been tested and proposed for screw-type connections between zirconia implants and abutments, offering a variety of options for abutment angulation and reversibility if necessary. Today manufacturers use titanium inserts in ceramic implants and corresponding screws made of titanium, carbon fiber, or even polyetheretherketone (PEEK), a colorless organic thermoplastic polymer in the polyaryletherketone family.[24]

In an experimental trial, Spies et al[25] investigated the long-term stability of metal-free zirconia two-piece implants assembled with a carbon fiber–reinforced screw by means of transformation propagation, potential changes in surface roughness, the gap size of the implant-abutment connection, and fracture load values. They found no fractures of carbon fiber–reinforced screws during static or dynamic loading and concluded that the metal-free implants were sufficiently stable.[25]

Nevertheless, the impact of low-temperature degradation (LTD) on the long-term stability of zirconia dental implants is still an intensively discussed topic. Besides the material that is used, the design of the implant with either an integrated abutment or a separate abutment seems to affect the fracture resistance of zirconia implants. As already discussed, one-piece ceramic implants are superior to two-piece implants in terms of fracture resistance in preclinical situations.[3] However, long-term clinical data on zirconia implants is scarce and mainly refers to one-piece implants used to replace up to three missing adjacent teeth.[21,26] Two-piece zirconia implants are still seldomly used and just starting to be represented in clinical trials due to the technical challenges of integrating the screw connection as part of the implant-abutment assembly.[6]

In one experimental trial[27] evaluating the influence of artificial aging on phase transformation propagation and fracture resistance of zirconia implants, the authors considered one-piece zirconia implants, two-piece 4.1-mm-diameter titanium implants and 5-mm-diameter zirconia implants. One subgroup of implants was loaded simultaneously, dynamically loaded, and hydrothermally aged, whereas the other subgroup remained untreated. Finally, specimens were statically loaded to the point of fracture. Potential crystal phase transformation was examined in cross section using scanning electron microscopy (SEM). A multivariate linear regression model was applied for statistical analyses. The fracture resistance of the tested implants was not affected significantly by loading or aging. However, a comparison between the systems revealed significant differences independent of loading/aging. Regarding the crystal structure, a transformation zone was observed in SEM images even before aging that increased in both tested zirconia implant systems. In the fracture analysis, the titanium control implants showed higher fracture resistance compared with both zirconia implants. Loading/aging had no significant impact on the fracture resistance of either zirconia implant type, though the wide-diameter zirconia implants were weaker than the regular one-piece zirconia implants.

CLINICAL STUDIES

Clinical data on two-piece zirconia implants is scarce. Systematic reviews on the clinical performance of zirconia implants in general include data and calculated survival rates of one-and two-piece commercially available implants ranging from 87% to 98.3% after 1 year of function, with an estimated 5-year survival rate of 97.2%.[23,28] However, there are only a few clinical publications reporting trials and follow-up publications on two-piece zirconia implants available in the literature.[6,22,24,29–31] In all studies and the follow-up publications, adhesive or cemented abutment fixation at a supracrestal level was performed.

In the study by Cionca et al,[29] 32 patients were treated with 49 implants restored with single-unit all-ceramic crowns. After a mean time of 82.2 months after loading, the cumulative survival rate was 83%. Reported causes for failure were lack of osseointegration, aseptic loosening at different timepoints, implant fracture, and peri-implantitis. The authors further reported six abutment fractures at the implant level and thus a cumulative technical complication rate of 13%, a biologic complication rate of 8%, and a success rate of only 63%. The zirconia implant system used in this trial has been withdrawn from the market.

In a prospective randomized pilot trial on two-piece zirconia and titanium implants conducted by Payer et al,[22] no difference in success rate was observed between the two types of implants. The behavior of the bonded zirconia abutment connection was adequate for the clinical application over the observed period.

Koller et al[6] published survival rates of 87.5% for zirconia implants and 93% for titanium implants after 80 months. The calculated mean marginal bone loss after 80 months was 1.38 mm for zirconia compared with 1.17 mm for titanium. There were no statistically significant differences between the two groups in terms of survival rates and bone loss after an observation time of 80 months.[6] The zirconia implant system used in this trial has also been withdrawn from the market.

Brüll et al[31] retrospectively evaluated 66 two-piece zirconia implants for up to 3 years and calculated an overall survival rate of 97% and a mean bone loss of 0.1 mm. In a study by Becker et al,[30] 60 patients with two-piece zirconia implants were included initially, and the authors reported an implant survival rate of 83.3% after a mean observation period of 26 months, with an estimated incidence of biologic complications of 37.5%.[30]

More recent systematic reviews[32–34] report promising longevity and success rate outcomes, especially for commercially available implants. However, there is still insufficient long-term clinical evidence to support the use of two-piece ceramic dental implants in daily practice. The popularity of two-piece zirconia implants will likely increase because they are more versatile than one-piece implants, though this versatility may also be tied to higher clinician and patient costs.[35] In general, the clinical performance of commercially available implants seems to be better than that of commercially unavailable systems, and rehabilitation with zirconia implants of either one- or two-piece designs leads to high patient satisfaction in clinical trials.

Conclusion

Due to the paucity of controlled clinical data on the design of zirconia implants, no clear conclusions can be drawn on the long-term performance and fracture resistance of two-piece zirconia implants compared with one-piece zirconia implants and standard titanium implants, especially with regard to wide-body zirconia implants with platform switching. Based on systematic reviews of clinical trials, the short- and medium-term survival rates for zirconia one-piece implants seem to be promising and in line with titanium two-piece implant systems. In general, the clinical performance of commercially available implants seems to be better than that of commercially unavailable systems. However, more randomized clinical trials are urgently needed to evaluate all aspects of the clinical application of both one-piece and especially two-piece zirconia implants to provide clinicians with solid guidelines and clinical recommendations.

References

1. Sandhaus S. Technic and instrumentation of the implant C.B.S. (Cristalline Bone Screw) [in Italian]. Inf Odontostomatol 1968;4:19–24.
2. Andreiotelli M, Kohal RJ. Fracture strength of zirconia implants after artificial aging. Clin Implant Dent Relat Res 2009;11:158–166.
3. Bethke A, Pieralli S, Kohal RJ, et al. Fracture resistance of zirconia oral implants in vitro: A systematic review and meta-analysis. Materials (Basel) 2020;13:562.
4. Wenz HJ, Bartsch J, Wolfart S, Kern M. Osseointegration and clinical success of zirconia dental implants: A systematic review. Int J Prosthodont 2008;21:27–36.
5. Payer M, Arnetzl V, Kirmeier R, Koller M, Arnetzl G, Jakse N. Immediate provisional restoration of single-piece zirconia implants: A prospective case series—Results after 24 months of clinical function. Clin Oral Implants Res 2013;24:569–575.
6. Koller M, Steyer E, Theisen K, Stagnell S, Jakse N, Payer M. Two-piece zirconia versus titanium implants after 80 months: Clinical outcomes from a prospective randomized pilot trial. Clin Oral Implants Res 2020;31:388–396.
7. Cionca N, Hashim D, Mombelli A. Zirconia dental implants: Where are we now, and where are we heading? Periodontol 2000 2017;73:241–258.
8. Steyer E, Herber V, Koller M, et al. Immediate restoration of single-piece zirconia implants: A prospective case series-long-term results after 11 years of clinical function. Materials (Basel) 2021;14:6738.
9. Zembic A, Johannesen L, Schou S, et al. Immediately restored one-piece single-tooth implants with reduced diameter: One-year results of a multi-center study. Clin Oral Implants Res 2012;23:49–54.
10. Hermann JS, Schoolfield JD, Schenk RK, Buser D, Cochran DL.J. Influence of the size of the microgap on crestal bone changes around titanium implants. A histometric evaluation of unloaded non-submerged implants in the canine mandible. J Periodontol 2001;72:1372–1383.
11. Hartman GA, Cochran DL. Initial implant position determines the magnitude of crestal bone remodeling. J Periodontol 2004;75:572–577.
12. Hermann JS, Cochran DL, Buser D, Schenk RK, Schoolfield JD. Biologic width around one-and two-piece titanium implants. Clin Oral Implants Res 2001;12:559–571.
13. Roehling S, Gahlert M, Janner S, Meng B, Woelfler H, Cochran DL. Ligature-induced peri-implant bone loss around loaded zirconia and titanium implants. Int J Oral Maxillofac Implants 2019;34:357–365.
14. Clever KA, Schlegel H, Kniha G, et al. Experimental peri-implant mucositis around titanium and zirconia implants in comparison to a natural tooth: Part 2—Clinical and microbiological parameters. Int J Oral Maxillofac Surg 2019;48:560–565.
15. Wilson TG Jr. The positive relationship between excess cement and peri-implant disease: A prospective clinical endoscopic study. J Periodontol 2009;80:1388–1392.
16. Linkevicius T, Vindasiute E, Puisys A, Linkeviciene L, Maslova N, Puriene A. The influence of the cementation margin position on the amount of undetected cement. A prospective clinical study. Clin Oral Implants Res 2013;24:71–76.

17. Korsch M, Robra BP, Walther W. Cement-associated signs of inflammation: Retrospective analysis of the effect of excess cement on peri-implant tissue. Int J Prosthodont 2015;28:11–18.
18. Squier RS, Agar JR, Duncan JP, Taylor TD. Retentiveness of dental cements used with metallic implant components. Int J Oral Maxillofac Implants 2001;16:793–798.
19. Wittneben JG, Joda T, Weber HP, Brägger U. Screw retained vs. cement retained implant-supported fixed dental prosthesis. Periodontol 2000 2017;73:141–151.
20. Zaugg LK, Zehnder I, Rohr N, Fischer J, Zitzmann NU. The effects of crown venting or pre-cementing of CAD/CAM-constructed all-ceramic crowns luted on YTZ implants on marginal cement excess. Clin Oral Implants Res 2018;29:82–90.
21. Pieralli S, Kohal RJ, Jung RE, Vach K, Spies BC. Clinical outcomes of zirconia dental implants: A systematic review. J Dent Res 2017;96:38–46.
22. Payer M, Heschl A, Koller M, Arnetzl G, Lorenzoni M, Jakse N. All-ceramic restoration of zirconia two-piece implants—A randomized controlled clinical trial. Clin Oral Implants Res 2015;26:371–376.
23. Roehling S, Schlegel KA, Woelfler H, Gahlert M. Performance and outcome of zirconia dental implants in clinical studies: A meta-analysis. Clin Oral Implants Res 2018;29(suppl 16):135–153.
24. Cionca N, Hashim D, Mombelli. Two-piece zirconia implants supporting all-ceramic crowns: Six-year results of a prospective cohort study. Clin Oral Implants Res 2021;32:695–701.
25. Spies BC, Fross A, Adolfsson E, Bagegni A, Doerken S, Kohal RJ. Stability and aging resistance of a zirconia oral implant using a carbon fiber-reinforced screw for implant-abutment connection. Dent Mater 2018;34:1585–1595.
26. Bormann KH, Gellrich NC, Kniha H, Schild S, Weingart D, Gahlert M. A prospective clinical study to evaluate the performance of zirconium dioxide dental implants in single-tooth edentulous area: 3-year follow-up. BMC Oral Health 2018;18:181.
27. Burkhardt F, Spies BC, Riemer L, Adolfsson E, Doerken S, Kohal RJ. Fracture resistance and crystal phase transformation of a one- and a two-piece zirconia implant with and without simultaneous loading and aging—An in vitro study. Clin Oral Implants Res 2021;32:1288–1298.
28. Hashim D, Cionca N, Courvoisier DS, Mombelli A. A systematic review of the clinical survival of zirconia implants. Clin Oral Investig 2016;20:1403–1417.
29. Cionca N, Müller N, Mombelli A. Two-piece zirconia implants supporting all-ceramic crowns: A prospective clinical study. Clin Oral Implants Res 2015;26:413–418.
30. Becker J, John G, Becker K, Mainusch S, Diedrichs G, Schwarz F. Clinical performance of two-piece zirconia implants in the posterior mandible and maxilla: A prospective cohort study over 2 years. Clin Oral Implants Res 2017;28:29–35.
31. Brüll F, van Winkelhoff AJ, Cune MS. Zirconia dental implants: A clinical, radiographic, and microbiologic evaluation up to 3 years. Int J Oral Maxillofac Implants 2014;29:914–920.
32. da Silva AMP, Horta dos Santos FA, Mota RF, Teixeira MKS, Telles DM, Lourenço EJV. Clinical and radiographic outcomes of a two-piece ceramic implant: One year results from a prospective clinical trial. Clin Oral Investig 2024;28:380.
33. Attard L, Lee V, Le J, et al. Mechanical factors implicated in zirconia implant fracture placed within the anterior region--A systematic review. Dent J (Basel) 2022;10:22.
34. Roehling S, Gahlert M, Bacevic M, Woelfler H, Laleman I. Clinical and radiographic outcomes of zirconia dental implants--A systematic review and meta-analysis. Clin Oral Implants Res 2023;34(suppl 26):112–124.
35. Arefnia B, Fakheran O, Jakse N, Payer M. Patient-reported outcomes of zirconia dental implants: A systematic review and future directions. J Patient Rep Outcomes 2025;9:7.

09

RATIONALE FOR USING ZIRCONIA DENTAL IMPLANTS

Jens Tartsch

Ceramic implants have already lost their reputation as a niche product and are increasingly finding their way into conventional implantology practices. This is partially due to an increased awareness about health among the general population and the associated rise in the demand for metal-free dental restorations. However, the development of ceramic materials, surface treatments, and application concepts making ceramic implants safe for use is also a major reason for the increased acceptance of ceramic implants on the part of implantologists. Ceramic implants offered alongside titanium ones (Fig 9-1) can provide advantages for daily clinical practice, especially because even gold standard titanium is not always entirely unproblematic. This chapter describes the potential risks associated with titanium intolerance and the benefits of using zirconia dental implants.

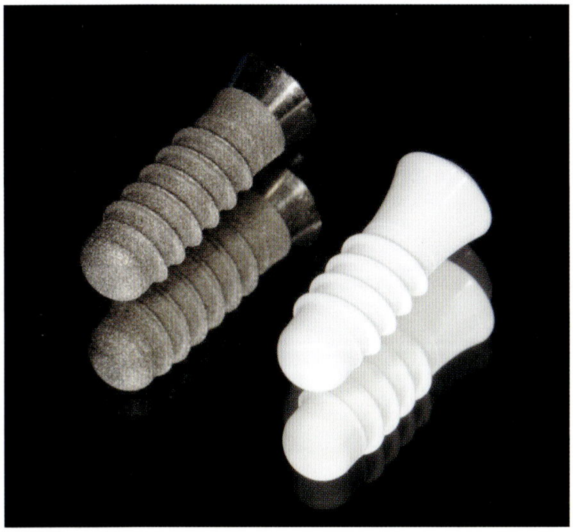

FIG 9-1 › Titanium and zirconia implants.

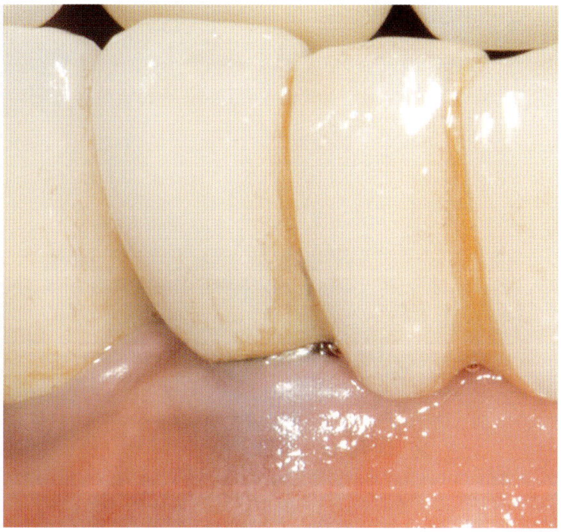

FIG 9-2 › Gray titanium showing through the peri-implant soft tissue.

Esthetics

Along with the increased health awareness of the population, the standard esthetic requirements for restorations have also risen. Ceramic implants are more esthetic than titanium thanks to the white color of zirconia, and they are especially beneficial for use in anterior areas in patients with thin gingival phenotypes. Although excellent esthetics can be achieved with titanium implants, the peri-implant mucosa must be at least 2 mm thick to prevent grayish-looking soft tissue[1] (Fig 9-2).In one study, titanium and ceramic specimens were placed under porcine jaw mucosal preparations of different thicknesses and evaluated spectrophotometrically. The gray show-through of the titanium specimens was present at mucosal thicknesses of up to 2 mm. The white zirconia specimens showed only up to a thickness of 1.5 mm.[2]

Several techniques have been suggested for improving the esthetics of titanium implants. Connective tissue grafts harvested from the palate can be used to increase mucosal thickness, but this entails performing another procedure with additional morbidity and extended risks. Thus, especially in patients with a thin mucosal phenotype, ceramic implants appear to have an esthetic advantage (Fig 9-3). In rare cases, ceramic implants may cause undesirable inflammation-free recession of the gingiva that exposes the implant shoulder, but the esthetic impairment is less severe than comparable recessions with titanium implants. These "white recessions" are usually barely noticed by patients and are tolerated much better than the dark margins of titanium implants (Fig 9-4).

FIG 9-3 › Esthetic examples of ceramic implants without a soft tissue graft.

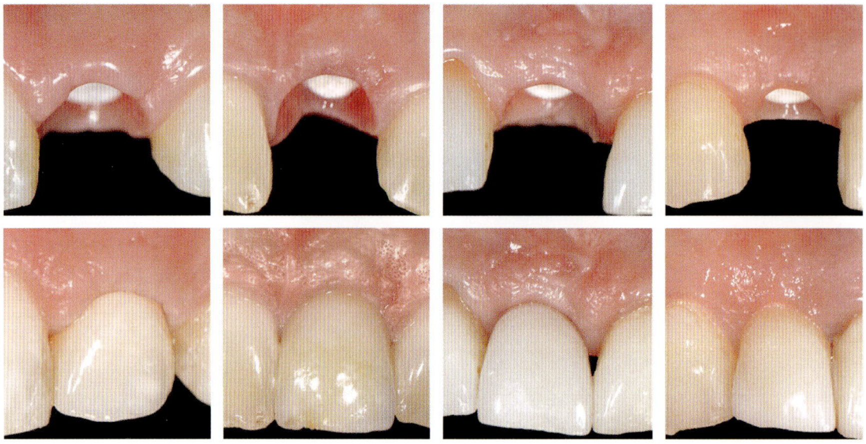

FIG 9-4 › Soft tissue recession around ceramic *(a)* and titanium *(b)* implants.

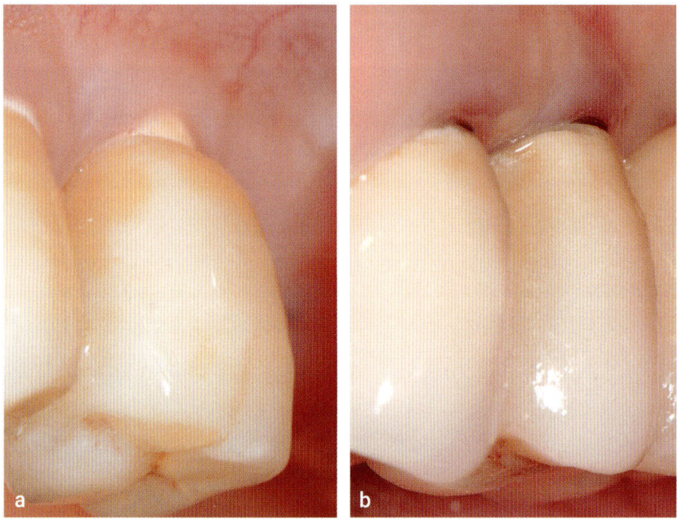

All-ceramic abutments are an alternative to titanium abutments and can prevent show-through at the abutment level when used with titanium implants. However, connections between all-ceramic abutments and titanium implants are subject to special problems. For example, the fracture rate of all-ceramic abutments ranges from 1% to 17% as reported in systematic reviews.[3] Furthermore, micromovements of the hard zirconia abutment against the softer titanium implant can lead to abrasion and even destruction of the implant-abutment connection.[4]

The wear of the interface between titanium implants and one-piece zirconia abutments was compared with that of titanium implants with titanium abutments. Six implants, three with one-piece zirconia abutments and three with titanium abutments, were cyclically loaded in epoxy resin blocks in a fatigue-testing machine for

1,200,000 cycles at 100 N. Scanning electron microscopy (SEM) of the implant interfaces was then performed for comparison and statistical analysis. The implants connected to zirconia abutments showed greater wear than the implants with titanium abutments. Although the clinical relevance of these results is unclear, damage to the internal implant connection could lead to prosthetic failures, including the need for implant removal.[5] Thus, the implant-abutment connection should be made of the same material as the implant. To meet esthetic requirements, a titanium adhesive base with an all-ceramic restoration is preferred for titanium implants.

In another study, 40 single implants in the incisor and premolar regions of 40 patients were examined 3 to 7 years after implant placement. The color difference between the peri-implant mucosa and natural gingiva was analyzed spectrophotometrically and rated visually by clinicians as "clinically visible" or "clinically invisible" from a speaking distance. Clinical examination revealed that the color difference between peri-implant mucosa and natural gingiva was clinically visible from a speaking distance in 60% of cases.[6]

To achieve esthetic results, it is recommended to position the shoulder of a titanium implant 2 to 3 mm inferior to the cementoenamel junction of an adjacent tooth in bone-level implants. In this way, an appropriate emergence profile with suitable support of the soft tissue can be achieved.[7] Ceramic implants, on the other hand, are usually tissue-level implants, with the implant shoulder placed at the gingival level because reliable cement removal is not possible if one-piece ceramic implants are placed deeper than 1 to 1.5 mm subgingivally.[8] Any remaining cement residue could lead to cementitis and associated peri-implant bone resorption. For esthetic reasons, however, the implant shoulder should be positioned slightly subgingivally in the anterior region, as visibility of even a white implant could have a poor esthetic effect. The position of the implant shoulder must also allow for an adequate emergence profile. Implants placed too far coronally lead to undesirable, balcony-like negative overhangs. Two-piece systems may offer advantages here, but the gingival height of the abutment must be added to the position of the implant shoulder.

In summary, when used correctly, ceramic implants have esthetic advantages over titanium implants, especially in patients with a thin mucosal phenotype.

Systemic Effects of Titanium Implants

Titanium has been the material of choice in both endoprosthetics and dental implantology for many years. The reasons for this are its anticorrosive behavior and corresponding biocompatibility. However, an increasingly emotional debate is now being held among experts about the effects of titanium on the human body. The systemic effects of metals on an organism are determined by toxicologic and immunologic mechanisms.

TOXICOLOGIC MECHANISMS

Toxicologic effects are dose dependent and usually based on the disruption of enzyme functions. In many cases, the toxic effects of heavy metals are due to their ability to form complexes with proteins. If metals are present in ionic form, they bind with proteins to form complexes known as *haptens*. Toxic metals can have a higher binding capacity to such enzyme complexes. Essential trace elements are displaced from their central position in the enzyme by heavy metals, resulting in the loss of the functional structure of the protein and thus deactivating the function of the enzyme.[9]

Fortunately, metallic titanium reacts with oxygen within a fraction of a nanosecond to form titanium dioxide (TiO_2).[10] Thus, free titanium ions are not available for further reactions with proteins. Binding to enzymes with a displacement effect is therefore physiologically impossible, as is a toxicologic effect caused by altered enzyme structures. However, nanoparticles (< 100 nm) can have toxicologic effects. For example, compared to titanium macroparticles, titanium nanoparticles induce higher cellular uptake efficiency and have toxic potential in periodontal ligament cells.[11] Acute colitis can also be exacerbated by oral administration of titanium dioxide nanoparticles. In relevant studies, increased titanium concentrations were also found in the blood of ulcerative colitis patients with active disease.[12] The toxicologic relevance of dental titanium implants has not yet been clinically proven.

IMMUNOLOGIC MECHANISMS

With metals, immunologic effects play a more important role than toxicologic effects. The term *sensitization* is generally equated with "allergy." However, a clear distinction must be made. Sensitization to a specific allergen means that the immune system is aware of the allergen and allergen-specific cells are present. A clinical reaction does not have to be present yet, but the risk for it exists because the patient has the immunologic prerequisite. One speaks of an "allergy" only when clinical symptoms occur as a result of exposure to the allergen. Strictly speaking, an allergy is nothing other than a mostly chronic inflammatory reaction.

Our immune system can be divided into the nonspecific innate immune system and the specific acquired immune system. Biologic reactions are induced by the release of different cytokines as inflammatory mediators. The nonspecific immune system is present from birth and is mediated by tissue macrophages (osteoclasts and connective tissue macrophages). It has no antigen specificity and no memory response. Anything recognized as foreign is eliminated by cells of the nonspecific immune system via phagocytosis and the release of cytokines. Tumor necrosis factor alpha (TNF-α) is the lead cytokine of nonspecific inflammation. Nonspecific foreign body reactions are thus reactions of the innate immune system.

The specific acquired immune system causes two forms of allergic reaction: the immunoglobulin E (IgE)–mediated type I immediate reaction and the cellular-mediated type IV delayed reaction. Antigen specificity and sensitization, as well as selective immune response, are the main features. The type I reaction is

FIG 9-5 › Allergic reaction to nickel. (Reprinted with permission from IMD Berlin.)

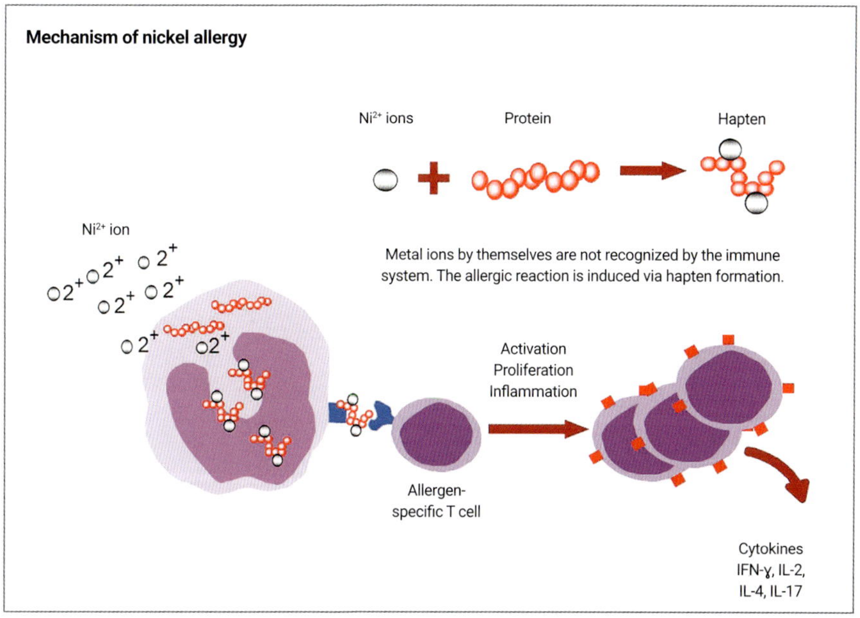

IgE antibody–mediated, with clinical manifestation occurring after seconds or minutes. The main mediator is histamine. Examples of type I allergic reactions include anaphylactic shock and allergic asthma. A prerequisite for triggering an IgE-mediated reaction is a complex structure and a certain size of allergen that can bind to an IgE antibody. Metal ions are too small to trigger a type I immune response. The most important immune reaction against metals is type IV delayed reaction. It is mediated by T lymphocytes and is therefore also called *cellular sensitization*. After initial contact with an allergen, allergen-specific T lymphocytes develop, which proliferate upon second contact and trigger appropriate immune responses by releasing interferon gamma (IFN-γ).

With metals, the type IV reaction is again based on the formation of hapten metal-protein complexes. The metal ion is too small to be recognized by the immune system, but it binds to endogenous proteins and changes their structure. The metal ion (hapten) thus becomes a true allergen only by binding to an endogenous protein. The modified proteins are recognized as foreign by the nonspecific immune cells and presented to the specific immune cells. If allergen-specific immune cells are present, a corresponding immune reaction is triggered[13] (Fig 9-5). A prerequisite for a type IV reaction is therefore the presence of allergen-specific immune cells and the presence of the metal in free ionic form. Otherwise, protein/hapten binding cannot take place.

In summary, metals can be present as either conglomerated particles or dissolved ions. Particles are regarded by the immune system as foreign bodies and are subject to phagocytosis by the nonspecific defense system. In ionic form, metals do not represent fully fledged antigens as they are not capable of triggering an immune response on their own.[14]

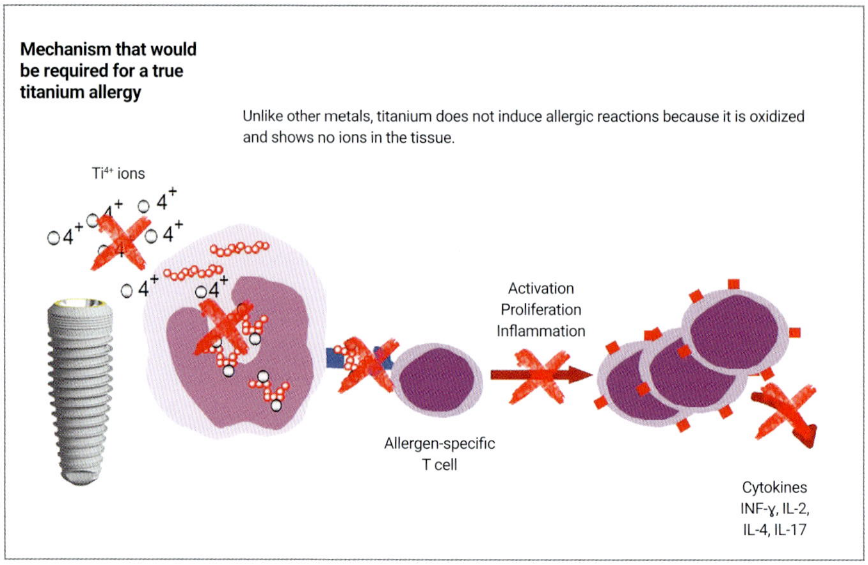

FIG 9-6 › Presentation of a titanium allergy is physiologically impossible. (Reprinted with permission from IMD Berlin.)

TITANIUM ALLERGY

In dentistry, when talking about problems related to titanium, reference is usually made to titanium allergy. The prevalence of titanium allergy has been estimated at 0.6%.[15] The term "titanium allergy" has also been used in the literature for all reactions in connection with titanium and is often misleading. As described in the previous section, sensitization and thus allergy to metals is based on the presence of free metal ions, which can form haptens. Titanium ions form titanium oxides immediately after their release due to their high oxygen affinity.[16] Unlike free ions, oxides cannot form protein bonds and are therefore not haptens and have no allergenic effect. Genuine allergies to titanium are therefore not physiologically presentable (Fig 9-6).

When allergies to titanium implants are described, they usually refer to sensitization to additives such as aluminum, vanadium, or chromium contained in titanium grade V alloys (used in endoprostheses and some dental implants). Impurities involving nickel due to the manufacturing process have been described even in pure grade IV titanium, which may well trigger sensitization.[17,18]

TITANIUM CORROSION

Animal studies have provided evidence that titanium dioxide particles are found in all peri-implant tissues following implant placement with titanium implants.[19]

FIG 9-7 › Titanium particles in the peri-implant tissue. (Courtesy of E. Jacobi-Gresser.)

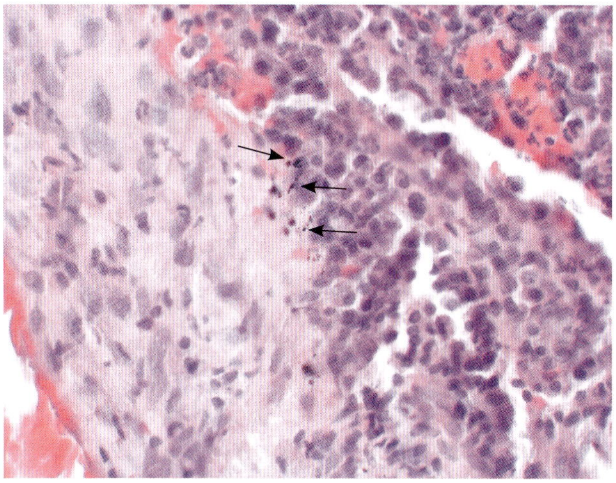

Mechanical friction during implant placement or micromovements during masticatory loading lead to particle abrasion in titanium implants.[20] With this micromovement, the thin oxide layers in the nanometer range are continuously abraded, with the debris infiltrating the surrounding tissue, as shown in Fig 9-7.

Particularly in a microbial environment, electrochemical mechanisms lead to chemical corrosion of titanium. In one study, titanium plates were placed in pure saline solution and stored at 37.6°C for 4 weeks. The solution was analyzed and no relevant titanium concentration was found. However, when bacterial lipopolysaccharides were added, the concentration increased significantly.[21] Thus, bacterial lipopolysaccharides have the potential to cause titanium implant corrosion.

Similarly, a combination of different metals used for the abutment and restoration seems to promote titanium corrosion via stress gradients. In an animal model, 24 titanium implants were randomly restored with precious metal alloy or titanium superstructures. It was shown that superstructures made of precious metal alloys led to titanium migration in the cervical direction after only 2 months and caused titanium corrosion.[22] Plaque samples taken from the periodontium around healthy implants and those with peri-implantitis showed that more plaque was consistently found around implants affected by peri-implantitis. Significantly more titanium was also found in this plaque. Thus, increased corrosion occurs in the presence of bacterial plaque and inflammation in an acidic environment.[23] Multiple other studies and reports have also shown the presence of titanium particles in the peri-implant tissues resulting from titanium corrosion (Figs 9-8 and 9-9).

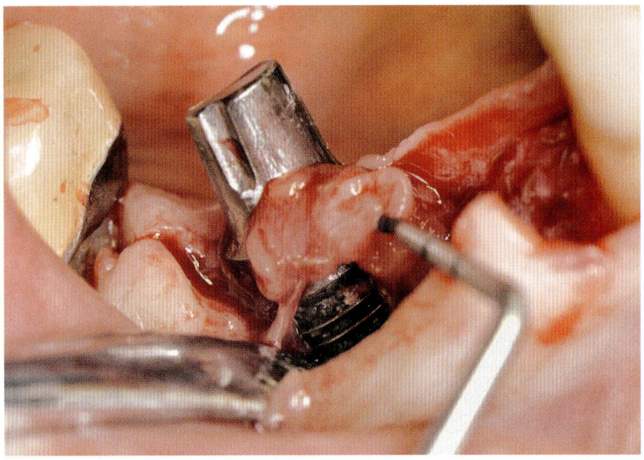

FIG 9-8 › Granulation tissue around a peri-implant defect. (Courtesy of E. Jacobi-Gresser.)

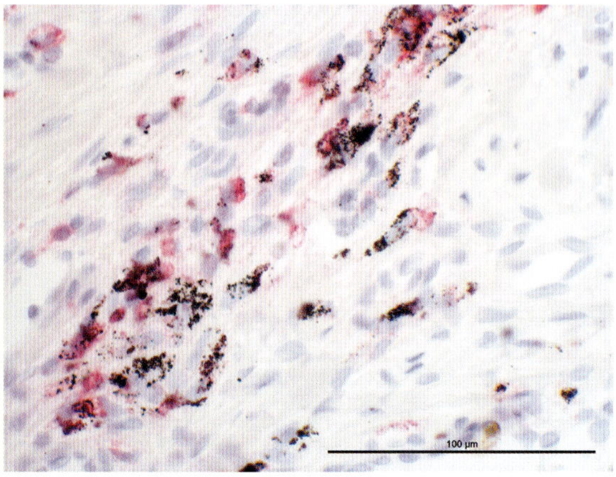

FIG 9-9 › Titanium particles in the tissue. (Courtesy of E. Jacobi-Gresser.)

TITANIUM INTOLERANCE

Titanium particles present in the peri-implant tissues are subject to the same immune reaction as all other foreign bodies—phagocytosis by macrophages as part of a nonspecific immune reaction and foreign body reaction. It has been demonstrated in animal experiments that titanium particles cleared in this way are found in the spleen after 16 weeks due to transport via macrophages.[24]

Depending on the phagocytized material, the activated macrophages secrete mainly the inflammatory cytokines TNF-α, interleukin 1 (IL-1), and IL-6 in varying amounts. The secretion rate is significantly higher with titanium dioxide particles than with zirconium dioxide particles, which could be an indication of good tissue tolerance of zirconium dioxide.[25] The released TNF-α leads to chemotaxis of more macrophages and thus to increased inflammation. It also activates osteoclasts via the RANK/RANKL mechanism, leading to bone resorption. IL-6 leads to activation and attraction of granulocytes and the release of metalloproteinases, including active matrix metalloproteinase 8 (aMMP-8), which promotes collagenolysis (Fig 9-10).

In principle, every titanium implantation is accompanied by these physiologic immune processes. However, there seems to be a certain subgroup of patients who react with an increased cytokine output and therefore tend to present an excessive inflammatory reaction.[26] When inflammatory reactions are described in connection with titanium, it is due to a foreign body reaction of the nonspecific immune system and not a sensitization or allergy. This excessive inflammatory reaction of the nonspecific immune system is referred to as *titanium intolerance*. Therefore, affected patients cannot be identified with an allergy test (eg, epicutaneous test, lymphocyte transformation test). However, a titanium whole blood

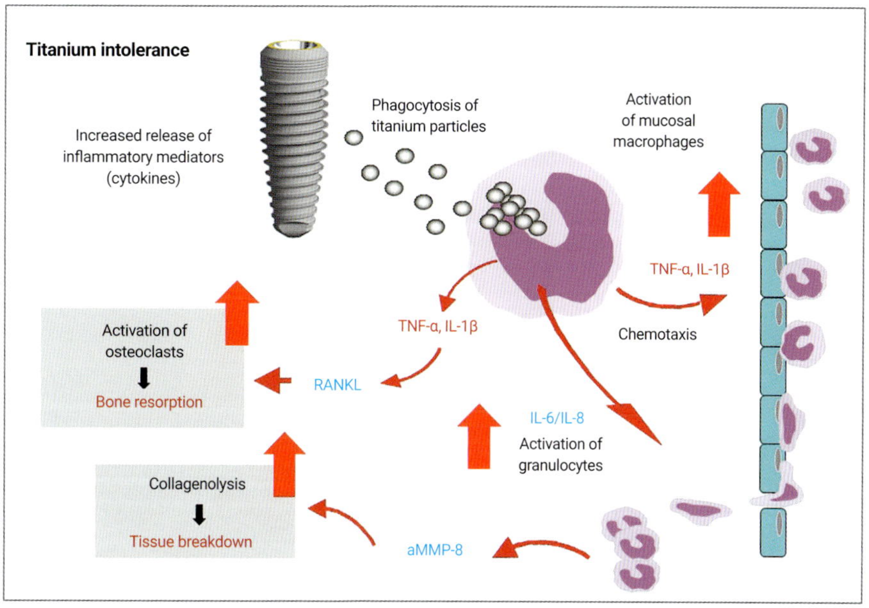

FIG 9-10 › Mechanism of titanium intolerance. (Reprinted with permission from IMD Berlin.)

stimulation test can be performed to detect an increased release of proinflammatory cytokines TNF-α and IL-1 on titanium particles.[26] Additional prospective studies on this topic are required.

Two studies[26,27] showed a significant association between titanium intolerance and implant loosening and peri-implantitis, though a third[28] did not. Therefore, it remains to be seen in future studies whether titanium intolerance can be considered an additional risk factor for peri-implantitis. Signs pointing in that direction should not be ignored.

Tissue Behavior

The favorable material properties of zirconia compared with titanium have a direct effect on the tissues it comes into contact with. Zirconia is considered more advantageous than titanium for peri-implant tissues for various reasons.

ZIRCONIA AS A BIOINERT MATERIAL

Dental implants are in direct contact with bone and soft tissue. Materials are considered biocompatible if they do not have any negative effects on the organism. Biocompatible materials can also be further classified as follows[29]:

- Biotolerant: The material can remain in the body for up to several years, although a minor, nontoxic tissue reaction may occur.
- Bioinert: There is no chemical and/or biologic interaction between the implant and the organism. (Although this can never be fully achieved, the lower the interaction is, the more suitable the material is.) No rejection reaction takes

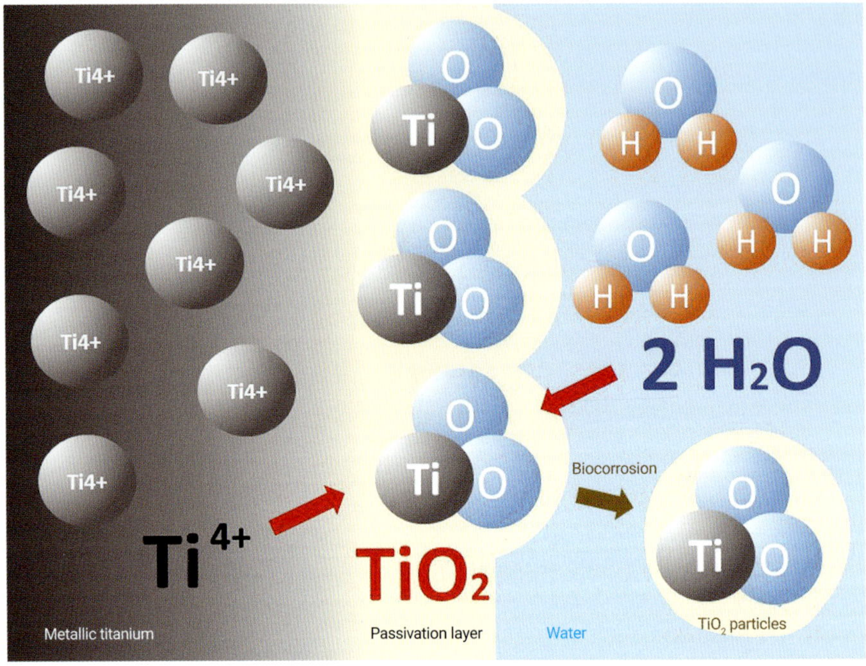

FIG 9-11 › Illustration of the passivation layer on titanium oxide.

place. Materials can be made bioinert by means of a surface coating (ie, a *passivation layer*).

- Bioactive: The organism reacts to the material. In arthroplasty, for example, some materials are referred to as "bioactive" because they promote a bone reaction to the material. Bioinert materials can be converted to bioactive materials with a coating. In such cases, the organism breaks down the bioactive layer and forms an intensive bond with the material.

Both titanium and zirconium are metals that react with oxygen to form metal oxides, which are ceramics. As a result of oxidation, the originally free, active electrons of the metal are firmly integrated into covalent, nonactive bonds. This chemical reaction is not reversible and makes ceramics only slightly reactive and gives them their bioinert properties. However, there is a significant difference between titanium dioxide and zirconium dioxide.

On titanium, only a very thin layer of titanium dioxide forms as a result of interaction with oxygen. This thin metal oxide layer coats the metal titanium (as seen in Fig 9-11) and gives it its bioinert properties. However, the metallic properties of a titanium implant, such as elasticity, are not affected by this thin passivation layer. Zirconia, on the other hand, is completely oxidized to zirconium dioxide, and the electrons are fully incorporated into a stable crystal lattice. Unlike in metals or metal alloys, electrons cannot escape from the material structure and cause undesirable interactions, such as corrosion. The high chemical inertness of zirconium dioxide is the reason for its high biologic compatibility.

The biocompatibility of zirconia implants can be summarized in terms of the response of lymphocytes, fibroblasts, chondrocytes, osteoblasts, and macrophages,[30] as discussed in detail in chapter 5 of this book. Against lymphocytes, zirconium dioxide shows a dose-dependent inhibitory effect, although at high concentrations the cytotoxic effect did not exceed 50% and was lower than that of titanium dioxide.[31] Against osteoblasts, zirconium dioxide shows no cytotoxicity, and the cells exhibit good adhesion and colonization.[32] As a bioinert material, zirconia exhibits lower inflammatory infiltrate within the peri-implant soft tissues and near-natural blood flow around the implants. Zirconia thus exhibits high chemical inertness and subsequent high biocompatibility with low reactivity with surrounding tissues.

PLAQUE/BACTERIAL ADHESION

Bacteria and plaque play an essential role in the development of inflammation around implants. Reduced bacterial adhesion to implants causes a lower risk of inflammation. Thus, titanium and zirconia disks with machined and microroughened surfaces were inoculated with a bacterial biofilm and incubated for 72 hours. Bacterial adhesion was subsequently investigated. Zirconia implant surfaces showed a statistically significant reduction in human plaque biofilm formation compared with titanium implant surfaces.[33]

In another study, plaque formation on titanium and zirconia specimens was investigated in vivo. Ten patients were fitted with a removable acrylic intraoral appliance, which was covered with titanium and zirconium dioxide platelets. After 24 hours, all platelets were examined via SEM. The zirconium dioxide platelets showed significantly less plaque accumulation than the titanium platelets.[34]

In terms of biofilm deposition, bioinert zirconia with its low reactivity may therefore have an advantage over titanium, which has only a thin bioinert layer.

BONE DEFECTS AND PERI-IMPLANTITIS

Peri-implantitis is playing an increasingly important role in implantology and is also being discussed in connection with ceramic implants. Ceramic implants are considered to have the advantage of exhibiting a lower tendency for peri-implantitis. A possible difference in the course of inflammation between zirconium dioxide and titanium could be due to the lower reactivity of the completely oxidized zirconium dioxide. Although hard scientific data is still lacking to support this theory, circumstantial evidence seems to confirm it. For example, significantly better blood flow has been found around zirconium dioxide material compared with titanium.[35] Also, significantly fewer inflammatory infiltrates were found in soft tissues around ceramics than in tissues around titanium.[36] Clinical observations also support a lower tendency for inflammation and healthier soft tissues around ceramic implants[37] (Fig 9-12).

FIG 9-12 › Soft tissue free of inflammation around a ceramic implant.

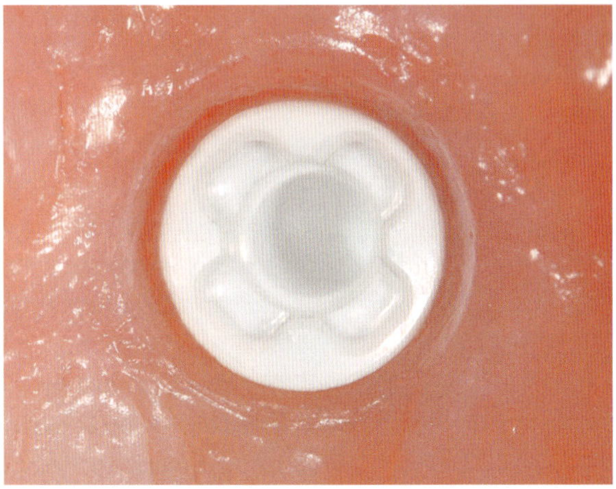

Peri-implant bone defects have been described with ceramic implants but at a significantly lower rate compared with titanium ones. To make a comparison with peri-implantitis in titanium implants, the causes of defect formation must be considered. Contrary to what happens with titanium implants, most of the factors causing defects around ceramic implants are iatrogenic. Therefore, they must be avoided.

Bone remodeling

Ceramic implants are mostly tissue-level implants and therefore have a machined, smooth neck area. If this neck area is countersunk subcrestally, bone remodeling occurs up to the beginning of the endosseous, microrough implant body, usually up to the first thread. This bone remodeling has already been described for titanium implants,[38] which exhibit the same behavior. However, bone remodeling occurs during only the first 3 months after implant placement, with bone levels remaining stable thereafter.[39] Ultimately, this bone remodeling is due to the biologic width.[40]

Cementitis

Restorations on ceramic implants are often cemented, especially on one-piece implant systems. However, if the implant shoulder is more than 1 to 1.5 mm subgingival, the cement cannot always be removed without leaving a residue that could lead to peri-implant defects.[41] Correct vertical positioning of the implant according to the implant system guidelines can prevent cementitis.

Oversized implant diameters

The known biologic principles of implantology should also be adhered to for ceramic implants. For example, at least 1 mm of residual bone is required around a ceramic implant to ensure long-term stability. Because thicker ceramic implants are often considered more stable, however, implants with a diameter of more

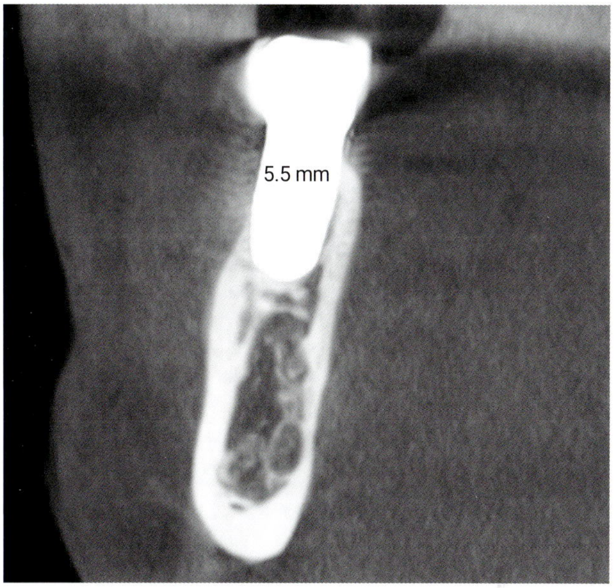

FIG 9-13 › Peri-implantitis caused by an oversized implant diameter.

than 5 mm are increasingly being used, especially for ceramic implants, even if the bone thickness is insufficient. This leads to buccal or palatal bone resorption and subsequent recession (Fig 9-13). To avoid this kind of complication, the ceramic implant diameter can be selected to match the appropriate diameter of a titanium implant if it were being used in the same clinical scenario.

Heat defects

The thermal conductivity of zirconia (2 W/mK) is significantly lower than that of titanium (22 W/mK). In addition, ceramic implants are usually not self-tapping, so a tap must be used. If a ceramic implant is inserted into the bone without a correct thread cut and with an insertion torque that is too high for the system being used, heat can be generated that is up to 18°C higher than the insertion temperature of titanium.[42] Due to the low thermal conductivity of ceramics, the heat is not dissipated and can lead to degeneration of the peri-implant bone. Crestal heat defects or a lack of osseointegration (aseptic loosening) are possible consequences. These complications can be avoided by using a thread cutter and performing careful implant placement that respects the insertion torque prescribed for the implant system.

Surface topography

The ideal surface roughness for a successful restoration is 1.0 to 2.0 µm.[43] A surface rougher than 2.0 nm or an additively coated surface may lead to peri-implant bone defects.[44,45] Heat or pressure defects and/or increased bacterial accumulation could be possible causes. The use of systems with modern and moderate surface treatment will not lead to these kinds of defects.

Conclusion

When the background and properties of zirconium dioxide materials are understood and the clinical guidelines are followed, modern ceramic dental implants show possible clinical advantages and are a reliable addition to the use of titanium implants.

References

1. van Brakel R, Noordmans HJ, Frenken J, de Roode R, de Wit GC, Cune MS. The effect of zirconia and titanium implant abutments on light reflection of the supporting soft tissues. Clin Oral Implants Res 2011;22:1172–1178.
2. Jung R, Sailer I, Hämmerle CH, Attin T, Schmidlin P. In vitro color changes of soft tissues caused by restorative materials. Int J Periodontics Restorative Dent 2007;27:251–257.
3. Gou M, Chen H, Fu M, Wang H. Fracture of zirconia abutments in implant treatments: A systematic review. Implant Dent 2019;28:378–387.
4. Almeida PJ, Silva CL, Alves JL, Silva FS, Martins RC, Sampaio Fernandes J. Comparative analysis of the wear of titanium/titanium and titanium/zirconia interfaces in implant/abutment assemblies after thermocycling and mechanical loading. Rev Portuguesa Estomatologia Med Dent Circugia Maxilofacial 2016;57:207–214.
5. Stimmelmayr M, Edelhoff D, Güth JF, Erdelt K, Happe A, Beuer F. Wear at the titanium-titanium and the titanium-zirconia implant-abutment interface. Dent Mater 2012;28:1215–1220.
6. Benic GI, Scherrer D, Sancho-Puchaes M, Thoma DS, Hämmerle CHF. Spectrophotometric and visual evaluation of peri-implant soft tissue color. Clin Oral Implants Res 2017;28:192–200.
7. Buser D, Martin W, Belser UC. Optimizing esthetics for implant restorations in the anterior maxilla: Anatomic and surgical considerations. Int J Oral Maxillofac Implants 2004;19:43–61.
8. Vindasiute E, Puisys A, Maslova N, Linkeviciene L, Peciuliene V, Linkevicius T. Clinical factors influencing removal of the cement excess in implant-supported restorations. Clin Implant Dent Relat Res 2015;17:771–778.
9. Gourlaounen C, Parisel O. Is an electronic shield at the molecular origin of lead poisoning? A computational modeling experiment. Angew Chem Int Ed Engl 2007;119:559–562.
10. Solar RJ, Pollack SR, Korostoff E. In vitro corrosion testing of titanium surgical implant alloys: An approach to understanding titanium release from implants. J Biomed Mater Res 1979;13:217–250.
11. He X, Hartlieb E, Rothmund L, et al. Intracellular uptake and toxicity of three different titanium particles. Dent Mater 2015;31:734–744.
12. Ruiz PA, Morón B, Becker HM, et al. Titanium dioxide nanoparticles exacerbate DSS-induced colitis: Role of the NLRP3 inflammasome. Gut 2017;66:1216–1224.
13. Saito M, Arakaki R, Yamada A, Tsunematsu T, Kudo Y. Molecular mechanisms of nickel allergy. Int J Mol Sci 2016;17:202.
14. Müller-Esterl W. Biochemie: Eine Einführung für Mediziner und Naturwissenschaftler. Spektrum Akademischer, 2004.
15. Sicilia A, Cuesta S, Coma G, et al. Titanium allergy in dental implant patients: A clinical study on 1500 consecutive patients. Clin Oral Implants Res 2008;19:823–835.
16. Liu X, Chu PK, Ding C. Surface modification of titanium, titanium alloys, and related materials for biomedical applications. Mater Sci Eng R Reports 2003;47(3-4):49–121.
17. Schuh A, Thomas P, Kachler W, et al. Allergic potential of titanium implants [in German]. Orthopade 2005;34:327–328,330–333.
18. Harloff T, Hönle W, Holzwarth U, Bader R, Thomas P, Schuh A. Titanium allergy or not? "Impurity" of titanium implant materials. Health 2010;2:306–310.
19. Guglielmotti MB, Olmedo DG, Cabrini RL. Research on implants and osseointegration. Periodontol 2000 2019;79:178–189.
20. Meyer U, Bühner M, Büchter A, Kruse-Lösler B, Stamm T, Wiesmann HP. Fast element mapping of titanium wear around implants of different surfaces. Clin Oral Implants Res 2006;17:206–211.
21. Yu F, Addison O, Baker SJ, Davenport AJ. Lipopolysaccharide inhibits or accelerates titanium biocorrosion depending on environmental acidity Int J Oral Sci 2015;7:179–186.
22. Foti B, Tavitian P, Tosello A, Bonfil JJ, Franquin JC. Polymetallism and osseointegration in oral implantology: Pilot study on primate. J Oral Rehabil 1999;26:495–502.
23. Safioti LM, Kotsakis GA, Pozhitkov AE, Chung WO, Daubert DM. Increased levels of dissolved titanium are associated with peri-implantitis—A cross-sectional study. J Periodontol 2017;88:436–442.

24. Unterer N. Verteilung von abriebpartikeln von titan und stahl in verschiedenen organen eine vergleichende in-vivo studie [thesis]. Ludwig Maximilian University of Munich, 2007.
25. Sterner T, Schütze N, Saxler G, Jakob F, Rader CP. Effects of clinically relevant alumina ceramic, zirconia ceramic and titanium particles of different sizes and concentrations on TNF-alpha release in a human macrophage cell line [in German]. Biomed Tech (Berl) 2004;49:340–344.
26. Jacobi-Gresser E, Huesker K, Schütt S. Genetic and immunological markers predict titanium implants failure: A retrospective study. Int J Oral Maxillofac Surg 2013;42:537–543.
27. Stolzer C, Müller M, Gosau M, et al. Do titanium dioxide particles stimulate macrophages to release proinflammatory cytokines and increase the risk for peri-implantitis? J Oral Maxillofac Surg 2023;81:308-317.
28. Sahrmann P, Tartsch J, Schmidlin PR. Comparison of clinical parameters of peri-implantitis and parameters related to tissue macrophage sensitization on TiO2. Clin Oral Investig 2024;28:499.
29. Schmalz G, Bindslev DA. Biocompatibility of Dental Materials. Springer, 2009.
30. Cerroni L. Ceramics for dentistry: Commercial devices and their clinical analysis. In: Palmero P, Cambier F, De Barra E (eds.) Advances in Ceramic Biomaterials: Materials, Devices and Challenges. Elsevier, 2017:181–248.
31. Bukat A, Fassina P, Greco F, Piantelli S, Piconi C, Zaghini N. GSP-made Ca-PSZ for biomedical applications. In: Hulbert JE, Hulbert SF, Society for Biomaterials (Minneapolis) (eds). Bioceramics. Vol 3: Proceedings of the 3rd International Symposium on Ceramics in Medicine, Terre Haute, Indiana, USA, November 1990. Rose-Hulman Institute of Technology, 1990:355–366.
32. Josset Y, Oum'Hamed Z, Zarrinpour A, Lorenzato M, Adnet JJ, Maquin D. In vitro reactions of human osteoblasts in culture with zirconia and alumina ceramics. J Biomed Mater Res 1999;47:481–493.
33. Roehling S, Astasov-Frauenhoffer M, Hauser-Gerspach I, et al. In vitro biofilm formation on titanium and zirconia implant surfaces. J Periodontol 2017;88:298–307.
34. Scarano A, Piattelli M, Caputi S, Favero GA, Piattelli A. Bacterial adhesion on commercially pure titanium and zirconium oxide disks: An in vivo human study. J Periodontol 2004;75:292–296.
35. Kajiwara N, Masaki C, Mukaibo T, Kondo Y, Nakamoto T, Hosokawa R. Soft tissue biological response to zirconia and metal implant abutments. Implant Dent 2015;24:37–41.
36. Degidi M, Artese L, Scarano A, Piattelli V, Gehrke P, Piatelli A. Inflammatory infiltrate, microvessel density, nitric oxide synthase expression, vascular endothelial growth factor expression, and proliferative activity in peri-implant soft tissues around titanium and zirconium oxide healing caps. J Periodontol 2006;77:73–80.
37. Chen A, Gahlert M, Özcan M, et al. Clinical approach of ceramic dental implants. European Society for Ceramic Implantology, 2022. https://esci-online.com/wp-content/uploads/2022/03/Result-ESCI-survey-ceramic-implants-final-web.pdf. Accessed 6 June 2024.
38. Buser D, Martin W, Belser U. Optimizing esthetics for implant restorations in the anterior maxilla: Anatomic and surgical considerations. Int J Oral Maxillofac Implants 2004;19:43–61.
39. Rohr N, Balmer M, Jung RE, et al. Influence of zirconia implant surface topography on first bone implant contact within a prospective cohort study. Clin Implant Dent Relat Res 2021;23:593–599.
40. Berglundh T, Lindhe J. Dimension of the periimplant mucosa. Biological width revisited. J Clin Periodontal 1996;23:971–973.
41. Ramer N, Wadhwani C, Kim A, Hershman D. Histologic findings within peri-implant soft tissue in failed implants secondary to excess cement. N Y State Dent J 2014;80:43–46.
42. Zipprich H, Weigl P, König E, Toderas A, Balaban Ü, Ratka C. Heat generation at the implant–bone interface by insertion of ceramic and titanium implants. J Clin Med 2019;8:1541.
43. Wennerberg A, Albrektsson T. Effects of titanium surface topography on bone integration: A systematic review. Clin Oral Implants Res 2009;20(suppl 4):172–184.
44. Kohal RJ, Patzelt SB, Butz F, Sahlin H. One-piece zirconia oral implants: One-year results from a prospective case series. 2. Three-unit fixed dental prosthesis (FDP) reconstruction. J Clin Periodontol 2013;40:553–562.
45. Schwarz F, John G, Hegewald A, Becker J. Non-surgical treatment of peri-implant mucositis and peri-implantitis at zirconia implants: A prospective case series. J Clin Periodontol 2015;42:783–788.

10

GUIDED SURGICAL TECHNIQUES

Andre Chen

Digital methods for planning implant placement and fabricating surgical guides have the potential to improve the accuracy and safety of implant procedures. Drilling protocols and surgical guides are tailored to individual patients based on their unique situations. This chapter describes the workflows and technologies used to plan implant surgeries and design various types of surgical guides.

Ceramic Implants and Digital Protocols

Ceramic-based implantology (Fig 10-1) has grown in the last few years with the introduction of new ceramic materials, stabilizing agents, sintering procedures, and fabrication processes such as injection molding and 3D printing.[1,2] Digital protocols and machinery in dentistry offer new possibilities for implant planning and clinical procedures,[3] allowing for more precise surgical planning and execution. CBCT, intraoral scanners (IOSs), and 3D printers and milling machines facilitate faster and more accurate procedures. Titanium implants, transitional anchorage devices, subperiosteal implants, and ceramic implants can all be used with these new technologies (Fig 10-2).

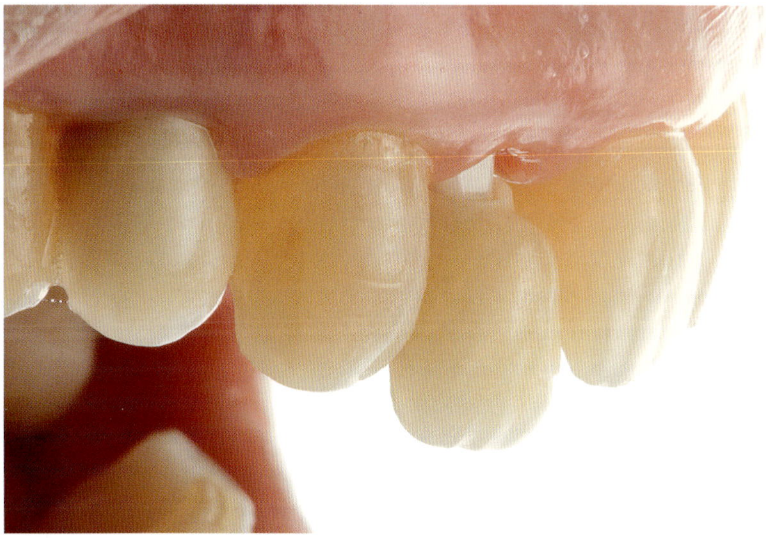

FIG 10-1 › An all-ceramic crown in a ceramic implant–supported restoration.

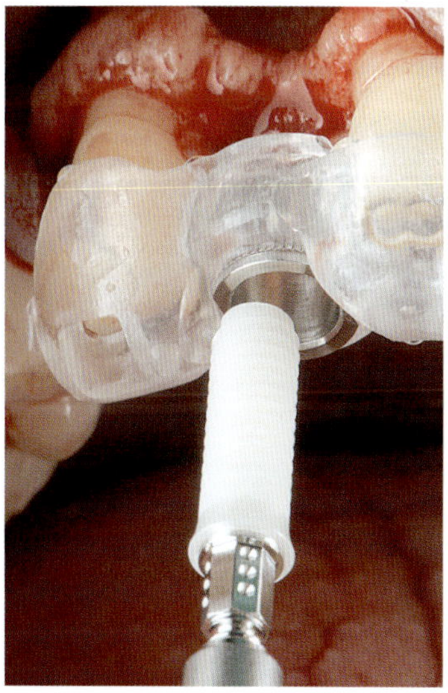

FIG 10-2 › Digital technology was used to create this surgical guide for a ceramic implant.

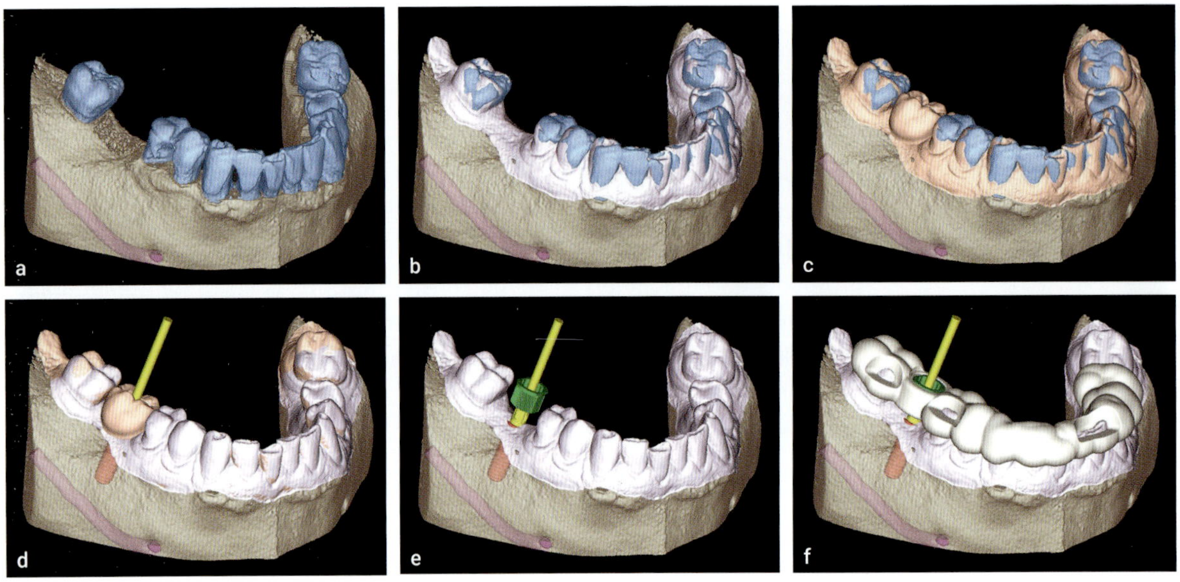

FIG 10-3 › Step-by-step surgical guide fabrication for ceramic implant placement. *(a)* Segmentation of the STL file. *(b)* Merging the STL file with data from the IOS *(pink)*. *(c)* Virtual diagnostic wax-up. *(d)* The planned implant position. *(e)* Designing the drill sleeve. *(f)* Assembled tooth-supported surgical guide.

Image and Data Acquisition for Implant Planning

Digital planning in dentistry entails collecting data and importing it into a computer to create a digital patient profile. Understanding how machines communicate—via STL, DCM, and DICOM files, etc—is essential. A digital workflow is followed to build a surgical guide from the gathered data (Fig 10-3). It all starts with importing DICOM files from the CBCT machine and STL files from the IOS into the implant planning software.

There are many digital implant planning software systems on the market, and mastering the specific workflows is critical for ensuring proper alignment of the IOS and CBCT data and avoiding inaccurate merging and poor superimpositions. Special care should be taken to acquire optimal CBCT image quality, which is dependent on a high-quality radiographic system/machinery, the skill of the operator, and the position of the patient. Always follow the guidelines recommended for the specific CBCT machine, and use cotton rolls to retract the patient's cheeks when taking the image, which will help to differentiate between soft and hard tissues. Next, bone availability is assessed, and ceramic implants are planned accordingly.

As with titanium implants, ceramic implants come with various microgeometries. The apicocoronal position of the implant in relation to the crestal bone can also vary, and it conditions the formation of the biologic width. It is important to know the type of ceramic implant and whether it should be placed subcrestally or supracrestally. With a supracrestal approach, the part of the implant with the rough surface, which usually corresponds with the implant body, is located inside the bone and the machined/polished collar is located at tissue level (Fig 10-4). With a subcrestal approach, the

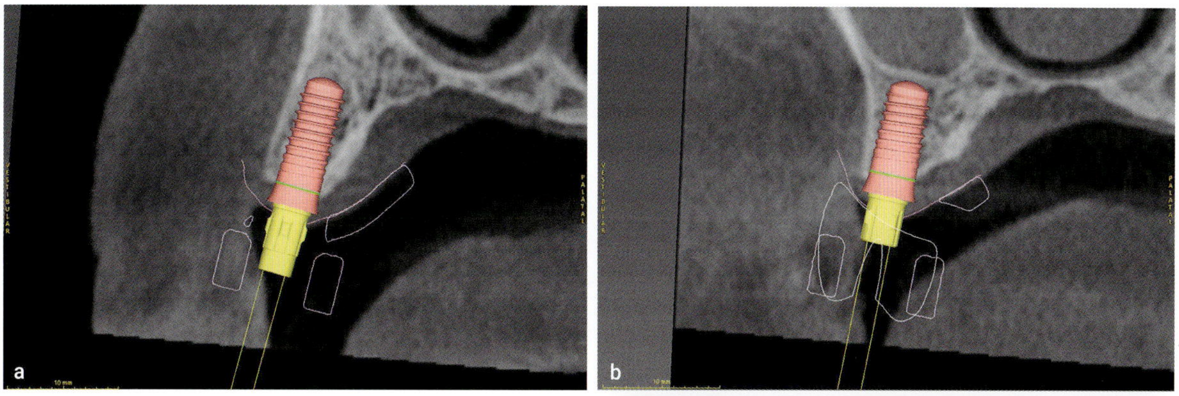

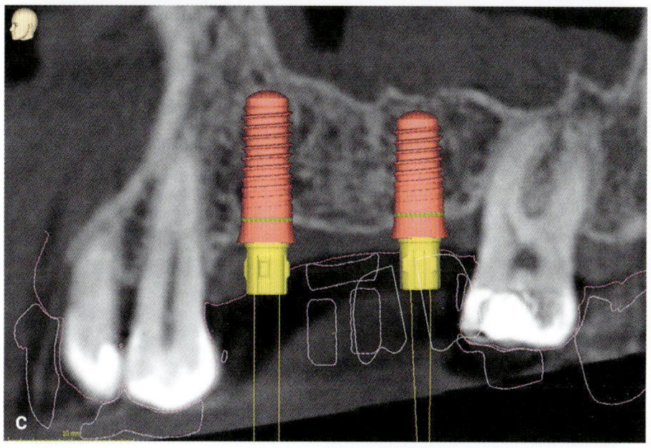

FIG 10-4 › Planning for supracrestal ceramic implants. Note the *green line* separating the rough surface from the smooth collar. *(a)* Planned implant in the position of the maxillary left first premolar. *(b)* Sagittal view of a ceramic implant in the position of the maxillary left first molar. *(c)* Lateral view of the planned implants.

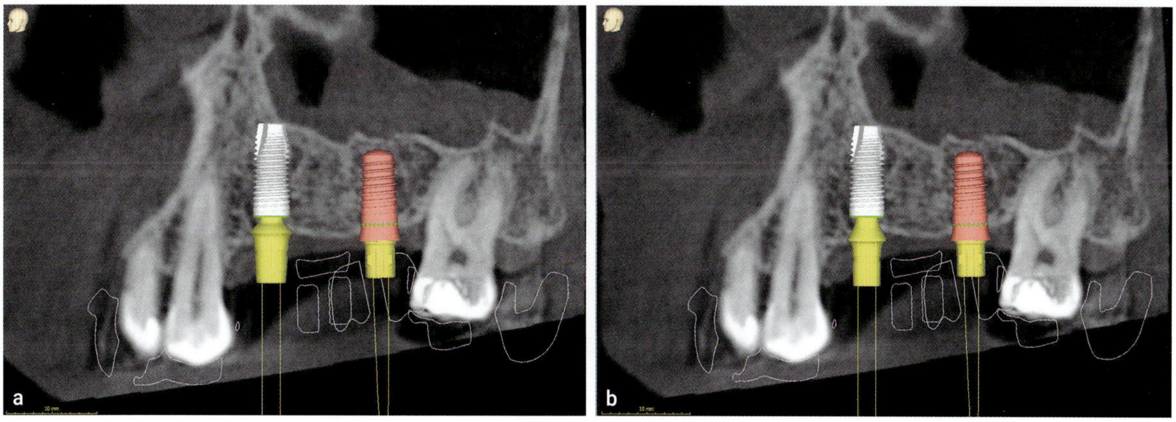

FIG 10-5 › Planning a subcrestal ceramic implant in the position of the maxillary left first premolar and a supracrestal implant in the position of the maxillary left first molar. The implant in the site of the first molar should be deep enough to allow for adequate prosthetic space and abutment insertion. Note that the *green line* of the subcrestal implant is at the top with no machined/polished 2-mm supracrestal part. *(a)* Inadequate height for the proper emergence profile of the provisional abutment, which may lead to peri-implant complications. *(b)* A higher abutment transgingival profile allows for the correct anatomical crown contour and respects the biologic width.

entire implant should be located within the bone, and care should be taken to insert the implant deep enough to allow for the correct crown emergence profile but not so deep as to create prosthetic difficulties with the intermediate abutments (Fig 10-5). Most implant software systems facilitate selection of the correct abutment and transfer of that information to the surgical guide.

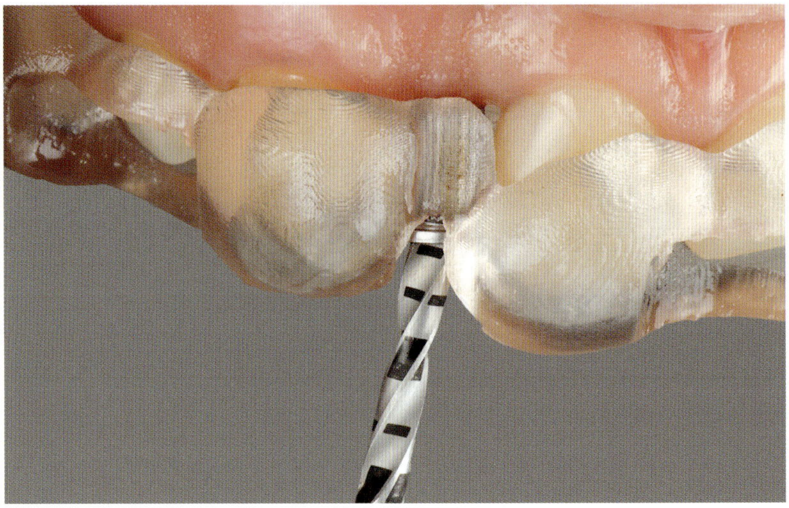

FIG 10-6 › Pilot drilling procedure with a 2-mm bur to mark and guide the correct osteotomy.

Surgical Guides

Transferring digitally planned ceramic implant positions to static surgical guides requires choosing the implant site preparation method. The most common methods are either a guided pilot osteotomy (ie, a *half-guided osteotomy*) or a fully guided osteotomy for implant placement.[4]

Pilot drilling is a technique used to pinpoint the correct 3D position of the implants to support the planned prosthesis and allows for guiding the first bur (2 mm) through a drill sleeve to outline the correct drill path (Fig 10-6). With most pilot drilling procedures, there is no restriction on the depth of the osteotomy. For some ceramic systems with implants longer than 14 to 16 mm, the bur will not be able to reach maximum depth if the clinician plans to submerge the implant 2 mm subcrestally, but pilot drilling can still be used as a tool for pinpointing the best implant position before finishing the implant site preparation via the traditional method. Fully guided implant protocols entail following a guided drilling sequence of burs before implant placement. The sequential drilling procedure is outlined by the planning software in PDF format and followed step by step by the clinician. Various drilling strategies call for different procedures for guide fabrication and assembly.

When performing static guided surgery with a fully digital workflow, be aware of the potential for lateral deviations in implant placement and discrepancies in implant depth between the digital plan and the actual procedure.[4] Deviations in implant angle are important, and erroneous implant depth can be especially

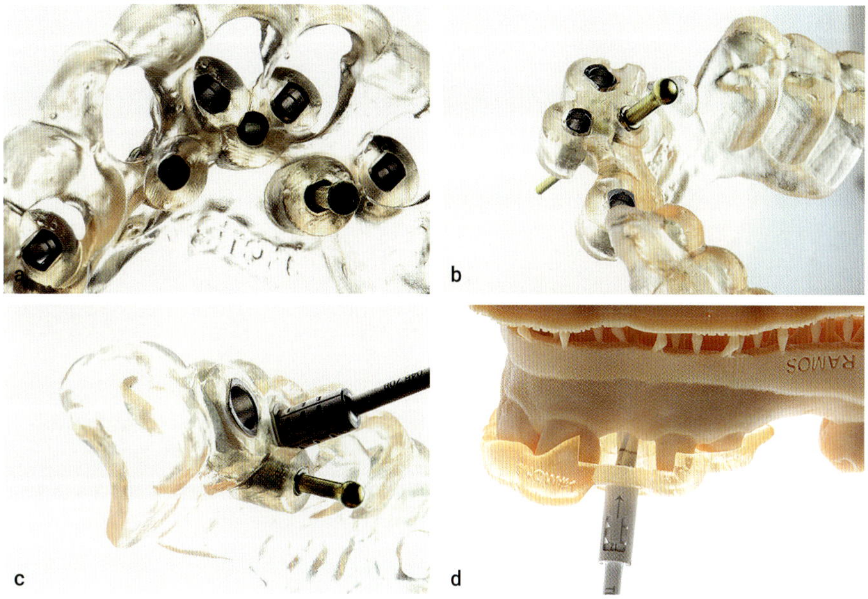

FIG 10-7 › Different types of surgical guides. *(a)* Tooth-supported surgical guide for pilot drilling. *(b)* Tooth and mucosa–supported pilot guide with palatal anchorage pins. *(c)* Surgical guide with a palatal fixation pin for a fully guided procedure. *(d)* Surgical guide with drill stops for a fully guided procedure.

problematic. An osteotomy of inadequate length can result in the implant not being fully apically seated, with its rough surface exposed to the oral environment. This affects implant survival and could cause peri-implant problems. Lateral deviations have a direct impact on the position of the prosthetic crown or partial denture. Avoiding lateral deviations depends on many factors, including achieving proper alignment of the intraoral scans and CBCT data during planning, good guide stability, and meticulous surgical execution.

Always perform a radiographic exam and assess the depth of the final implant position. If required, the implant position should be corrected. It is better to correct faulty implant positioning on the day of the surgery than to wait for short- or medium-term complications to occur in an osseointegrated implant.

TYPES OF SURGICAL GUIDES

When using a static surgical guide, whether for fully guided surgery or just as a pilot guide, clinicians can choose from several supporting structures for guide stability and retention: bone, mucosa, teeth, bone anchors/pins, or a combination (Fig 10-7). Tooth-supported guides are common and rank second best for accuracy of transferring the planned implant position.[4] When using tooth-supported guides, it is important to open windows to allow for visual confirmation of correct tooth seating (Fig 10-8).

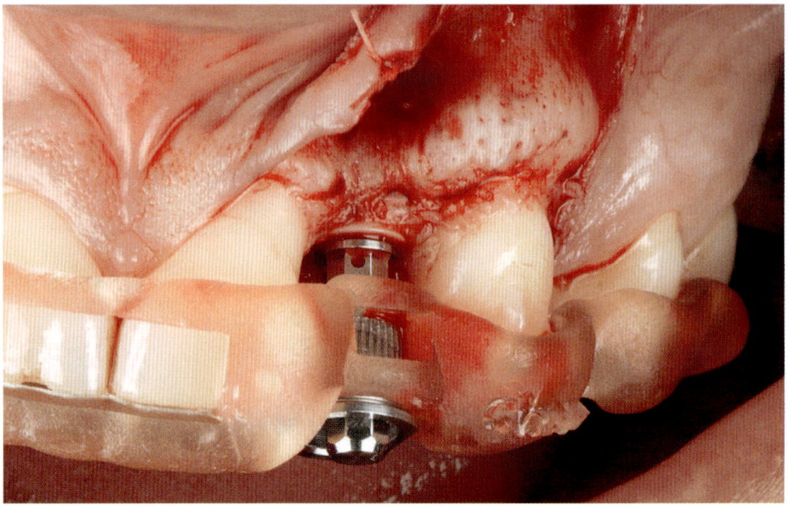

FIG 10-8 › Tooth-supported surgical guide for a two-piece implant in a fully guided procedure. This guide has windows for visualization and reduced bulkiness to facilitate adequate saline irrigation.

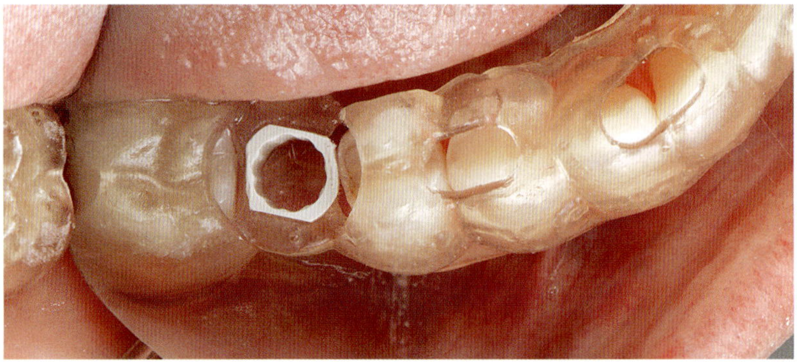

FIG 10-9 › Tooth-supported static surgical guide for a fully guided procedure in a case with limited interproximal space.

When used with fully guided surgical techniques, most implant systems require drill sleeves with a minimum diameter of 5 mm. Evaluate the interdental space during the presurgical appointment. If there is none, it's a good opportunity to see if interproximal guides can be designed for the adjacent teeth to optimize the contact points and at the same time provide space for the surgical guide and drill sleeve (Fig 10-9). This factor is one (of many) that can be responsible for guide misfit. If there is no space and interproximal enameloplasty is not an option, consider using only a pilot drill guide (since the drill sleeves are narrower), using a traditional approach without a surgical guide, or revising the treatment plan to include orthodontics to open a space.

Pin-supported guides with bone anchorage (Fig 10-10) are reported to result in the most accurate transfer of the planned implant position to the surgical site.[4] Although this type of guide was once used only for full-arch implant therapy, any

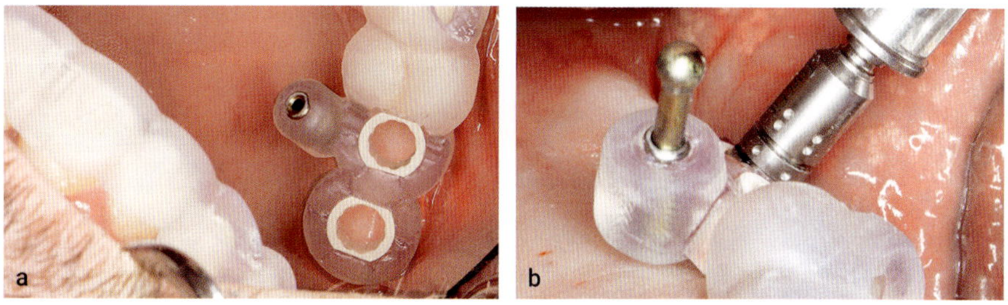

FIG 10-10 › *(a and b)* Fully digital workflow using a surgical guide with a palatal anchorage pin to avoid excessive buccal rotation.

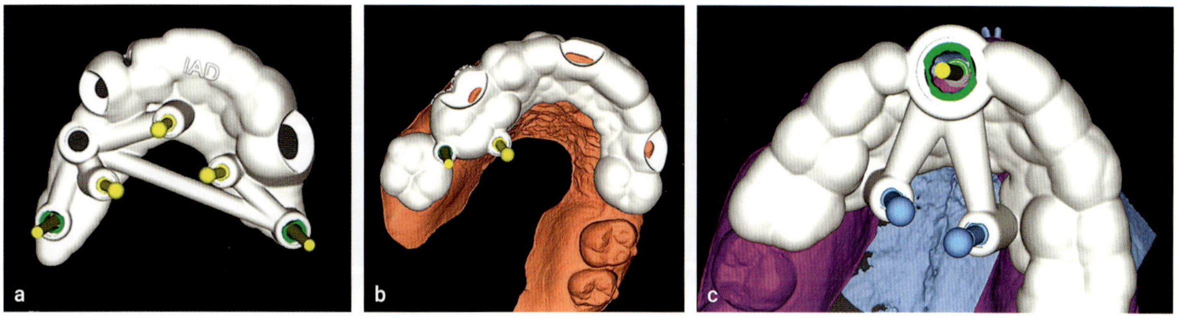

FIG 10-11 › Palatal bone anchorage pins used to support the surgical guide. *(a)* Tooth and mucosa–supported surgical guide for a partial-arch rehabilitation. *(b)* Tooth-supported pilot guide with a palatal anchorage pin. *(c)* Surgical guide with two bilateral anchorage pins for a fully guided procedure.

guide can have a bone-stabilized anchorage pin. Surgical guides for single-tooth restorations and partial dentures can also benefit from this increased stability. Place an anchorage pin if guide stability will be jeopardized. In maxillary arches, pins can be placed on the palatal side of the guide, on the buccal side adjacent to the surgical site, or in a mixed situation. Palatal pins (Fig 10-11) have several advantages. They do not take up buccal space, they can compensate for the buccal force of the surgical instruments as they travel through the guide, and they allow for buccal opening of the guide.

In the mandible, the interforaminal buccal bone is a stable and safe place to anchor a drill guide, but there are also other strategies for stabilization. Short stability "arms" that embrace adjacent teeth are common, especially as a substitute for anchorage pins on the lingual aspect of the mandibular central incisors (Fig 10-12). This is done when lingual concavities and the mental foramen do not allow for proper pin anchorage (Fig 10-13).

There are many bone anchorage pins with various diameters on the market, and almost all implant brands have their own pins that must be used when designing the drill guide. A good trick is to use the slimmest anchorage pin possible to avoid additional morbidity and difficulties when inserting it into cortical bone.

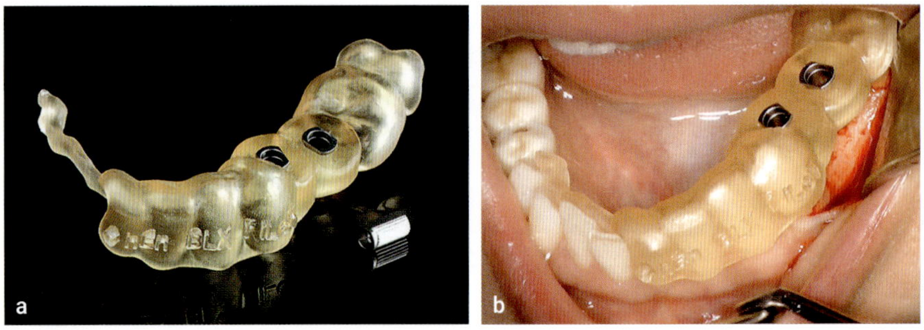

FIG 10-12 › Mandibular surgical guide for a pilot drilling protocol with a resistance arm on the lingual side to avoid lateral displacement. *(a)* Pilot drill guide before incorporation of the 2.2-mm-diameter sleeve. *(b)* Clinical overview of the guide fit.

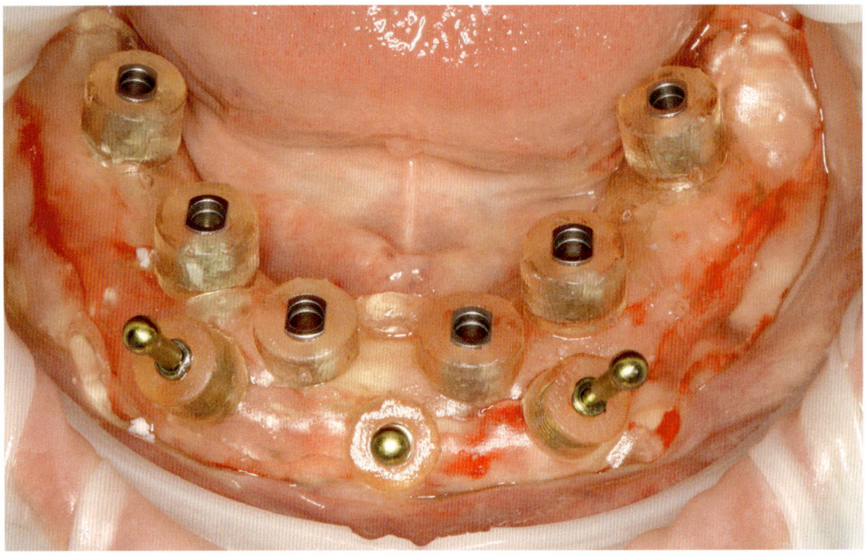

FIG 10-13 › Mandibular pin-supported guide for a pilot drilling protocol. Note the buccal position of the anchorage pins in the interforaminal region.

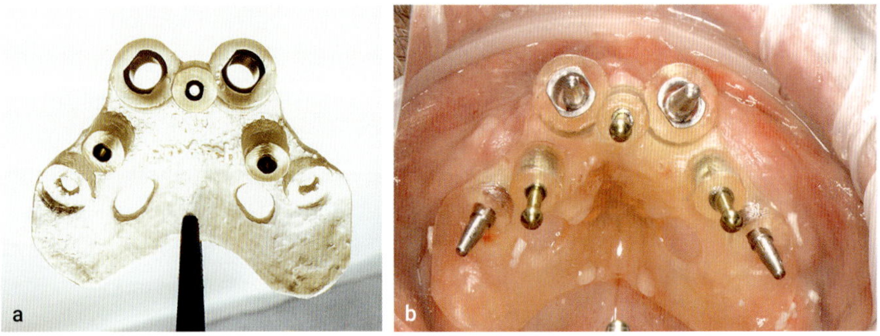

FIG 10-14 › *(a)* 3D-printed guide for a full-arch case. *(b)* Mucosa-supported surgical guide with three palatal anchorage pins for stabilization. The two anterior implants were placed via a fully guided procedure, and the posterior implants were placed with only a pilot guide.

Mucosa-supported surgical guides can be used, but the literature reports that they present some degree of misfit and are some of the most unstable guides. Thus, they are rarely used alone but rather together with anchorage pins for full-arch procedures (Fig 10-14) or for partial-arch restorations together with tooth support.[4,5]

Bone-supported guides are also rarely used for implant placement. They are predominately used for bone reduction with stackable guides and are reported

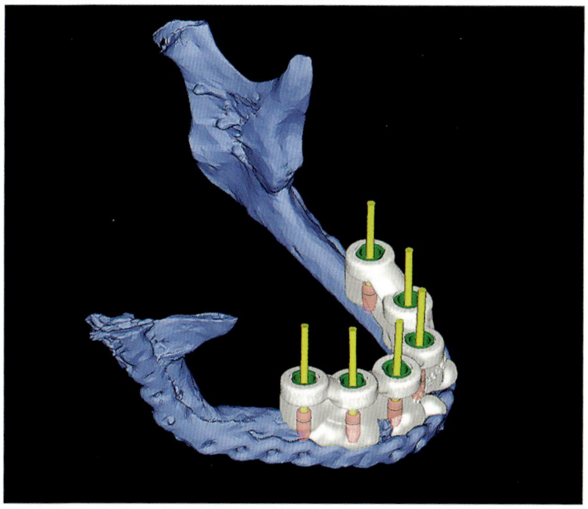

FIG 10-15 › Bone-supported surgical guide for implant placement in an oncologic patient.

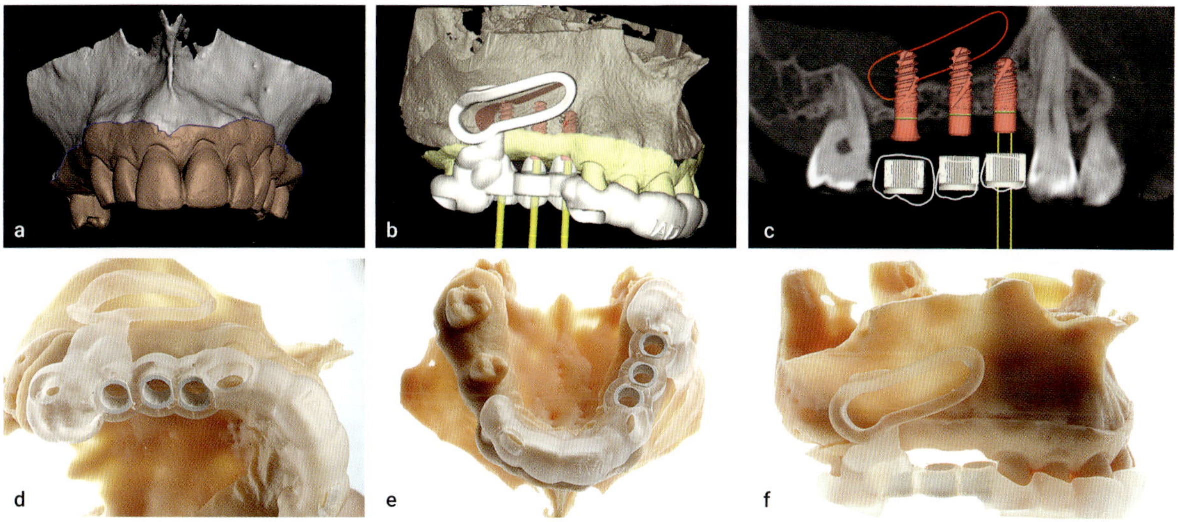

FIG 10-16 › Integrating DICOM files from the CBCT machine with the STL files from the IOS to create a guide with tooth- and bone-supported regions. *(a)* Merging the STL file with the DICOM file. *(b)* Development of the surgical guide for a lateral window sinus elevation procedure and simultaneous ceramic implant placement. *(c)* Radiologic overview. *(d to f)* 3D-printed model and surgical guide try-in for a fully guided surgical approach.

in the literature as one of the most unstable types of guides, resulting in great discrepancies in implant placement. They are often used in oncologic patients (Fig 10-15), in cases of tumor resection, and in case of other conditions that impair good mucosa- or tooth-seating ability.

When several surgical procedures are being performed simultaneously, a surgical guide with both tooth and bone support can be used. One example is for implant placement with simultaneous sinus elevation. These complex guided procedures require mastering the process of combining the DICOM files with the STL files and 3D printing (Fig 10-16).

The best treatment strategy is determined by the clinician, and the design of the surgical guide is adapted to individual requirements. The choice is almost always based upon professional decision making and clinical expertise.

Surgical Guide Fabrication

Traditional vacuum and thermoformable methods can be used to fabricate simple surgical guides. However, fast-paced technologic developments have led to workflows in which drill guides are designed virtually and fabricated with computer-aided technologies (Fig 10-17). Either subtractive technology (milling machinery) or additive technology (3D printing) can be used to fabricate surgical guides of acceptable quality (Fig 10-18), but additive technology offers better detail, passive seating, and the possibility for recreating angles that even a milled system with five axes cannot provide. There are numerous advantages to 3D printing. One of them is the fact that most implant planning software systems are calibrated with 3D printers, allowing for an interconnected workflow for producing high-quality guides.

FIG 10-17 › A 3D-printed surgical guide developed from an STL file.

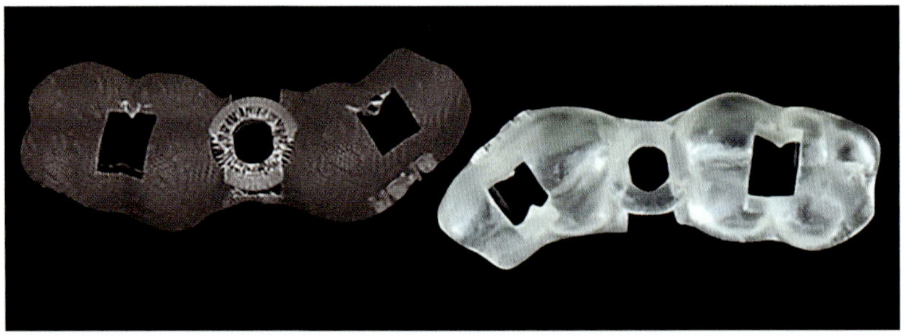

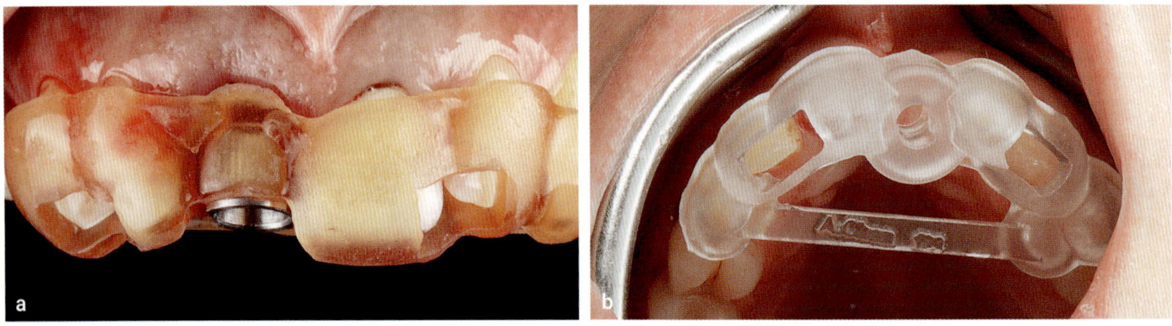

FIG 10-18 › *(a)* 3D-printed surgical guide. *(b)* CAD/CAM-milled surgical guide.

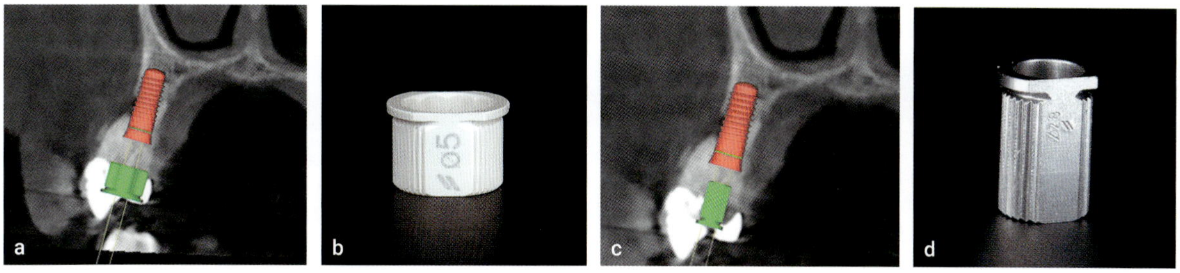

FIG 10-19 › *(a)* Planning for ceramic two-piece implant placement with a 5-mm drill sleeve for a fully guided workflow. *(b)* A 5-mm polyetheretherketone (PEEK) drill sleeve for a fully guided drilling protocol. *(c)* Planning for ceramic two-piece implant placement with a 2.2-mm drill sleeve for use with a pilot guide. *(d)* A 2.2-mm drill sleeve for use with a pilot guide.

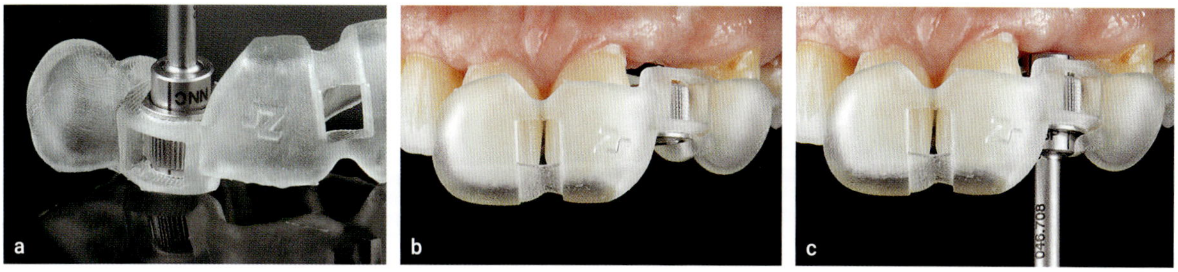

FIG 10-20 › *(a)* 3D-printed surgical guide with a 5-mm drill sleeve for a fully guided procedure. *(b)* Good seating of a surgical guide and drill sleeve for a two-piece ceramic implant in a fully guided procedure. *(c)* Implant mount try-in.

DRILL SLEEVES AND GUIDE ASSEMBLY

For most ceramic implant systems, there are two separate parts to the surgical guide: the guide itself and the drill sleeve. The guide is produced via additive or subtractive computer-aided manufacturing (CAM); the drill sleeve is prefabricated and provided by implant companies. The two parts must fit together perfectly to ensure a smooth and precise surgical procedure. Different sizes and shapes of drill sleeves are required for performing various drilling strategies (Fig 10-19). The choice of drill sleeve depends on which drill the clinician wants to stop at and if the procedure is fully guided.

When a drill sleeve is placed into a surgical guide, it is crucial that it has sufficient and secure retention to allow for free movement of the drill with the greatest possible operator control. The sleeve must be correctly calibrated to provide space for a passive fit with friction when inserted. To avoid misfits and the need for additional bur refinement of the sleeve hole (which could lead to imperfections and imprecision), always print calibration sleeve guides to calibrate the implant planning software with the 3D printer. The surgical guide and drill sleeve should work well together as one unit (Fig 10-20).

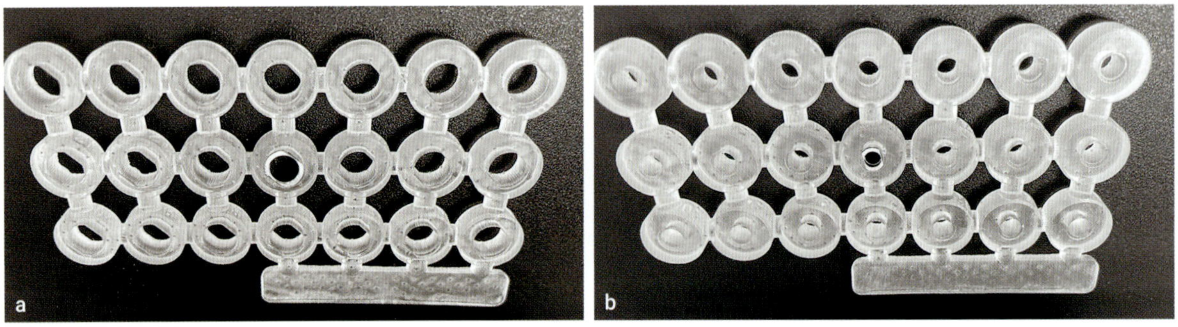

FIG 10-21 › Sleeve calibration template for ensuring 3D printer accuracy. *(a)* Calibration sleeves in sizes of 0.1-mm increments for the correct calibration of the 3D printer for fully guided procedures. *(b)* Calibration template for pilot guides.

FIG 10-22 › Sleeveless surgical guide for pilot drilling. *(a)* Implant position according to the prosthetic plan. *(b)* Extraction socket. *(c and d)* Pilot drilling protocol for immediate placement of a one-piece ceramic implant. *(e)* Final restoration with a veneered feldspathic ceramic crown.

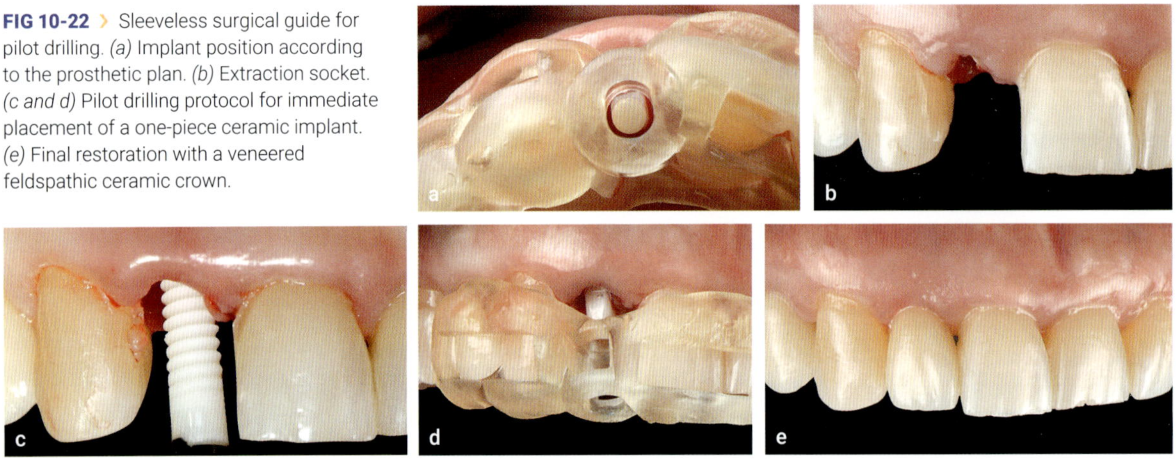

A calibration guide consists of a series of holes sized in increments of 0.1 mm (Fig 10-21). The clinician tests which hole offers sufficient retention for proper surgery. After choosing the correct size, the 3D printer parameters are set in the planning software and the guide is calibrated. It is important to calibrate all the sleeves—the 5-mm sleeves for a fully guided workflow and the 2.2- and 2.8-mm sleeves for pilot guide drilling, as well as the sleeves for the bone anchorage pins. There is no rule for how many times to print the calibration guides. In the author's opinion, it should be done regularly along with liquid changes in the 3D printer or when there are software or hardware changes.

Another option for pilot drilling is to go sleeveless (Fig 10-22), meaning that the bur passes directly through the 3D-printed hole. This provides some freedom but reduced accuracy and is sometimes done to facilitate visualization of the crestal bone.

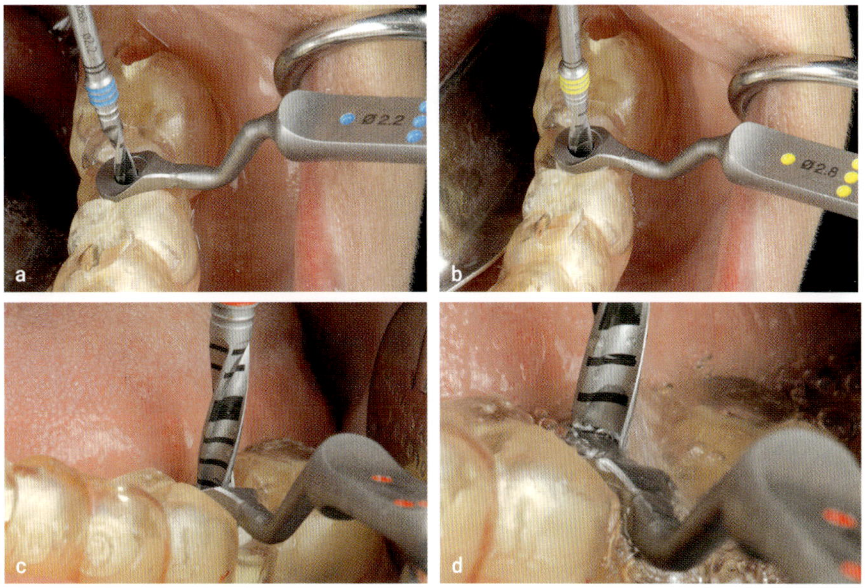

FIG 10-23 › Overview of fully guided implant bed preparation for a ceramic implant. Drills with smaller diameters are used first before sequentially enlarging the implant bed with wider burs: *(a)* pilot drill with a 2.2-mm bur; *(b)* 2.8-mm bur; *(c)* 3.5-mm bur; *(d)* 3.7-mm bur.

Digitally Planned Drilling Protocols for Ceramic Implants

Ceramic implant placement does not differ much from placing traditional root-form cylindrical implants. Ceramic implants differ mainly in biomaterial rather than macrogeometry. As with any titanium implant, ceramic implants are placed after performing a sequential drilling protocol (Fig 10-23). The last bur used always has a smaller diameter than the implant for the purpose of fostering primary stability. In self-tapping implant systems, the difference in diameter between the last drill and the implant is usually greater than the difference in cylindrical systems.

Guided osteotomy and implant placement protocols have had a very positive impact on the overall quality and accuracy of transferring planned implant positions to the surgical site (Fig 10-24). However, some anatomical limitations that are not visible during digital implant planning can have a direct impact on the clinical procedure. Mouth opening, muscle impairments, and malpositioned teeth are the most common factors that interfere with guided implant placement, drilling protocols, and instrument insertion. It is important to check the interocclusal space prior to implant placement, especially in the posterior mandible and maxilla. The length of the drills may compromise the execution of guided osteotomy preparation, sometimes making it impossible to perform guided surgery.

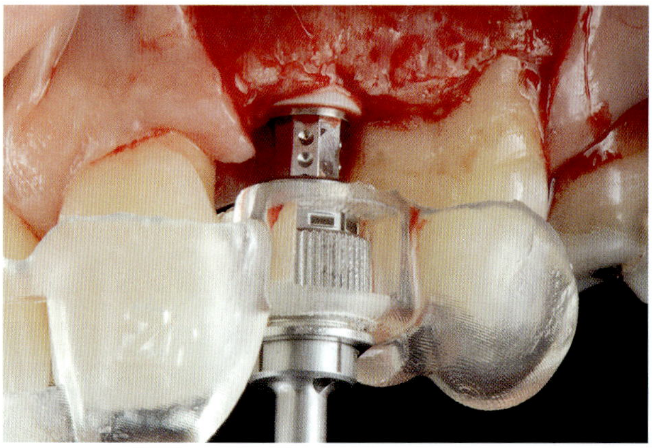

FIG 10-24 › Ceramic implant placement with a fully digital workflow. This workflow allows for more accurate implant placement than freehand procedures.

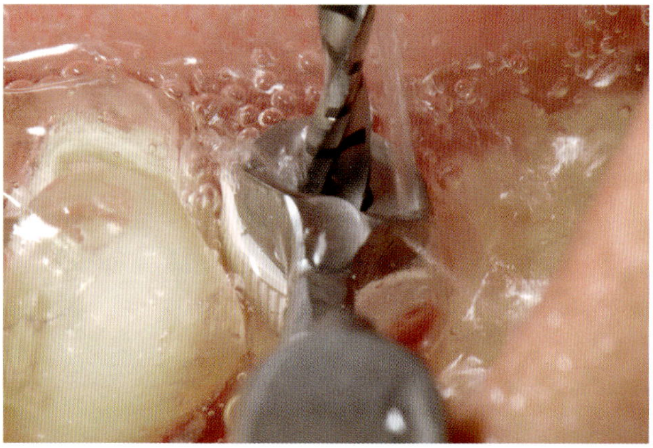

FIG 10-25 › Saline solution irrigation in a fully digital workflow.

When planning a posterior implant, always have a plan A, a plan B, and a plan C. Plan A should be fully guided surgery in cases that allow for the use of guided drilling and implant placement. Plan B is implemented when reduced interocclusal space is diagnosed preoperatively. In this case, plan to use a shorter drill and change to a guided pilot drill protocol to mark the best prosthetic site. After guided pilot drilling, implant site preparation is performed freehand without a guide. Plan C applies when guided drilling is impossible. In this scenario, a traditional procedure is performed without a surgical guide of any kind.

Ceramic implant placement carries irrigation and insertion torque concerns that differ from those associated with titanium implants. This is due to the low thermal conductivity of ceramic implants. Insertion torques should be kept from 25 to 30 Ncm, and good irrigation is required (Fig 10-25), especially if ceramic drills are used.

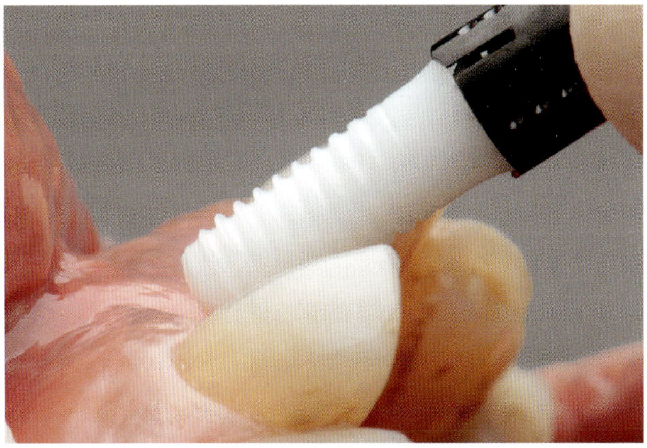

FIG 10-26 › One-piece ceramic implant placed in a healed ridge.

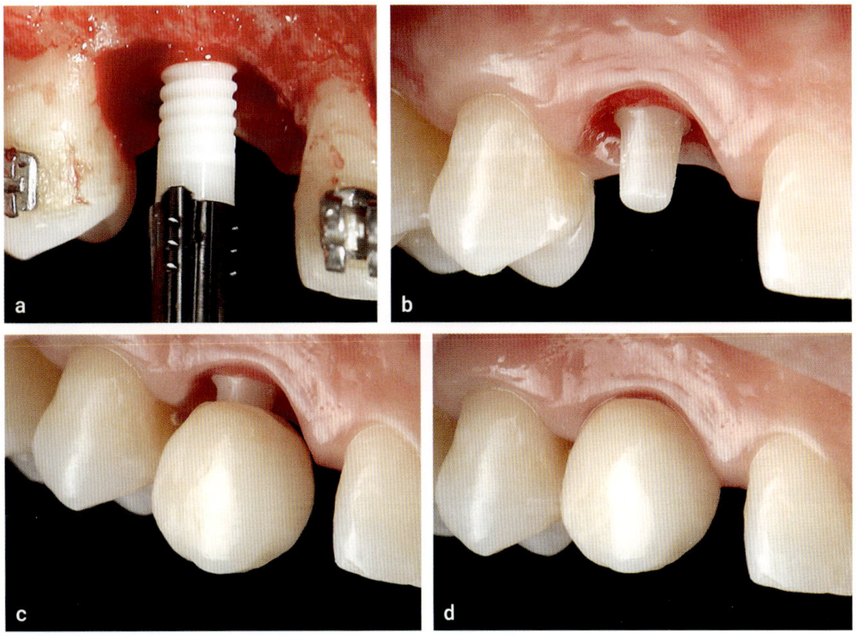

FIG 10-27 › One-piece implant placement according to a classic analog procedure. *(a)* Day of insertion. *(b)* Three-month follow-up. *(c and d)* Definitive prosthesis delivery.

ONE-PIECE CERAMIC IMPLANTS PLACED IN HEALED RIDGES

Ceramic implants placed in healed ridges (Fig 10-26) have proven biocompatibility and osseointegration patterns, as assessed via bone-to-implant contact (BIC).[6,7] One-piece implants are known to present clinical challenges because there is no option for correcting improper implant angulation or using prosthetic components for screw access channel correction. This makes achieving perfect prosthetic positioning of the implant even more difficult. When using an analog protocol without a surgical guide, adjacent teeth are crucial for guiding implant placement in a cemented situation (Fig 10-27).

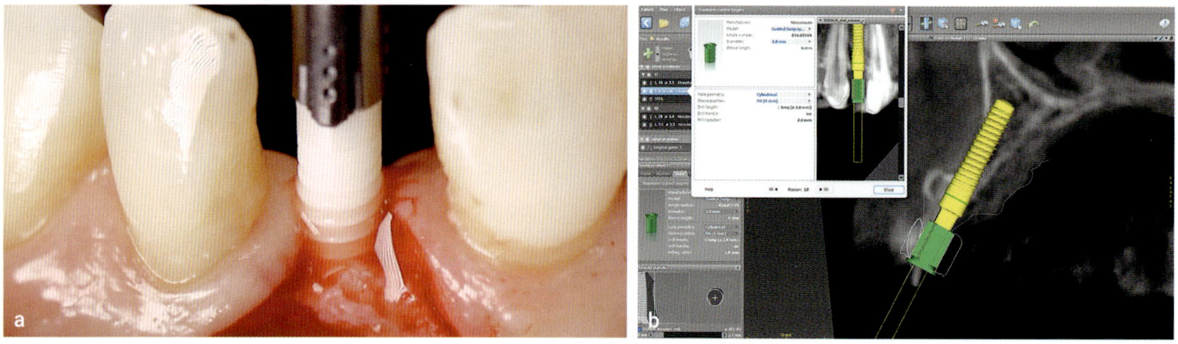

FIG 10-28 › *(a)* Placement of a one-piece ceramic implant. *(b)* Planning a supracrestal one-piece ceramic implant.

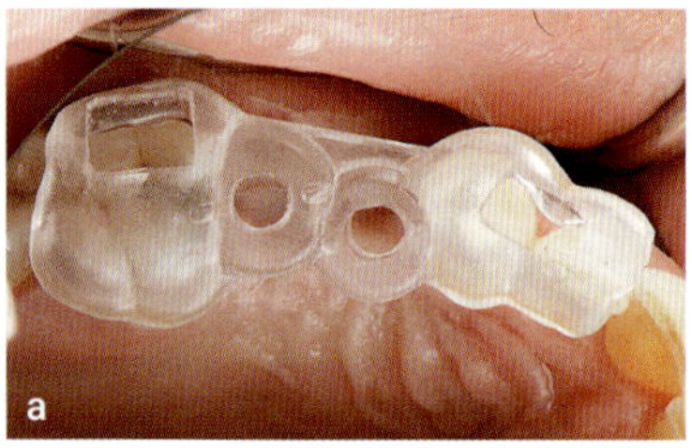

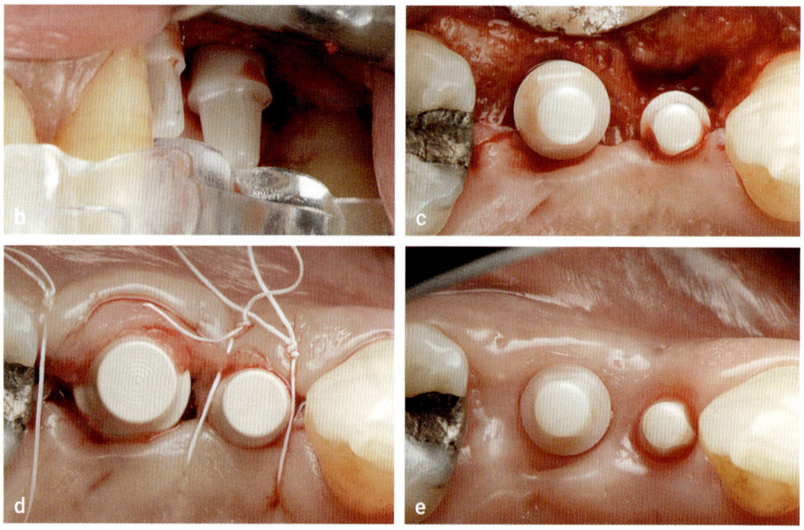

FIG 10-29 › Supracrestal placement of one-piece ceramic implants. *(a)* Pilot surgical guide. *(b)* Implants placed and positions evaluated. *(c)* Placement of ceramic one-piece implants—a 3.3-mm-diameter implant in the site of the maxillary right first premolar and a 4.1-mm-diameter implant in the site of the maxillary right second premolar. *(d)* Wound closure. *(e)* Healing at the 3-month follow-up.

As detailed in other chapters, there are several biomechanical and biologic advantages to one-piece implants. There is no two-piece metal interface and no microgap, meaning there is reduced bacterial contamination and no micromovement between the prosthodontic components. In one systematic review of 11 studies with follow-ups up to 7 years,[8] healed ridges with one-piece ceramic implants showed a mean bone loss of 0.98 mm, and this number was confirmed in 19 publications examined in a separate review.[9]

When placing one-piece ceramic implants, the use of a surgical guide is of extreme importance for achieving the best implant position possible. One-piece ceramic implants require correct buccolingual and apicocoronal positioning and enough room for supracrestal biologic width formation (Fig 10-28). One option is to use only a pilot guide to define the trajectory for the subsequent drills (Fig 10-29). Another option is to go fully guided and control the entire process from drilling to implant placement. With most one-piece ceramic systems, however,

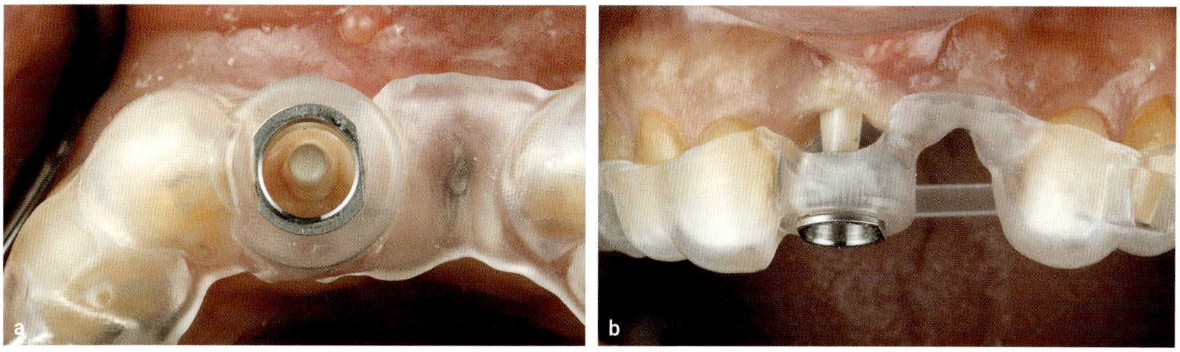

FIG 10-30 › One-piece ceramic implant placed with a fully guided workflow. *(a)* Occlusal view of the accurate placement of the ceramic implant. *(b)* Frontal view of the correct apicocoronal position.

implant depth is not controllable with implant mounts, so ensure that there is good visibility of the bone/soft tissue to identify where drilling should stop. Implant depth can be difficult to correct and sometimes depends on whether there is bone available apically to place the implant. If implants are placed deeper than planned, none of the provisional parts that were previously planned and fabricated can be used, so it is important to place implants correctly (Fig 10-30).

The literature reports that primary stability is one of the key factors for success of an implant-supported restoration. With the advancement of guided surgery, implant site preparation protocols have changed and created new challenges. On one hand, drill sleeves and handles increase stability. On the other hand, the clinician's ability to perceive bone quality is diminished. This may result in overpreparation of the implant site, which would not easily happen with a freehand approach. Overpreparation of the implant site jeopardizes provisionalization and the possibility of immediate loading. A lack of primary implant stability after removing the surgical guide can be difficult to solve.

When primary implant stability is lacking, an implant with a wider diameter can be placed to increase BIC and thus insertion torque and primary stability. Most titanium implant systems have a set of "one-connection-fits-all" prosthetic parts that make it possible to use the same connection with a larger implant at the same depth so that the planned screw-retained provisional restoration can still be used. Because the implant driver and drill sleeve are the same for all implant dimensions, it is a simple matter to switch the implant diameter. However, this is rarely the case with ceramic implant systems.

ONE-PIECE CERAMIC IMPLANTS PLACED IN FRESH EXTRACTION SOCKETS

The osseointegration and histologic parameters of ceramic implants placed immediately in fresh extraction sockets show a tendency toward at least equality with titanium implants in preclinical studies,[10] and they are prone to the same limitations and complications. The use of digital technology for ceramic or titanium implant placement is very important for ensuring proper engagement of the native bone and still being able to place the implant with the proper prosthetic position.

Placing immediate one-piece implants is difficult because most immediate implants in the esthetic area require a closed approach without raising a full-thickness mucoperiosteal flap. Placing an implant in a position that is too buccal makes the area prone to gingival recession, bone resorption, and prosthetic difficulties. An implant placed too far palatally will impair speech and cause discomfort. Again, there is no way to correct implant angulation with one-piece implants or adjust the depth with provisional abutments. Placing an immediate implant requires clinical expertise and thorough knowledge of the socket healing cascade and expected tissue volume changes. The implant should be placed palatally and apically to compensate for buccal and apical tissue loss but still be in the best prosthetic position. A pilot surgical guide or a fully guided protocol are both options for immediate implant placement. Guided surgery is very helpful for marking the correct implant position (Fig 10-31).

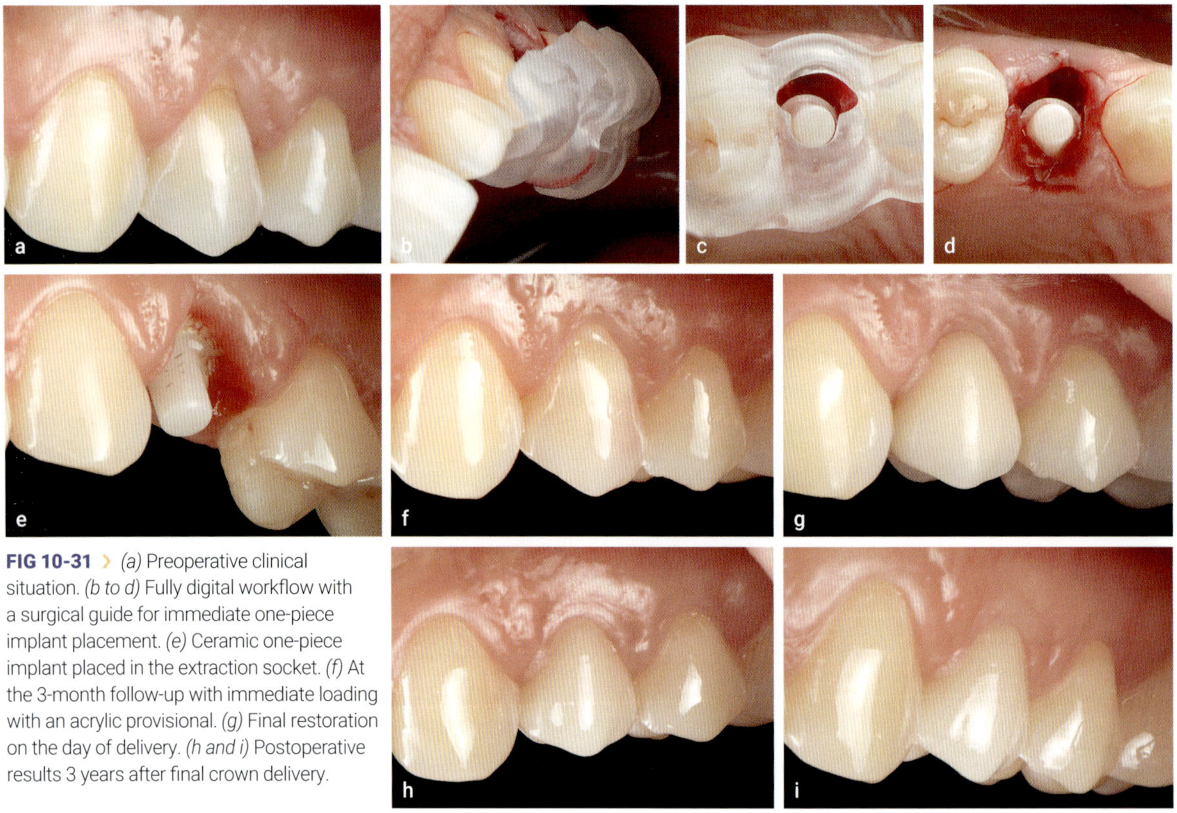

FIG 10-31 › *(a)* Preoperative clinical situation. *(b to d)* Fully digital workflow with a surgical guide for immediate one-piece implant placement. *(e)* Ceramic one-piece implant placed in the extraction socket. *(f)* At the 3-month follow-up with immediate loading with an acrylic provisional. *(g)* Final restoration on the day of delivery. *(h and i)* Postoperative results 3 years after final crown delivery.

To ensure clinical success with immediately placed ceramic implants, specific clinical steps must be performed, just like with titanium dental implants: atraumatic extraction that maintains the alveolar socket, buccal plate, and soft tissue with no open flap surgery[11]; correct apicocoronal and buccolingual 3D implant positioning; primary implant stability; adequate buccal gap management; and a proper emergence profile from day 1.[12]

Managing the buccal gap in cases involving ceramic implants is open to discussion because there is almost no data on biomaterial selection and outcomes when compared with titanium implants. Biomaterial grafting performed simultaneously with immediate implant placement has been used to treat the gap between the buccal bone and implant surface, reducing the risk of esthetic complications.[13] The decision on whether to fill this gap is based on alveolar extraction socket physiology. Some reports show good healing and BIC in type 1 sockets with no grafting,[14] but most publications (according to systematic reviews and consensus proceedings) show a reduction in the volume of bone and soft tissue that can result in esthetic compromise.[15,16] Placing inorganic hydroxyapatite in a socket gap is a predictable technique for titanium implants for single-root tooth replacement[17] and for the replacement of teeth with multiple roots in posterior areas.[18]

The final and crucial clinical step is placement of the provisional restoration. When using a one-piece ceramic implant, primary stability is almost always a requirement because there is no room for submerged healing. There is also no option to use healing abutments, so in most cases, a provisional crown is used to seal the socket and provide the best emergence profile possible (see Fig 10-31).

TWO-PIECE CERAMIC IMPLANTS PLACED IN HEALED RIDGES

The protocol for placing two-piece ceramic implants (Fig 10-32) resembles that for titanium implant placement, where everything is the same except the biomaterial composition of the implant. In a healed ridge, a fully guided protocol or a pilot guide can be used. For supracrestal implants, polyetheretherketone (PEEK) or ceramic healing abutments are used. Immediate provisionalization is also allowed if there are no occlusal contacts in centric or eccentric movements (Fig 10-33).

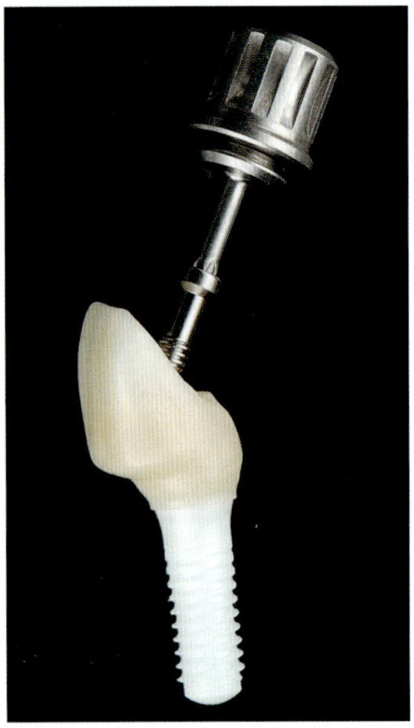

FIG 10-32 › A two-piece, screw-retained ceramic implant.

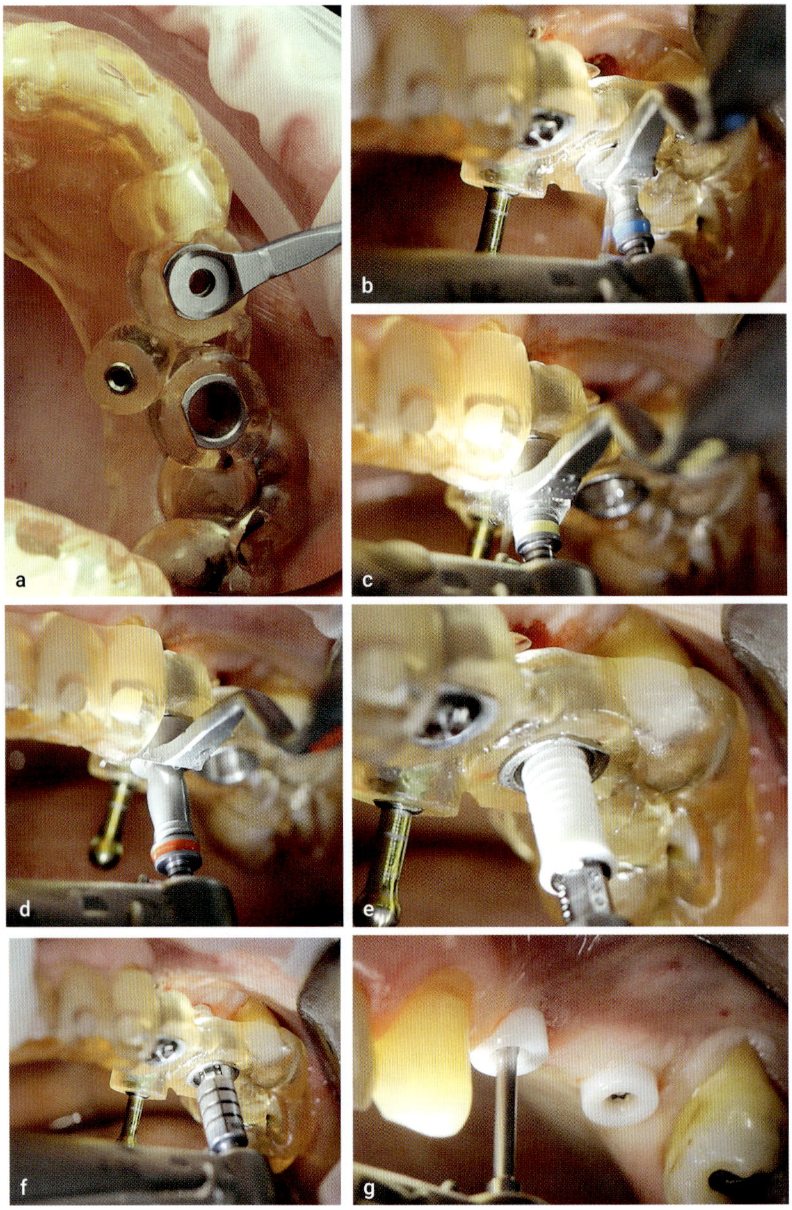

FIG 10-33 › Fully guided workflow using a surgical guide for a two-piece zirconia implant. *(a)* Tooth-supported surgical guide with a palatal anchorage pin. *(b to g)* Sequential drilling protocol and fully guided implant placement with transgingival healing and a two-piece ceramic healing abutment.

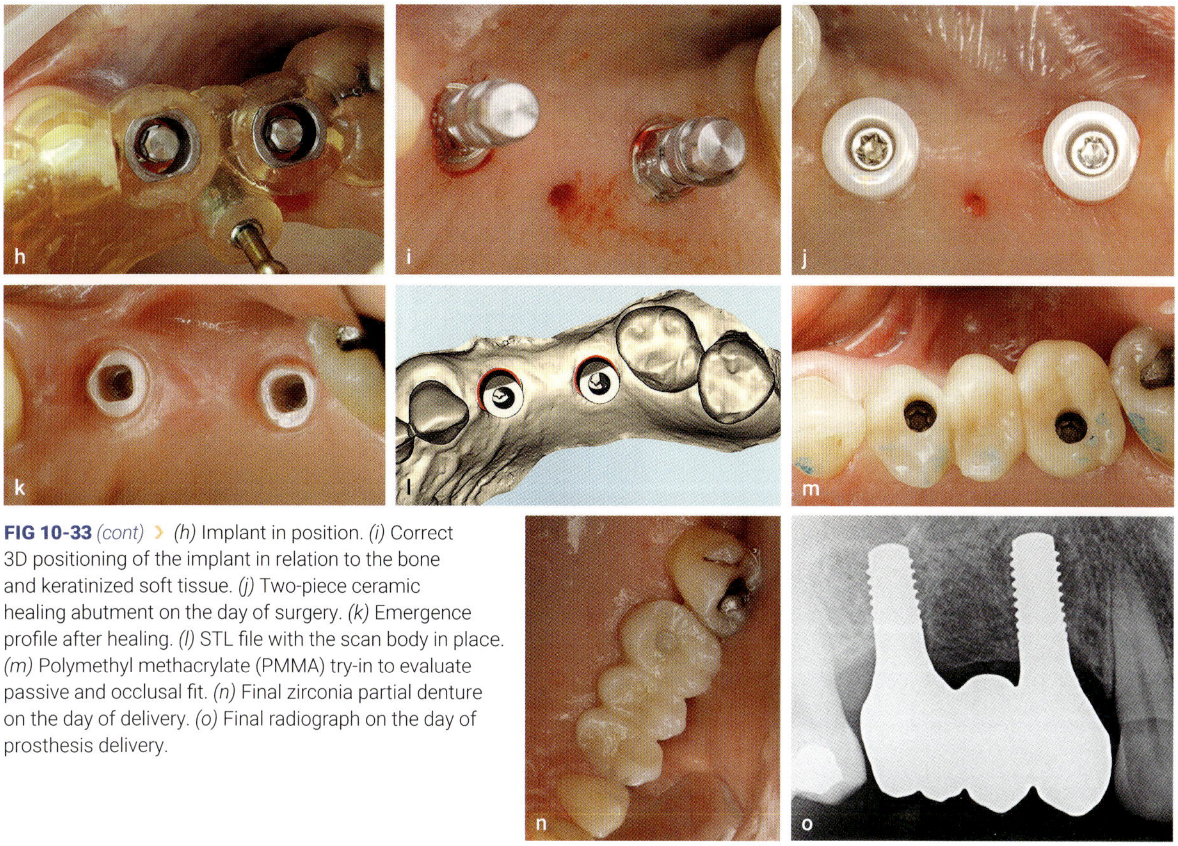

FIG 10-33 *(cont)* › *(h)* Implant in position. *(i)* Correct 3D positioning of the implant in relation to the bone and keratinized soft tissue. *(j)* Two-piece ceramic healing abutment on the day of surgery. *(k)* Emergence profile after healing. *(l)* STL file with the scan body in place. *(m)* Polymethyl methacrylate (PMMA) try-in to evaluate passive and occlusal fit. *(n)* Final zirconia partial denture on the day of delivery. *(o)* Final radiograph on the day of prosthesis delivery.

TWO-PIECE CERAMIC IMPLANTS PLACED IN FRESH EXTRACTION SOCKETS

Placing two-piece ceramic implants immediately in fresh extraction sockets follows much the same methodology as for one-piece ceramic implants. The main difference is that the clinician and lab technician have better control of the supracrestal area because a two-piece restoration allows for flexibility and freedom of choice rather than restricting users to a prefabricated abutment. The drilling technology and the surgical guide use are the same (Fig 10-34).

The possibility of using customized healing abutments to seal the socket of immediate sites optimizes the biologic response of the transmucosal area without compromising the stability of the implant during healing.[19] The prosthetic

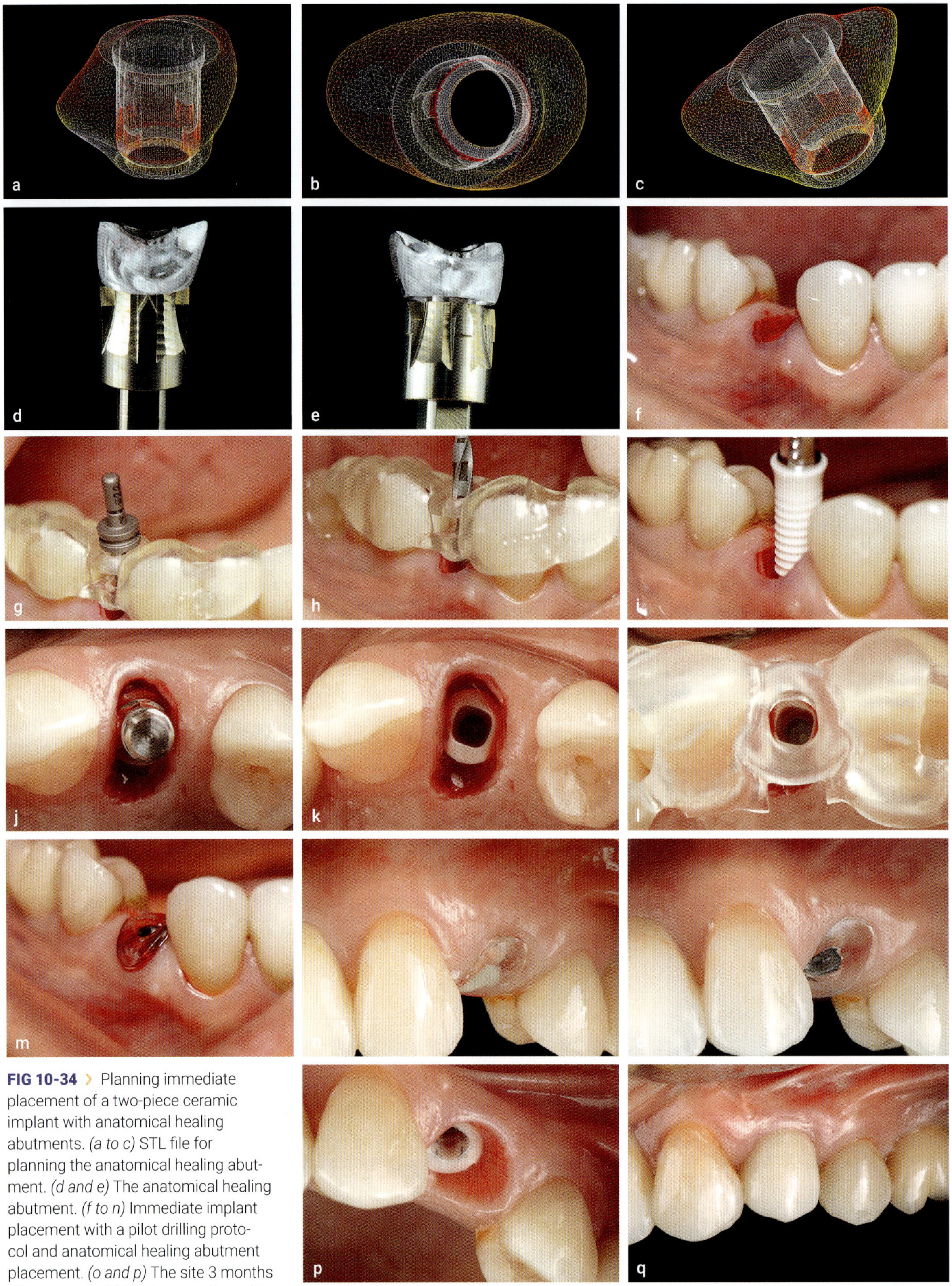

FIG 10-34 › Planning immediate placement of a two-piece ceramic implant with anatomical healing abutments. *(a to c)* STL file for planning the anatomical healing abutment. *(d and e)* The anatomical healing abutment. *(f to n)* Immediate implant placement with a pilot drilling protocol and anatomical healing abutment placement. *(o and p)* The site 3 months after surgery. *(q)* Final restoration with a monolithic all-ceramic crown.

flexibility of two-piece ceramic implants is one of the most important features that opens the future possibility of 3D-printed ceramic healing abutments in various colors according to the gingival phenotype and a vast array of technology that will eventually make treatment faster, more individualized, and biocompatible. This will also open the possibility of brands to have "twin" ceramic and titanium implant systems with the same drilling protocols, digital solutions, surgical kits, and mountings, enabling clinicians to choose the system that best suits the specific patient needs.

Conclusion

Implant dentistry is a prosthetically driven therapy that requires accurate spatial orientation to transfer planning from the implant software to the clinical arena. Guided implant surgery and ceramic implants have evolved over the years, and today the same digital tools used for titanium implants are used for their ceramic counterparts.

References

1. Holländer J, Lorenz J, Stübinger S, et al. Zirconia dental implants: Investigation of clinical parameters, patient satisfaction, and microbial contamination. Int J Oral Maxillofac Implants 2016;31:855–864.
2. Roehling S, Schlegel KA, Woelfler H, Gahlert M. Performance and outcome of zirconia dental implants in clinical studies: A meta-analysis. Clin Oral Implants Res 2018;29(suppl 1):135–153.
3. Joda T, Zarone F, Ferrari M. The complete digital workflow in fixed prosthodontics: A systematic review. BMC Oral Health 2017;17:124.
4. Tahmaseb A, Wu V, Wismeijer D, Coucke W, Evans C. The accuracy of static computer-aided implant surgery: A systematic review and meta-analysis. Clin Oral Implants Res 2018;29(suppl 1):416–435.
5. Ajami E, Bell S, Liddell RS, Davies JE. Early bone anchorage to micro- and nano-topographically complex implant surfaces in hyperglycemia. Acta Biomaterialia 2016;39:169–179.
6. Pieralli S, Kohal RJ, Jung RE, Vach K, Spies BC. Clinical outcomes of zirconia dental implants. J Dent Res 2017;96:38–46.
7. Roehling S, Schlegel KA, Woelfler H, Gahlert M. Zirconia compared to titanium dental implants in preclinical studies—A systematic review and meta-analysis. Clin Oral Implants Res 2019;30:365–395.
8. Haro Adánez M, Nishihara H, Att W. A systematic review and meta-analysis on the clinical outcome of zirconia implant-restoration complex. J Prosthodont Res 2018;62:397–406.
9. Borges H, Correia ARM, Castilho RM, de Oliveira Fernandes GV. Zirconia implants and marginal bone loss: A systematic review and meta-analysis of clinical studies. Int J Oral Maxillofac Implants 2020;35:707–720.
10. Calvo-Guirado JL, Aguilar-Salvatierra A, Gomez-Moreno G, Guardia J, Delgado-Ruiz RA, Mate-Sanchez de Val JE. Histological, radiological and histomorphometric evaluation of immediate vs. non-immediate loading of a zirconia implant with surface treatment in a dog model. Clin Oral Implants Res 2014;25:826–830.
11. Fickl S, Zuhr O, Wachtel H, Bolz W, Huerzeler M. Tissue alterations after tooth extraction with and without surgical trauma: A volumetric study in the beagle dog. J Clin Periodontol 2008;35:356–363.
12. Gallucci GO, Hamilton A, Zhou W, Buser D, Chen S. Implant placement and loading protocols in partially edentulous patients: A systematic review. Clin Oral Implants Res 2018;29(suppl 1):106–134.

13. Perez A, Caiazzo A, Valente NA, Toti P, Alfonsi F, Barone A. Standard vs customized healing abutments with simultaneous bone grafting for tissue changes around immediate implants. 1-year outcomes from a randomized clinical trial. Clin Implant Dent Relat Res 2020;22:42–53.
14. Tarnow DP, Chu SJ. Human histologic verification of osseointegration of an immediate implant placed into a fresh extraction socket with excessive gap distance without primary flap closure, graft, or membrane: A case report. Int J Periodontics Restorative Dent 2011;31:515–521.
15. Chen ST, Buser D. Esthetic outcomes following immediate and early implant placement in the anterior maxilla—A systematic review. Int J Oral Maxillofac Implants 2014;29(suppl):186–215.
16. Hämmerle CHF, Chen ST, Wilson TGJ. Consensus statements and recommended clinical procedures regarding the placement of implants in extraction sockets. Int J Oral Maxillofac Implants 2004;19(suppl):26–28.
17. Tarnow DP, Chu SJ, Salama MA, et al. Flapless postextraction socket implant placement in the esthetic zone: Part 1. The effect of bone grafting and/or provisional restoration on facial-palatal ridge dimensional change—A retrospective cohort study. Int J Periodontics Restorative Dent 2014;34:323–331.
18. Ragucci GM, Elnayef B, Criado-Cámara E, Del Amo FSL, Hernández-Alfaro F. Immediate implant placement in molar extraction sockets: A systematic review and meta-analysis. Int J Implant Dent 2020;6:40.
19. Finelle G, Sanz-Martín I, Knafo B, Figué M, Popelut A. Digitalized CAD/CAM protocol for the fabrication of customized sealing socket healing abutments in immediate implants in molar sites. Int J Comput Dent 2019;22:187–204.

11

CERAMIC RESTORATIVE MATERIALS FOR ZIRCONIA DENTAL IMPLANTS

Mutlu Özcan, Bruno Freitas Mello, André Luiz Berbel, Levy Rau, and Claudia Angela Maziero Volpato

The lifespan of zirconia implants is greatly influenced by the materials selected for restoring them. It's important to control excess cement in one-piece implants and to select an adequate connection type, screw geometry, and design and material for securing two-piece implants. Both types of implant are frequently restored with metal-free, single-unit ceramic materials, but when multiple units are present, fixed dental prostheses made of zirconia or metal frameworks veneered with feldspathic porcelain may be considered. This chapter provides an overview of the strategies for restoring zirconia implants and describes material selection and limitations for various clinical indications. Chapter 12 provides more details about zirconia frameworks.

Overview of Zirconia Implants

With the advancement of esthetic dentistry and the introduction of metal-free prostheses, zirconia-based ceramic implants have become a viable alternative to titanium implants.[1,2] Favorable results found with clinical and preclinical studies on zirconia implants are increasingly reported in the literature, reinforcing evidence of zirconia implant efficacy and clinical feasibility.[3–8] Yttria-stabilized tetragonal zirconia polycrystal (Y-TZP) has high flexural strength, excellent corrosion and wear resistance, a high elastic modulus, a color and radiopacity similar to that of teeth, low thermal conductivity, low affinity for bacterial plaque, high biocompatibility, and a degree of osseointegration comparable to that of titanium implants.[9–14] For the industrial production of ceramic implants, Y-TZP is treated with hot isostatic pressing (HIP) in an argon atmosphere to optimize its mechanical properties, increase its density, and reduce its porosity and material defects.[15,16]

Zirconia implants have esthetic advantages over titanium implants, especially when they are placed in anterior areas in patients with thin periodontal phenotypes. In these situations, titanium implants can often be seen through the peri-implant mucosa due to their grayish color, thus impairing the esthetic results.[17] In addition, studies have shown concerns regarding titanium particles and their implications in inflammatory reactions in peri-implant tissues[18,19] (see chapter 9).

Zirconia implants can be produced as one- or two-piece systems. One-piece systems do not require abutments, as the transmucosal part of the implant is integrated with the implant body. In two-piece systems, one part is inserted during surgery and the transmucosal part is joined to the implant in a second clinical procedure after osseointegration.[20,21]

ONE-PIECE ZIRCONIA IMPLANTS

One-piece implant systems consist of an endosseous part, a prefabricated abutment, and a transmucosal profile lying in between so that the provisional prosthesis can be immediately loaded. Recent studies show survival rates of 94.3% to 98.4% after 5 years of use.[7,8] One-piece implants allow clinicians to perform minimally invasive surgical procedures that preserve adjacent soft tissues by avoiding the creation of tissue flaps.[5,22] Because one-piece implants are visible after surgery, they are also exposed to the oral environment and masticatory forces during the healing process.[23,24] Due to the absence of an abutment fixation screw, there is no loosening of the components, and an esthetic result can be achieved immediately after surgery with the placement of a provisional crown as long as the implant has achieved primary stability.[11] As widely known and reported in the literature, primary stability of the implant is essential for successful immediate loading.[25]

An aspect of one-piece systems that must be considered is the possibility of excess cement remaining after fixation of the definitive prosthesis, which may result in a peri-implant inflammatory reaction.[26] This occurs mainly in anterior areas, where there is a tendency to place implants more apically to hide the margins of the prosthetic restoration. It is also important to highlight that the intraoral cementation protocol is a technique-sensitive process and that cemented prostheses make removal of the implant-supported prosthesis unfeasible.

The surgical positioning of one-piece implants is also critical. Clinicians must pay close attention when placing implants to ensure ideal prosthetic positioning. Correcting misalignment with an angulated abutment is not possible with one-piece systems. Any errors in surgical placement require adjustment via bur preparation.[27,28] Intraoral preparation with diamond burs with adequate cooling can be performed to define the location of the implant-supported restoration. However, wear on zirconia can result in tetragonal to monoclinic phase transformation as a consequence of grinding, resulting in microcracks and compromised mechanical properties.[27] Studies have reported a reduction in fracture strength in prepared zirconia implants of around 40%. However, according to the authors, the fracture resistance values found in prepared implants would still be able to withstand average occlusal forces.[28]

TWO-PIECE ZIRCONIA IMPLANTS

Two-piece implants are composed of an intraosseous implant and a custom abutment that is connected to the implant after osseointegration. The first commercial implant systems used abutments cemented to the implants.[29,30] Screw-retained prostheses were developed later. However, this type of system may be susceptible to fracture due to the presence of the metallic screw.[31] Studies show superior survival rates of two-piece implants with cemented implant-abutment connections compared with screw-retained one-piece systems.[32]

When compared with one-piece implants, two-piece implant systems offer individualized transmucosal designs, which certainly have a positive impact on soft tissue contour and implant stability. Despite being marketed with advanced asymmetric designs, one-piece implant systems have limitations and, in most cases, require intraoral preparation.[33]

Two-piece implants are generally used when the primary stability of the implant cannot be ensured during surgical placement and when more time is needed for osseointegration. They minimize the transmission of unwanted loads to bone and adjacent tissues during the healing phase,[34] and the risk of infection is also reduced because they are submerged in the soft tissue.[35] The literature reports a failure rate of 13.7% for two-piece zirconia implants.[36]

Prosthetic Restorations on Zirconia Dental Implants

The number of published studies focusing on the use of zirconia dental implants has increased by about 180% in the last 5 years.[37] These one- or two-piece implants have been largely restored with zirconia prostheses—either single crowns or fixed dental prostheses—which is in line with the concept of metal-free treatment.[3,38–41]

One study on one-piece zirconia implants restored with cemented zirconia single crowns or fixed dental prostheses reported a high survival rate and stable marginal bone and mucosal margin levels after 5 years in function. The authors concluded that these implants are safe and reliable in the medium term.[7] Similar studies report a median survival rate of 98% for zirconia prostheses cemented over zirconia implants after 5 years, with low marginal bone loss.[42] The most common biologic complication is failure to osseointegrate, with subsequent implant loss within the first 6 months.[6,7,43–46]

Monolithic zirconia prostheses and zirconia frameworks for bilayered prostheses can be obtained using CAD/CAM technology. Digital workflows using zirconia-based ceramics offer patients a metal-free treatment alternative with improved esthetics and good laboratory efficiency, considering cost and working time. However, due to the possibility of failures such as chipping of the veneering ceramic in bilayered prostheses, monolithic zirconia prostheses made from conventional or translucent zirconia blocks are increasingly being preferred.[47]

In 2015, Spies et al[48] evaluated the behavior of ceramic restorations on ceramic implants where zirconia single crowns and fixed dental prostheses with zirconia frameworks were veneered manually with a silicate ceramic. Although the authors did not observe framework fractures or decementation of the ceramic restorations, the number of complications such as chipping was very high, ranging between 42.8% and 62%. In 11 clinical situations, the authors had to replace the single crowns due to severe chipping. According to the authors, this represents a major problem from an economic point of view and may mean that this type of ceramic prosthesis on implants is unfeasible.[48] Similar chipping rates of 24.5% have been reported for implant-supported zirconia-based single crowns after 2 years, especially when located in posterior areas.[49]

It is also important to note that thick layers of veneering ceramic on zirconia frameworks are highly susceptible to generating high tensile subsurface residual stresses, which can result in cracks.[50] Due to the risk of failure, zirconia-based bilayered restorations on implants are technically material-sensitive pieces that require very thorough work from the professionals involved.[51] In these cases, it is important to employ anatomical frameworks rather than frameworks with uniform layer thickness, along with improved layering techniques and slower cooling procedures after the sintering process.[52,53]

Monolithic restorations, which do not present with an interface between materials and are made of a single material, are an alternative. The main advantage of monolithic crowns is the possibility of obtaining them by milling high-quality prefabricated blocks. Such blocks are currently available with gradient colors and/or translucency to mimic the characteristics of natural teeth, which considerably reduces the need for laboratory techniques for corrective staining. Although cement-retained zirconia crowns are currently the most commonly used CAD/CAM monolithic restorations used with zirconia implants,[54–57] other monolithic solutions have been described in the literature, including crowns made of CAD/CAM feldspathic ceramics and lithium disilicate, and even more elastic materials, such as polymers or polymer-infiltrated ceramics.[58–63]

Monolithic single crowns made of milled lithium disilicate for restoring zirconia implants have demonstrated promising survival rates after 3 years of observation. No restorations failed during the observation period, resulting in 100% survival. Chipping and fracture were also not observed, confirming the positive results.[51] Other studies reported that one-piece zirconia implants restored with lithium disilicate crowns showed promising clinical results in the short and medium term,[7,8] with rates of survival of up to 100% after 5 years.[64] In the study by Steyer et al,[65] zirconia implants were restored with provisional CAD/CAM crowns made of monolithic lithium disilicate shortly after implantation. The crowns were cemented onto the prepared implant abutment with the aid of an adhesive resin cement. They were adjusted so that no centric or eccentric occlusal contact was present to avoid functional loading, as well as to ensure a stress-free healing period. However, the implants were still exposed to indirect forces from mastication and tongue movements. After 4 months, these crowns were ground and served as abutments for the final CAD/CAM lithium disilicate restorations, which were also adhesively cemented to the prepared lithium disilicate framework.[65] According to the authors, the use of immediate provisional restorations facilitates formation of a favorable emergence profile for the final restoration and reduces the risk of peri-implant disease that is associated with the presence of excess cement.

Another strategy to minimize excess cement in one-piece implants is to cement a mesostructure on the implant abutment, which allows for the removal of excess cement under visual control.[55] Traditionally, because the margins of implant-supported crowns are located subgingivally, removing excess cement from this area is a major challenge. The cemented mesostructure over the abutment can be prepared intraorally and restored with a cemented crown. Nueesch et al[66] made mesostructures with polymer-infiltrated ceramics and crowns with CAD/CAM feldspathic ceramics that have the potential to be adhered to the mesostructure through acid etching techniques. According to the authors, this restorative approach can be classified as a biomimetic approach, as polymer-infiltrated ceramics have a modulus of elasticity (35.5 GPa) similar to that of dentin (12–45 GPa) and feldspathic ceramics have a modulus of elasticity (72.1 GPa) similar to that of enamel (40–130 GPa).[66] Polymer-infiltrated ceramic may also be a better choice to restore zirconia implants than a material with a high modulus of elasticity (zirconia) to prevent crown chipping. This is because a material with greater elasticity is able to compensate for the high stiffness of the zirconia implant.[60]

A representative case of a zirconia implant placed in the anterior region after trauma-induced root fracture is presented here (Fig 11-1). To preserve and restore the gingival architecture, a bone graft with biomaterial filling the buccal gap was applied after implant placement, followed by a subepithelial connective tissue graft. After 12 months, osseointegration and satisfactory esthetics were noted, with no metal show-through from the zirconia implant.

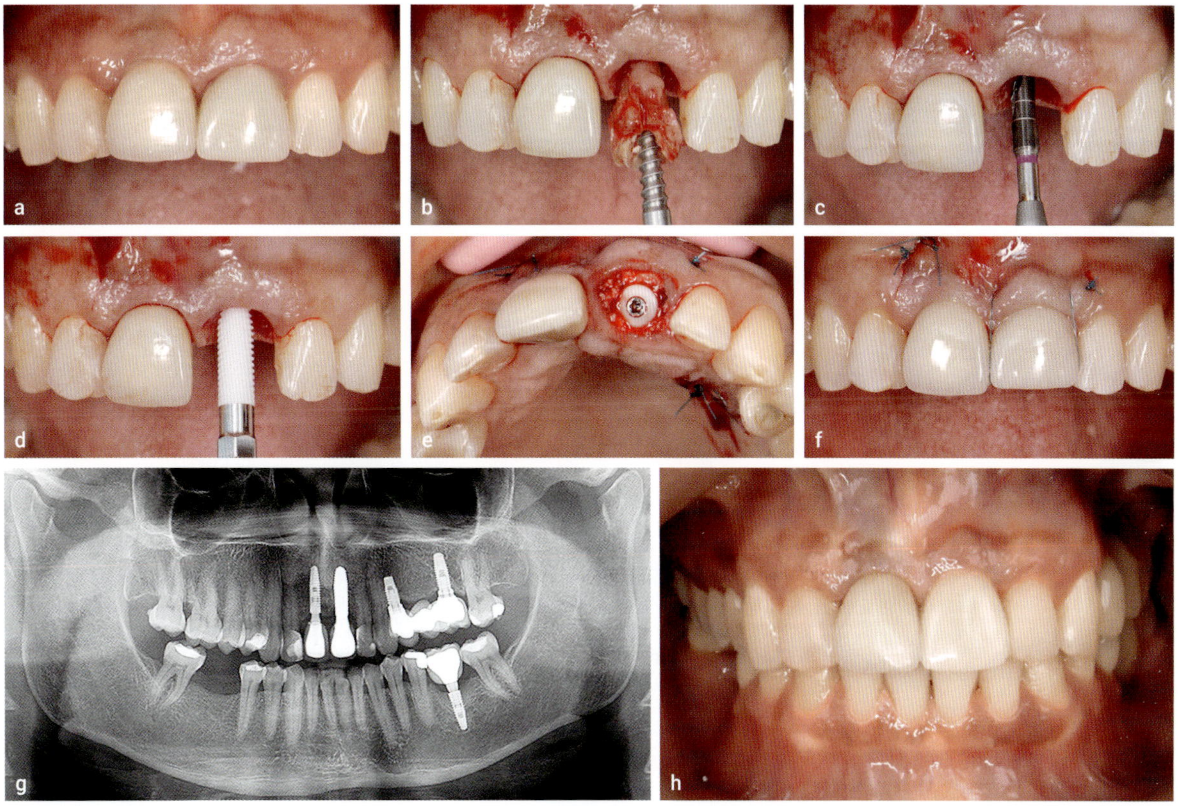

FIG 11-1 › *(a)* Initial clinical situation. The maxillary left central incisor has a root fracture, with indication for extraction and placement of a zirconia implant. *(b)* Atraumatic extraction of the left central incisor with a dental root extractor. The bone and gingival architecture are preserved as well as possible. *(c)* Surgical bone preparation for implant placement. *(d)* Placement of the zirconia implant (Neodent Zi Ceramic Implant System, Straumann). *(e)* Bone graft with biomaterial filling the buccal gap after implant placement and a subepithelial connective tissue graft used to preserve the gingival architecture. *(f)* Provisional prosthesis screwed over the implant with the area sutured to keep the tissues and graft in an optimal position. *(g)* Panoramic radiograph of the zirconia implant and prosthesis after 12 months. *(h)* Clinical view of the zirconia implant and prosthesis after 12 months.

Conclusion

One- and two-piece zirconia implants can be restored with bilayered or monolithic ceramic prostheses. Although bilayered prostheses possess excellent esthetics, failures such as chipping of the veneering ceramic can occur. During the manufacture of these prostheses, the use of anatomical frameworks[1] is strongly recommended, as well as control of the veneering ceramic thickness and slow cooling after sintering. On the other hand, monolithic prostheses do not have an interface and can be made of zirconia, feldspathic ceramic, lithium disilicate, or polymer-infiltrated ceramic. These prostheses are made by milling CAD/CAM blocks, which is versatile and fast, and the prosthesis is finished in the laboratory with polishing or staining.

References

1. Gahlert M, Gudehus T, Eichhorn S, Steinhauser E, Kniha H, Erhardt W. Biomechanical and histomorphometric comparison between zirconia implants with varying surface textures and a titanium implant in the maxilla of miniature pigs. Clin Oral Implants Res 2007;18:662–668.
2. Gahlert M, Röhling S, Wieland M, Eichhorn S, Küchenhoff H, Kniha H. A comparison study of the osseointegration of zirconia and titanium dental implants. A biomechanical evaluation in the maxilla of pigs. Clin Implant Dent Relat Res 2010;12:297–305.
3. Brull F, van Winkelhoff AJ, Cune MS. Zirconia dental implants: A clinical, radiographic, and microbiologic evaluation up to 3 years. Int J Oral Maxillofac Implants 2014;29:914–920.
4. Cionca N, Müller N, Mombelli A. Two-piece zirconia implants supporting all-ceramic crowns: A prospective clinical study. Clin Oral Implants Res 2015;26:413–418.
5. Payer M, Heschl A, Koller M, Arnetzl G, Lorenzoni M, Jakse N. All-ceramic restoration of zirconia two-piece implants—A randomized controlled clinical trial. Clin Oral Implants Res 2015;26:371–376.
6. Becker J, John G, Becker K, Mainusch S, Diedrichs G, Schwarz F. Clinical performance of two-piece zirconia implants in the posterior mandible and maxilla: A prospective cohort study over 2 years. Clin Oral Implants Res 2017;28:29–35.
7. Balmer M, Spier BC, Kohal RJ, Hämmerle CHF, Vach K, Jung RE. Zirconia implants restored with single crowns or fixed dental prostheses: 5-year results of a prospective cohort investigation. Clin Oral Implants Res 2020;31:452–462.
8. Kohal RJ, Spies BC, Vach K, Balmer M, Pieralli S. A prospective clinical cohort investigation on zirconia implants: 5-year results. J Clin Med 2020;9:2585.
9. Rimondini L, Cerroni L, Carrassi A, Torricelli P. Bacterial colonization of zirconia ceramic surfaces: An in vitro and in vivo study. Int J Oral Maxillofac Implants 2002;17:793–798.
10. Scarano A, Di Carlo F, Quaranta M, Piattelli A. Bone response to zirconia ceramic implants: An experimental study in rabbits. J Oral Implantol 2003;29:8–12.
11. Wenz HJ, Bartsch J, Wolfart S, Kern M. Osseointegration and clinical success of zirconia dental implants: A systematic review. Int J Prosthodont 2008;21:27–36.
12. Gahlert M, Burtscher D, Grunert I, Kniha H, Steinhauser E. Failure analysis of fractured dental zirconia implants. Clin Oral Implants Res 2012;23:287–293.
13. Möller B, Terheyden H, Acil Y, et al. A comparison of biocompatibility and osseointegration of ceramic and titanium implants: An in vivo and in vitro study. Int J Oral Maxillofac Surg 2012;41:638–645.
14. Kohal RJ, Weng D, Bächle M, Strub JR. Loaded custom-made zirconia and titanium implants show similar osseointegration: An animal experiment. J Periodontol 2004;75:1262–1268.
15. Iijima T, Homma S, Sekine H, Sasaki H, Yajima Y, Yoshinari M. Influence of surface treatment of yttria-stabilized tetragonal zirconia polycrystal with hot isostatic pressing on cyclic fatigue strength. Dent Mater J 2013;32:274–280.
16. Koyama T, Sato T, Yoshinari M. Cyclic fatigue resistance of yttria-stabilized tetragonal zirconia polycrystals with hot isostatic press processing. Dent Mater J 2012;31:1103–1110.
17. Lorenz J, Giulini N, Hölscher W, Schwiertz A, Schwarz F, Sader R. Prospective controlled clinical study investigating long-term clinical parameters, patient satisfaction, and microbial contamination of zirconia implants. Clin Implant Dent Relat Res 2019;21:263–271.
18. Mombelli A, van Oosten MA, Schurch E, Land NP. The microbiota associated with successful or failing osseointegrated titanium implants. Oral Microbiol Immunol 1987;2:145–151.

19. Fretwurst T, Nelson K, Tarnow DP, Wang HL, Giannobile WV. Is metal particle release associated with peri-implant bone destruction? An emerging concept. J Dent Res 2018;97:259–265.
20. Heydenrijk K, Raghoebar GM, Meijer HJ, Van Der Reijden WA, Van Winkelhoff AJ, Stegenga B. Two-part implants inserted in a one-stage or a two-stage procedure. A prospective comparative study. J Clin Periodontol 2002;29:901–909.
21. Kohal RJ, Finke HC, Klaus G. Stability of prototype two-piece zirconia and titanium implants after artificial aging: An in vitro pilot study. Clin Implant Dent Relat Res 2009;11:323–329.
22. Andreiotelli M, Wenz HJ, Kohal RJ. Are ceramic implants a viable alternative to titanium implants? A systematic literature review. Clin Oral Implants Res 2009;20:32–47.
23. Zembic A, Johannesen LH, Schou S, et al. Immediately restored one-piece single-tooth implants with reduced diameter: One-year results of a multi-center study. Clin Oral Implants Res 2012;23:49–54.
24. Payer M, Arnetzl V, Kirmeier R, Koller M, Arnetzl G, Jakse N. Immediate provisional restoration of single-piece zirconia implants: A prospective case series—Results after 24 months of clinical function. Clin Oral Implants Res 2013;24:569–575.
25. Esposito M, Grusovin MG, Maghaireh H, Worthington HV. Interventions for replacing missing teeth: Different times for loading dental implants. Cochrane Database Syst Rev 2013;2013:CD003878.
26. Hashimi D, Cionca N, Courvoisier DS, Mombelli A. A systematic review of the clinical survival of zirconia implants. Clin Oral Investig 2016;20:140–317.
27. Andreiotelli M, Kohal RJ. Fracture strength of zirconia implants after artificial aging. Clin Implant Dent Relat Res 2009;11:158–166.
28. Kohal RJ, Wolkewitz M, Tsakona A. The effects of cyclic loading and preparation on the fracture strength of zirconium-dioxide implants: An in vitro investigation. Clin Oral Implants Res 2011;22:808–814.
29. Kammermeier A, Rosentritt M, Behr M, Schneider-Feyrer S, Preis V. In vitro performance of one- and two-piece zirconia implant systems for anterior application. J Dent 2016;53:94–101.
30. Nevins M, Camelo M, Nevins ML, Schupbach P, Kim DM. Pilot clinical and histologic evaluations of a two-piece zirconia implant. Int J Periodontics Restorative Dent 2011;31:157–163.
31. Preis V, Kammermeier A, Handel G, Rosentritt M. In vitro performance of two-piece zirconia implant systems for anterior application. Dent Mater 2016;32:765–774.
32. Koller M, Steyer E, Theisen K, Stagnell S, Jakse N, Payer M. Two-piece zirconia versus titanium implants after 80 months: Clinical outcomes from a prospective randomized pilot trial. Clin Oral Implants Res 2020;31:388–396.
33. VanDooren E, Calamita M, Calgaro M, et al. Mechanical, biological and clinical aspects of zirconia implants. Eur J Esthet Dent 2012;7:396–471.
34. Thoma DS, Benic GI, Muñoz F, et al. Marginal bone-level alterations of loaded zirconia and titanium dental implants: An experimental study in the dog mandible. Clin Oral Implants Res 2016;27:412–420.
35. Cionca N, Hashim D, Mombelli A. Two-piece zirconia implants supporting all-ceramic crowns: Six-year results of a prospective cohort study. Clin Oral Implants Res 2021;32:695–701.
36. Adánez MH, Nishihara H, Att W. A systematic review and meta-analysis on the clinical outcome of zirconia implant-restoration complex. J Prosthodont Res 2018;62:397–406.
37. Lorusso L, Noumbissi S, Francesco I, Rapone B, Khater AGA, Scarano A. Scientific trends in clinical research on zirconia dental implants: A bibliometric review. Materials 2020;13:5534.
38. Siddiqi A, Kieser JA, Silva RK, Thomson WM, Duncan WJ. Soft and hard tissue response to zirconia versus titanium one-piece implants placed in alveolar and palatal sites: A randomized control trial. Clin Implant Dent Relat Res 2015;17:483–496.
39. Jung RE, Grohmann P, Sailer I, et al. Evaluation of a one-piece ceramic implant used for single-tooth replacement and three-unit fixed partial dentures: A prospective cohort clinical trial. Clin Oral Implants Res 2016;27:751–761.
40. Bömicke W, Gabbert O, Koob A, Krisam J, Rammelsberg P. Comparison of immediately loaded flapless-placed one-piece implants and flapped-placed conventionally loaded two-piece implants, both fitted with all-ceramic single crowns, in the posterior mandible: 3-year results from a randomised controlled pilot trial. Eur J Oral Implantol 2017;10:179–195.
41. Balmer M, Spies BC, Vach K, Kohal RJ, Hämmerle CHF, Jung RE. Three-year analysis of zirconia implants used for single-tooth replacement and three-unit fixed dental prostheses: A prospective multicenter study. Clin Oral Implants Res 2018;29:290–299.

42. Spies BC, Balmer M, Jung RE, Sailer I, Vach I, Kohal RJ. All-ceramic single crowns supported by zirconia implants: 5-year results of a prospective multicenter study. Clin Oral Implants Res 2019;30:466–475.
43. Cannizzaro G, Torchio C, Felice P, Leone M, Esposito M. Immediate occlusal versus non-occlusal loading of single zirconia implants. A multicentre pragmatic randomised clinical trial. Eur J Oral Implant 2010;3:111–120.
44. Kohal RJ, Patzelt SBM, Butz F, Sahlin H. One-piece zirconia oral implants: One-year results from a prospective case series. 2. Three-unit fixed dental prosthesis (FDP) reconstruction. J Clin Periodontol 2013;40:553–562.
45. Bormann KH, Gellrich NC, Kniha H, Schild S, Weingart D, Gahlert M. A prospective clinical study to evaluate the performance of zirconium dioxide dental implants in single-tooth edentulous area: 3-year follow-up. BMC Oral Health 2018;18:181.
46. Kohal RJ, Spies BC, Bauer A, Butz F. One-piece zirconia oral implants for single-tooth replacement: Three-year results from a long-term prospective cohort study. J Clin Periodontol 2018;45:114–124.
47. Sailer I, Strasding M, Valente NA, Zwahlen M, Liu S, Pjetursson BE. A systematic review of the survival and complication rates of zirconia-ceramic and metal-ceramic multiple-unit fixed dental prostheses. Clin Oral Implants Res 2018;29:184–198.
48. Spies BC, Stamp S, Kohal RJ. Evaluation of zirconia-based all-ceramic single crowns and fixed dental prosthesis on zirconia implants: 5-year results of a prospective cohort study. Clin Implant Dent Relat Res 2015;17:1014–1028.
49. Schwarz S, Schröder C, Hassel A, Bömicke W, Rammelsberg P. Survival and chipping of zirconia-based and metal-ceramic implant-supported single crowns. Clin Implant Dent Relat Res 2012;14:e119–e125.
50. Swain MV. Unstable cracking (chipping) of veneering porcelain on all-ceramic dental crowns and fixed partial dentures. Acta Biomater 2009;5:1668–1677.
51. Spies BC, Patzelt SBM, Vach K, Kohal RJ. Monolithic lithium-disilicate single crowns supported by zirconia oral implants: Three-year results of a prospective cohort study. Clin Oral Implants Res 2016;27:1160–1168.
52. Baldassarri M, Zhang Y, Thompson VP, Rekow ED, Stappert CF. Reliability and failure modes of implant-supported zirconium-oxide fixed dental prostheses related to veneering techniques. J Dent 2011;39:489–498.
53. Preis V, Letsch C, Handel G, Behr M, Schneider-Feyrer S, Rosentritt M. Influence of substructure design, veneer application technique, and firing regime on the in vitro performance of molar zirconia crowns. Dent Mater 2013;29:e113–e121.
54. Joos M, Sailer I, Filippi A, Mukaddam K, Rosentritt M, Kühl S. Stability of screw-retention in two-piece zirconia implants: An in vitro study. Clin Oral Implants Res 2020;31:607–614.
55. Nueesch R, Märtin S, Rohr N, Fisher J. In vitro investigations in a biomimetic approach to restore one-piece zirconia implants. Materials (Basel) 2021;14:4361.
56. Albiol JG, Böhm K, Wang HL. Clinical and radiographic outcomes of zirconia dental implants—A clinical case series study. Materials (Basel) 2022;25:15:2437.
57. Rohr N, Nüesch R, Greune R, et al. Stability of cantilever fixed dental prostheses on zirconia implants. Materials (Basel) 2022;15:3633.
58. Rohr N, Coldea A, Zitzmann NU, Fischer J. Loading capacity of zirconia implant supported hybrid ceramic crowns. Dent Mater 2015;31:e279–e288.
59. Zaugg LK, Meyer S, Rohr N, Zehnder I, Zitzmann NU. Fracture behavior, marginal gap width, and marginal quality of vented or pre-cemented CAD/CAM all-ceramic crowns luted on Y-TZP implants. Clin Oral Implants Res 2018;29:175–184.
60. Rohr N, Märtin S, Fischer J. Correlations between fracture load of zirconia implant supported single crowns and mechanical properties of restorative material and cement. Dent Mater J 2018;37:222–228.
61. Rohr N, Balmer M, Müller JA, Märtin S, Fischer J. Chewing simulation of zirconia implant supported restorations. J Prosthodont Res 2019;63:361–367.
62. Nueesch R, Conejo J, Mante F, et al. Loading capacity of CAD/CAM-fabricated anterior feldspathic ceramic crowns bonded to one-piece zirconia implants with different cements. Clin Oral Implants Res 2019;30:178–186.
63. Rohr N, Märtin S, Fischer J. Fracture load of zirconia implant supported CAD/CAM resin crowns and mechanical properties of restorative material and cement. J Prosthodont Res 2021;65:502–508.

64. Spies BC, Pieralli S, Vach K, Kohal RJ. CAD/CAM-fabricated ceramic implant-supported single crowns made from lithium disilicate: Final results of a 5-year prospective cohort study. Clin Implant Dent Relat Res 2017;19:876–833.
65. Steyer E, Herber V, Koller M, et al. Immediate restoration of single-piece zirconia implants: A prospective case series—Long-term results after 11 years of clinical function. Materials (Basel) 2021;14:6738.
66. Nueesch R, Karlin S, Fisher J, Rohr N. In vitro investigation of material combinations for meso- and suprastructures in a biomimetic approach to restore one-piece zirconia implants. Materials 2023;16:1355.

12

DESIGNING ZIRCONIA FRAMEWORKS

Mutlu Özcan, Luis Gustavo D´Altoé Garbelotto, and Claudia Angela Maziero Volpato

Due to its excellent mechanical properties, high flexural strength, and fracture toughness, zirconia is increasingly indicated for the fabrication of monolithic crowns and frameworks for bilayered crowns and fixed dental prostheses supported by teeth and implants. Frameworks support the glassy matrix ceramic veneering and provide mechanical reinforcement to the prosthesis during oral function. The ideal zirconia framework is 0.5 to 0.8 mm thick, has rounded edges to avoid stress concentration, and has a connector with a size of 9 to 16 mm^2.

Achievement of optimal framework parameters is guided by computer-aided design (CAD) systems. After computer-aided manufacturing (CAM) milling of the zirconia framework, a compatible ceramic material is selected based on thermal expansion coefficients. Because zirconia frameworks support ceramic veneering with bilayered structures, an interface free of stress zones is required to prevent the formation of cracks. Controlling sintering parameters by slow heating and cooling without external stresses is essential during fabrication and processing of zirconia crowns and fixed dental prostheses. Several mechanical surface conditioning methods for zirconia frameworks have been suggested to improve retention, along with the application of heat treatments to reduce the compressive mechanical stresses present at this interface. This chapter provides guidelines for adequate framework design and describes laboratory strategies to ensure the long-term clinical survival of tooth- and implant-supported zirconia restorations.

CAD/CAM for Framework Fabrication

The increasing use of zirconia-based crowns, fixed dental prostheses, implants, and abutments is due to the introduction of CAD/CAM technology, which has improved and accelerated laboratory procedures.[1,2] Zirconia is a unique material in restorative dentistry because, in addition to its excellent mechanical properties (greater strength, rigidity, and fracture toughness compared with other glassy matrix ceramics),[3] its optical properties have been improved considerably with the development of translucent and colored zirconia,[4,5] which has certainly contributed to its use for monolithic crowns. Yttria partially stabilized zirconia (Y-PSZ) shows high fracture toughness (5 to 10 MPa $m^{1/2}$) and a flexural strength of 900 to 1,440 MPa.[6] Thus, this zirconia-based material is promising for the fabrication of restoration frameworks and abutments for implants, especially for use under functional loads.

Partially sintered zirconia blocks are milled via CAM to a size that is about 20% to 30% larger than desired to compensate for shrinkage that will occur during the sintering process. The shrinkage rate depends on the composition of the zirconia and the density of the presintered block that will be machined.[7] These blocks have a chalk-like consistency and can be easily milled in CAM units.[8] After machining, the frameworks are sintered in a furnace at high temperatures to obtain the desired final dimensions, density, and strength.

Although the framework must be veneered via conventional ceramic layering techniques performed by a laboratory technician, there are advantages to obtaining frameworks with CAD/CAM machining technology. Among these advantages are the introduction of new, safe, esthetic, and durable materials; the improved efficiency of laboratory processing; and greater control of the quality of the restorations with improved fit.[2] However, variables such as the scanning process, milling parameters and process, and shrinkage ratio of zirconia during sintering may affect the accuracy of zirconia restorations obtained with CAD/CAM. All these factors must therefore be carefully controlled throughout the digital workflow.[9]

Main Features of Zirconia Frameworks

Adequate design of the zirconia framework is essential to support the glassy matrix veneering ceramic during oral function. Studies indicate that zirconia frameworks have sufficient mechanical strength to support posterior fixed prostheses on natural teeth,[10,11] and low failure rates (0% to 2.2%) have been reported in clinical studies.[11,12] To guarantee a good design, the laboratory technician should master the dental anatomy and proper handling of all the prosthetic materials.

The thickness of a zirconia framework can vary from 0.4 to 0.7 mm, with a minimum thickness of 0.5 mm recommended for posterior areas.[13–15] An excessive increase in these values can compromise esthetics by leading to opacity of the final prosthesis. However, these values are based on empirical data rather than clinical research.[13,14] Studies have made various suggestions regarding framework thickness and margins, including a 2-mm-thick cervical margin[16]; a framework with a 1-mm-thick lingual aspect and a proximal extension and cervical margin that is 2.5 mm in height[17]; a 0.3-mm-thick framework with a palatal cervical margin 2.0 mm high and 1.0 mm thick[15]; and a 0.5-mm-thick framework covering either one- or two-thirds of the palatal surface.[18] The introduction of cervical margins in zirconia frameworks seems to improve fracture resistance of the veneering ceramic, especially when it is extended to the proximal areas.[17,19]

Framework customization achieved by waxing the anatomical contour of the prosthesis has been reported in the literature.[14] Uniform and controlled thickness of the veneering ceramic, which is more prone to failure than the framework, can be more easily obtained this way, resulting in a framework with an "anatomical design." Studies have reported that this design shows favorable survival rates of the zirconia frameworks after 3 and 5 years in function.[20,21] Other studies have reported that anatomically designed frameworks resulted in a lower fracture rate of the veneering ceramic,[22,23] especially when sharp angles were not present.

In zirconia frameworks for fixed prostheses, the size of the connector can vary from 9 to 16 mm^2,[24] although 9 mm^2 is the most common.[25] The design of the connector area is critical for the success of the framework, as this is the weakest region of the prosthetic restoration,[24,26] especially in the posterior areas, where there are greater masticatory forces and often reduced coronal height.[27] To avoid fracture during masticatory function, the framework design must include space in the gingival embrasures to receive the gingival papillae and space on the occlusal surface for application of the veneering ceramic while not compromising the size of the connector.[28,29] Finite element analyses (FEAs) have shown that the shape and size of the connector affect the stress distribution, fracture resistance, and failure of implant-supported fixed zirconia prostheses,[30] further reinforcing the importance of proper framework design.

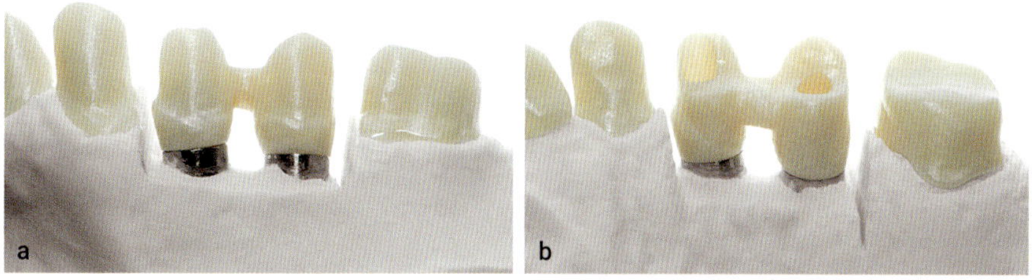
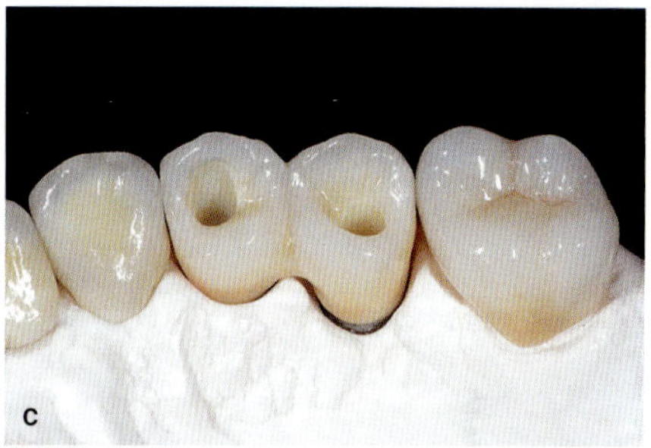

FIG 12-1 › *(a and b)* Zirconia frameworks on teeth and dental implants before ceramic layering. Note the anatomical form and step-like shoulder preparations at the margins to support the veneering ceramic. *(c)* Zirconia prosthesis after veneering with feldspathic porcelain.

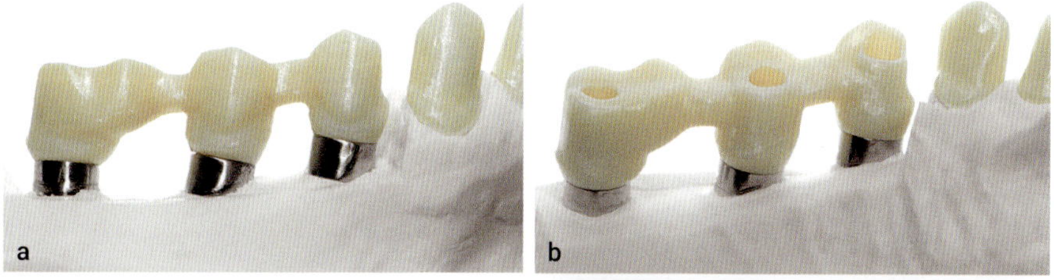
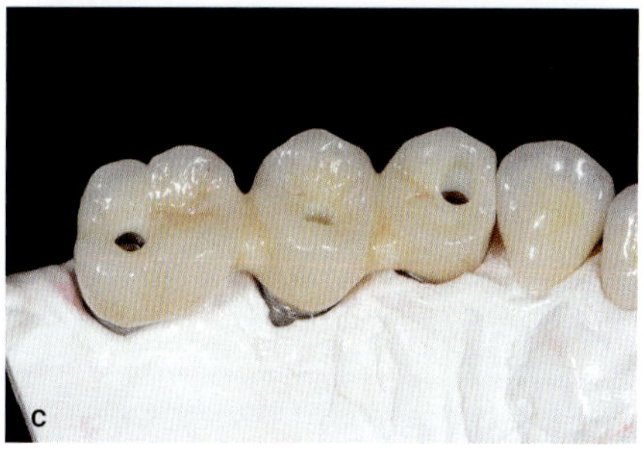

FIG 12-2 › *(a and b)* Zirconia frameworks on teeth and dental implants before ceramic layering. *(c)* Zirconia prosthesis after veneering with feldspathic porcelain.

Laboratory Steps

With the digital design prepared, the laboratory technician can proceed with milling and ceramic layering (Figs 12-1 and 12-2). The framework is fabricated using CAM equipment with special burs for milling zirconia blocks in a process that is completely guided by the computer. The milled framework is tested in the mouth to evaluate its fit and is then veneered with a glassy matrix ceramic. Studies have recommended that the zirconia surface be prepared prior to veneering to improve the bond strength between the framework and the veneering ceramic.[31–33] However, zirconia is highly susceptible to surface modifications and to changes induced by laboratory and clinical handling.[34] Therefore, the fewer changes that are made to the surface of sintered zirconia, the better its clinical performance will be over time.[33]

Airborne-particle abrasion with aluminum oxide is a strategy for increasing the surface roughness of zirconia.[32] It is a well-established technique that is easily accessible to laboratory technicians. However, studies suggest that it can lead to surface failures and induce tetragonal to monoclinic phase transformation, which affects the bonding strength between zirconia and the veneering ceramic.[33,35] In addition, surface failures can lead to the formation of stress concentration points, which can result in delamination of the veneering ceramic.[36]

Microretentions (discrete wear in the form of undulations) have also been leveraged to improve the adhesion between different materials.[37–39] To minimize the risk of damage to the zirconia surface, however, it is essential to use new burs with a fine grain[39] and to perform an adequate heat treatment followed by slow cooling to release stresses produced on the zirconia surface during mechanical surface conditioning methods. As a consequence of heat treatment, a new surface restructuring is achieved on zirconia.[40]

Clinical Steps

After the laboratory procedures are completed, a fixed prosthesis should be tried on the teeth or implants to evaluate the clinical fit and identify any necessary marginal and occlusal adjustments (Fig 12-3). Poor marginal fit of a fixed prosthesis can lead to plaque retention, cement solubility, and the possibility of secondary caries and endodontic complications.[41,42] In implant-supported zirconia dental prostheses, screw loosening and screw loss are the most common types of failures.[43,44]

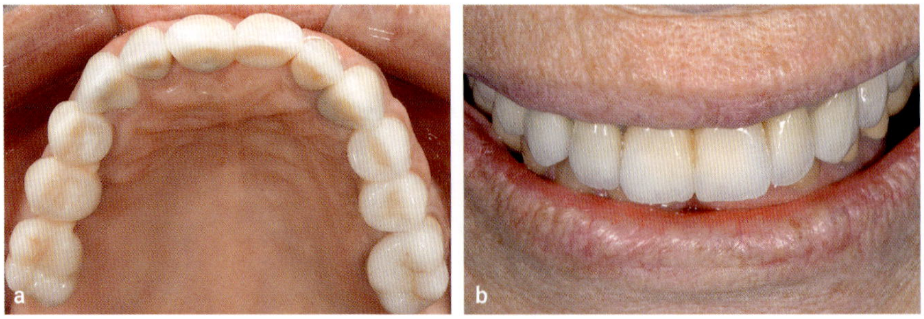

FIG 12-3 › *(a)* Intraoral view of a zirconia prosthesis on teeth and dental implants. *(b)* Extraoral view of the veneered zirconia prosthesis.

Studies recommend that marginal gaps should be between 50 and 75 µm,[45,46] although marginal gaps below 120 µm have been considered clinically acceptable.[47] Whenever possible, however, clinicians should aim for the best possible fit to reduce future complications.[48] During the digital workflow, digitization allows the framework to be built with an ideal predetermined internal space to be filled with adhesive cement. The accuracy of the scan directly affects the accuracy of the marginal fit.[49] Accurate scanning, precise CAD, and obtaining this internal space for the adhesive cement results in a reduced marginal gap between the framework and the tooth/implant abutment. A seal is then obtained after securing the fixed prosthesis with adhesive cement to achieve the desired marginal adaptation.

Fracture of the Veneering Ceramic

The most frequent technical complication of fixed prostheses with zirconia-based frameworks is chipping of the veneering ceramic.[25,50] This is because zirconia frameworks are veneered by glassy matrix ceramics with lower flexural strength and a higher coefficient of thermal expansion. The interface between these two materials is an area of tension that can result in failures within the veneering ceramic such as chipping or even lead to larger fractured areas (ie, delamination).[51] Several factors are related to this phenomenon, including framework design, thickness of the veneering ceramic, the type of glassy matrix ceramic that is used, the sintering process, differences in coefficients of thermal expansion, and cooling speed.[52–55]

A lack of uniform veneering ceramic thickness due to inadequate framework design contributes to chipping.[56] When an adequate design is used, the veneering ceramic can support oral function.[57] In anatomical frameworks, the thickness of the veneering ceramic is standardized more effectively, which reduces the chances of fracture and chipping.[14] Studies confirm that a consistent thickness of the veneering porcelain results in a more uniform distribution of residual stresses.[22,58]

The bond strength between a zirconia framework and the veneering ceramic depends on the type of ceramic that is used.[59,60] This is probably because the framework and veneering ceramic have different coefficients of thermal expansion, and therefore the behavior of each material is different, resulting in a challenge for the laboratory technician.[61] During the sintering process, the temperature differences in the heating and cooling cycles associated with different coefficients of thermal expansion tend to result in a stress gradient across the entire ceramic framework layer, with higher compressive stresses at the framework interface/surface and slight tensile stresses at the coating interface/surface.[62] Researchers agree that residual stresses resulting from coefficient of thermal expansion incompatibility can be very harmful, affecting both the veneering ceramic and the framework.[63] To minimize damage resulting from the difference in thermal expansion coefficients of the different materials used in zirconia prostheses, this difference should be kept small—at most the coefficient of thermal expansion of the veneering ceramic should be 10% smaller than that of the zirconia used in the framework.[62]

In addition, controlled techniques for cooling the framework to room temperature must be observed to minimize the development of stress, as residual stresses are modified by heat treatment in the glass transition phase and as a function of the change in cooling rate.[64] The relatively low thermal conductivity of zirconia may also explain failures in all-ceramic prostheses. The delay in cooling inherent to this ceramic introduces residual thermal stresses.[65,66] Nevertheless, faster cooling results in lower thermal conductivity of zirconia, and the greater the temperature difference is between the veneering ceramic and zirconia framework, the greater are the residual stresses generated within the veneering ceramic.[67]

Conclusion

Proper framework design is critical for the long-term success of zirconia restorations. The literature recommends the fabrication of zirconia frameworks with an average thickness of 0.5 mm and cervical shoulder margins to strengthen the veneering ceramic. It is also recommended to customize the framework by waxing the anatomical contour of the future prosthesis to standardize the thickness of the veneering ceramic. In zirconia frameworks, the most commonly employed connector diameter is 9 mm^2, which can help guarantee resistance to masticatory forces in this fragile area, along with facilitating oral hygiene in pontic areas. Laboratory and clinical steps for zirconia crowns and fixed prostheses must be performed with meticulous care to minimize damage to the zirconia surface, which can be detrimental to its clinical performance and result in failures such as chipping of the veneering ceramic. In addition to these precautions, proper surface preparation of the zirconia prior to ceramic veneering should be performed with fine-grain burs, adequate heat treatment, slow cooling, minimal marginal and internal gap design, and controlled occlusal adjustment with low-speed burs or polishing instruments to ensure successful tooth- or implant-supported zirconia restorations.

References

1. Miyazaki T, Hotta Y. CAD/CAM systems available for the fabrication of crown and bridge restorations. Aust Dent J 2011;56:97–106.
2. Miyazaki T, Nakamura T, Matsumura H, Ban S, Kobayashi T. Current status of zirconia restoration. J Prosthodont Res 2013;57:236–261.
3. Kelly JR, Denry I. Stabilized zirconia as a structural ceramic: An overview. Dent Mater 2008;24:289–298.
4. Zhang Y, Lawn BR. Novel zirconia materials in dentistry. J Dent Res 2018;97:140–147.
5. Tabatabaian F. Color aspect of monolithic zirconia restorations: A review of the literature. J Prosthodont 2019;28:276–287.
6. Guazzato M, Albakry M, Ringer SP, Swain MV. Strength, fracture toughness and microstructure of a selection of all-ceramic materials. Part II. Zirconia-based dental ceramics. Dent Mater 2004;20:449–456.
7. Kohorst P, Brinkmann H, Li J, Borchers L, Stiesch M. Marginal accuracy of four-unit zirconia fixed dental prostheses fabricated using different computer-aided design/computer-aided manufacturing systems. Eur J Oral Sci 2009;117:319–325.

8. Denry I, Kelly JR. State of the art of zirconia for dental applications. Dent Mater 2008;24:299–307.
9. Beuer F, Schweiger J, Edelhoff D. Digital dentistry: An overview of recent developments for CAD/CAM generated restorations. Br Dent J 2008;204:505–511.
10. Beuer F, Stimmelmayr M, Gernet W, Edelhoff D, Güth JF, Naumann M. Prospective study of zirconia-based restorations: 3-year clinical results. Quintessence Int 2010;41:631–637.
11. Sailer I, Pjetursson BE, Zwahlen M, Hämmerle CH. A systematic review of the survival and complication rates of all-ceramic and metal-ceramic reconstructions after an observation period of at least 3 years. Part II: Fixed dental prostheses. Clin Oral Implants Res 2007;18(suppl 3):86–96.
12. Edelhoff D, Florian B, Florian W, Johnen C. HIP zirconia fixed partial dentures—Clinical results after 3 years of clinical service. Quintessence Int 2008;39:459–471.
13. McLaren EA, White SN. Glass-infiltrated zirconia/alumina-based ceramic for crowns and fixed partial dentures. Pract Periodontics Aesthet Dent 1999;11:985–994.
14. Marchack BW, Futatsuki Y, Marchack CB, White SN. Customization of milled zirconia copings for all-ceramic crowns: A clinical report. J Prosthet Dent 2008;99:169–173.
15. Omori S, Komada W, Yoshida K, Miura H. Effect of thickness of zirconia-ceramic crown frameworks on strength and fracture pattern. Dent Mater J 2013;32:189–194.
16. Cho HY, Won HY, Choe HC, Son MK. Fracture characteristics of dental ceramic crown according to zirconia coping design. Procedia Engineering 2011;10:1561–1566.
17. Silva NRFA, Bonfante EA, Rafferty BT, et al. Conventional and modified veneered zirconia vs. metal ceramic: Fatigue and finite element analysis. J Prosthodont 2012;21:433–439.
18. Jo EH, Huh YH, Ko KH, Park CJ, Cho LR. Effect of different ceramic materials and substructure designs on fracture resistance in anterior restorations. J Prosthet Dent 2022;127:785–792.
19. Pogoncheff CM, Duff RE. Use of zirconia collar to prevent interproximal porcelain fracture: A clinical report. J Prosthet Dent 2010;104:77–79.
20. Tinschert J, Schulze KA, Natt G, Latzke P, Heussen N, Spiekermann H. Clinical behavior of zirconia-based fixed partial dentures made of DC-Zirkon: 3-year results. Int J Prosthodont 2008;21:217–222.
21. Molin MK, Karlsson SL. Five-year clinical prospective evaluation of zirconia-based Denzir 3-unit FPDs. Int J Prosthodont 2008;21:223–227.
22. Rosentritt M, Steiger D, Behr M, Handel G, Kolbeck C. Influence of substructure design and spacer settings on the in vitro performance of molar zirconia crowns. J Dent 2009;37:978–983.
23. Keough BE, Kay HB, Sager RD, Keen E. Clinical performance of scientifically designed, hot isostatic-pressed (HIP'd) zirconia cores in a bilayered all-ceramic system. Compend Contin Educ Dent 2011;32:58–68.
24. Motta AB, Pereira LC, Cunha ARCC. All-ceramic and porcelain-fused-to-metal fixed partial dentures: A comparative study by 2D finite element analyses. J Appl Oral Sci 2007;15:399–405.
25. Raigrodski AJ, Hillstead MB, Meng GK, Chung KH. Survival and complications of zirconia based fixed dental prostheses: A systematic review. J Prosthet Dent 2012;107:170–177.
26. Ha SR, Kim SH, Han JS, et al. The influence of various core designs on stress distribution in the veneered zirconia crown: A finite element analysis study. J Adv Prosthodont 2013;5:187–197.
27. Lee JY, Choi SJ, Kim MS, Kim HY, Kim YS, Shin SW. Effect of span length on the fit of zirconia framework fabricated using CAD/CAM system. J Adv Prosthodont 2013;5:118–125.
28. Oh WS, Anusavice KJ. Effect of connector design on the fracture resistance of all-ceramic fixed partial dentures. J Prosthet Dent 2002;87:536–542.
29. Mahmood DJH, Linderoth EH, Von Steyern PV, Wennerberg A. Fracture strength of all-ceramic (Y-TZP) three- and four-unit fixed dental prostheses with different connector design and production history. Swed Dent J 2013;37:179–187.
30. Tsumita M, Kokubo Y, von Steyern PV, Fukushima S. Effect of framework shape on the fracture strength of implant-supported all-ceramic fixed partial dentures in the molar region. J Prosthodont 2008;17:274–285.
31. Guazzato M, Quach L, Albakry M, Swain MV. Influence of surface and heat treatments on the flexural strength of Y-TZP dental ceramic. J Dent 2005;33:9–18.
32. Nakamura T, Wakabayashi K, Zaima C, Nishida H, Kinuta S, Yatani H. Tensile bond strength between tooth-colored porcelain and sandblasted zirconia framework. J Prosthodont Res 2009;53:116–119.
33. Tada K, Sato T, Yoshinari M. Influence of surface treatment on bond strength of veneering ceramics fused to zirconia. Dent Mater J 2012;31:287–296.
34. Luthardt RG, Holzhuter MS, Rudolph H, Herold V, Walter MH. CAD/CAM-machining effects on Y-TZP zirconia. Dent Mater 2004;20:655–662.

35. El-Shrkawy ZR, El-Hosary MM, Saleh O, Mandour MH. Effect of different surface treatments on bond strength, surface and microscopic structure of zirconia ceramic. Future Dent J 2016;2:41–53.
36. Kosmac T, Oblak C, Jevnikar P, Funduk N, Marion L. Strength and reliability of surface treated Y-TZP dental ceramics. J Biomed Mater Res 2000;53:304–313.
37. Casucci A, Osorio E, Osorio R, et al. Influence of different surface treatments on surface zirconia frameworks. J Dent 2009;37:891–897.
38. Kim HJ, Lim HP, Park YJ, Vang MS. Effect of zirconia surface treatments on the shear bond strength of veneering ceramic. J Prosthet Dent 2011;105:315–322.
39. Garbelotto LGD, Volpato CAM, Rocha M, Maranghello CA, Calasans A, Özcan M. Laboratory and clinical considerations on prosthetic zirconia infrastructures for implants. Implant Dent 2013;22:578–583.
40. Zhang Y, Chai H, Lee JJ, Lawn BR. Chipping resistance of graded zirconia ceramics for dental crowns. J Dent Res 2012;91:311–315.
41. Gavelis JR, Morency JD, Riley ED, Sozio RB. The effect of various finish line preparations on the marginal seal and occlusal seat of full crown preparations. J Prosthet Dent 1981;45:138–145.
42. Jacobs MS, Windeler AS. An investigation of dental luting cement solubility as a function of the marginal gap. J Prosthet Dent 1991;65:436–442.
43. Karl M, Graef F, Wichmann M, Krafft T. Passivity of fit of CAD/CAM and copy-milled frameworks, veneered frameworks, and anatomically contoured, zirconia ceramic, implant-supported fixed prostheses. J Prosthet Dent 2012;107:232–238.
44. Huang Y, Wang J. Mechanism of and factors associated with the loosening of the implant abutment screw: A review. J Esthet Restor Dent 2019;31:338–345.
45. Conrad HJ, Seong WJ, Pesun IJ. Current ceramic materials and systems with clinical recommendations: A systematic review. J Prosthet Dent 2007;98:389–404.
46. Azarbal A, Azarbal M, Engelmeier RL, Kunkel TC. Marginal fit comparison of CAD/CAM crowns milled from two different materials. J Prosthodont 2018;27:421-428.
47. McLean JW, von Fraunhofer JA. The estimation of cement film thickness by an in vivo technique. Br Dent J 1971;131:107–111.
48. Abduo J, Judge RB. Implications of implant framework misfit: A systematic review of biomechanical sequelae. Int J Oral Maxillofac Implants 2014;29:608–621.
49. Ahlholm P, Sipilä K, Vallittu P, Jakonen M, Kotiranta U. Digital versus conventional impressions in fixed prosthodontics: A review. J Prosthodont 2018;27:35–41.
50. Komine F, Blatz MB, Matsumura H. Current status of zirconia-based fixed restorations. J Oral Sci 2010;52:531–539.
51. Mosharraf R, Rismanchian M, Savabi O, Ashtiani AH. Influence of surface modification techniques on shear bond strength between different zirconia cores and veneering ceramics. J Adv Prosthodont 2011;3:221–228.
52. Salimi H, Mosharraf R, Savabi O. Effect of framework design on fracture resistance of zirconium oxide posterior fixed partial dentures. Dent Res J (Isfahan) 2012;9:764–769.
53. Kou W, Sjögren G. Fracture behaviour of zirconia FPDs substructures. J Oral Rehabil 2010;37:292–299.
54. Tholey MJ, Swain MV, Thiel N. Thermal gradients and residual stresses in veneered Y-TZP frameworks. Dent Mater 2011;27:1102–1110.
55. Nakamura K, Adolfsson E, Milleding P, Kanno T, Örtengren U. Influence of grain size and veneer firing process on the flexural strength of zirconia ceramics. Eur J Oral Sci 2012;120:249–254.
56. Donovan TE. Factors essential for successful all-ceramic restorations. J Am Dent Assoc 2008;139(suppl):14S–18S.
57. Raigrodski AJ, Yu A, Chiche GJ, Hochstedler JL, Mancl LA, Mohamed SE. Clinical efficacy of veneered zirconium dioxide-based posterior partial fixed dental prostheses: Five-year results. J Prosthet Dent 2012;108:214–222.
58. Kokubo Y, Tsumita M, Kano T, Fukushima S. The influence of zirconia coping designs on the fracture load of all-ceramic molar crowns. Dent Mater J 2011;30:281–285.
59. Cömlekoglu ME, Dündar M, Özcan M, Güngor MA, Gorce B, Artunç C. Evaluation of bond strength of various margin ceramics to a zirconia ceramic. J Dent 2008;36:822–827.
60. Fazi G, Vichi A, Ferrari M. Microtensile bond strength of three different veneering porcelain systems to a zirconia core for all ceramic restorations. Am J Dent 2010;23:347–350.
61. Göstemeyer G, Jendras M, Borchers L, Bach FW, Stiesch M, Kohorst P. Effect of thermal expansion mismatch on the Y-TZP/veneer interfacial adhesion determined by strain energy release rate. J Prosthodont Res 2012;56:93–101.

62. Swain MV. Unstable cracking (chipping) of veneering porcelain on all-ceramic dental crowns and fixed partial dentures. Acta Biomater 2009;5:1668–1677.
63. Lawn B, Bhowmick S, Bush MB, Qasim T, Rekow ED, Zhang Y. Failure modes in ceramic-based layer structures: A basis for materials design of dental crowns. J Am Ceram Soc 2007;90:1671–1683.
64. Taskonak B, Borges GA, Mecholsky JJ Jr, Anusavice KJ, Moore BK, Yan J. The effects of viscoelastic parameters on residual stress development in a zirconia/glass bilayer dental ceramic. Dent Mater 2008;24:1149–1155.
65. Guess PC, Kulis A, Siegbert Witkowski S, Wolkewitz M, Zhang Y, Strub RJ. Shear bond strengths between different zirconia cores and veneering ceramics and their susceptibility to thermocycling. Dent Mater 2008;24:1556–1567.
66. Guess PC, Schultheis S, Bonfante EA, Coelho PG, Ferencz JL, Silva NRFA. All-ceramic systems: Laboratory and clinical performance. Dent Clin North Am 2011;55:333–352.
67. Choi JE, Waddell JN, Swain MV. Pressed ceramics onto zirconia. Part 2: Indentation fracture and influence of cooling rate on residual stresses. Dent Mater 2011;27:1111–1118.

13

CASE REPORTS FROM THE EUROPEAN SOCIETY FOR CERAMIC IMPLANTOLOGY

Jens Tartsch, Sebastian Horvath, Juan Blanco Carrión, Thomas Mehnert, Franco Giancola, and Jochen Mellinghoff

Case reports offer insight into the diverse applications of ceramic implants and the challenges faced by both clinicians and manufacturers. This chapter describes the practical clinical use of ceramic implants and provides a detailed look at some of the very different ceramic implant systems available on the market today. We look behind the scenes and highlight the innovations that have contributed to the continuous improvement of implant technology. Keep in mind that the case studies presented in this chapter are not only success stories but also reflect clinician and manufacturer learning curves. They highlight both the challenges of using ceramic implants and the progress toward increasingly reliable ceramic implant technologies.

The cases in this chapter were provided by European Society for Ceramic Implantology (ESCI) company partners who were invited to present their systems by means of case studies. Submissions were made on a purely voluntary basis without financial compensation or commercial interests. To maintain neutrality, the submitted manuscripts were not selected or modified by the ESCI or the authors of this book. The responsibility for the individual contributions lies exclusively with the respective case authors.

Long-Term Restoration of Mandibular Teeth with Zirconia Implants with a 5-Year Follow-up

Company partner: Nobel Biocare
Product: NobelPearl
Clinician: Jens Tartsch

Nobel Biocare™

Ceramic dental implants are now established as a serious option within general implant dentistry. There is increasing patient demand for metal-free solutions, and the development of new materials, microrough surface treatments, and improved treatment protocols enables clinicians to leverage the advantages of ceramic dental implants as a reliable alternative to titanium implants. Patients should be informed about the advantages and disadvantages of both material options and be involved in decision making any time ceramic implants are considered as a treatment option. This case report demonstrates the standard procedure for using ceramic implants in our dental office.

INITIAL PRESENTATION AND TREATMENT PLANNING

A 57-year-old woman presented to our clinic in May 2018. She requested restorations for her mandibular right second premolar and first molar following extraction. The teeth had been extracted at another practice 3 months (second premolar) and 1 year (first molar) prior to her visit (Fig 13-1a). Radiographic examination revealed a single lateral dehiscence defect at the site of the second premolar and a fully healed first molar site (Fig 13-1b). The patient was informed of ceramic implants and the NobelPearl Tapered ceramic dental implant system (Nobel Biocare) as a metal-free alternative to titanium implants. After a detailed discussion, the patient provided informed consent for this treatment option. The main reason for her decision was the advantage of reduced inflammation in the peri-implant tissue with ceramic implants.

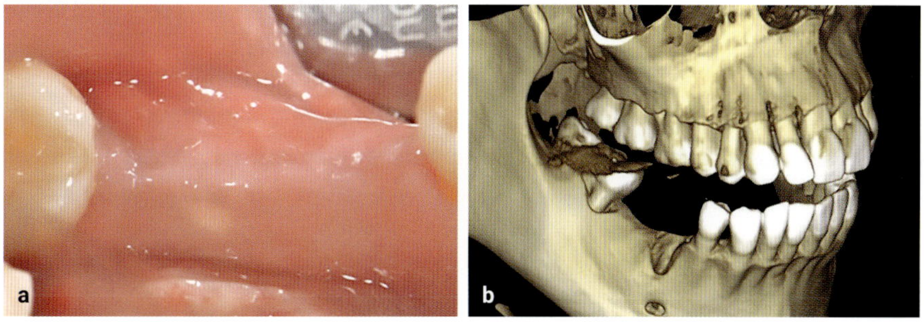

FIG 13-1 › *(a)* Healed site following extraction of the mandibular right second premolar and first molar 3 months and 1 year before surgery, respectively. *(b)* Preoperative CBCT showing a lateral defect near the site of the second premolar.

SURGICAL AND RESTORATIVE PROTOCOLS

After an initial hygiene phase and periodontal treatment of the adjacent second molar by root planing, the implant surgery was performed in July 2018. The alveolar bone was cleaned, and a suitable bone level for implant placement was found in the site of the first molar, with a lateral defect observed in the site of the second premolar (Fig 13-1c).

NobelPearl Tapered dental implants with a 4.2 × 10–mm diameter and NobelPearl Straight Inter-X abutments were used in the clinical procedure (Fig 13-1d). Both implants were inserted 0.6 mm supracrestal with torque of 30 Ncm. Primary implant stability was good. The implants were then covered with Inter-X cover screws (Fig 13-1e). The buccal surface of the implant in the site of the second premolar remained within the bone contour (a three-wall defect), so the lateral defect could be augmented easily with deproteinized bovine bone (Bio-Oss, Geistlich) and membrane (Bio-Gide, Geistlich) according to the standard clinical procedure (Fig 13-1f). After a smooth periosteal incision, primary wound closure was achieved (Fig 13-1g).

The restorative process was initiated 3 months after surgery with reentry via small single-roll flaps at each implant site to place 3-mm NobelPearl healing abutments. The soft tissue was healthy and keratinized around the healing abutments when the open tray impression was performed 2 weeks later (Figs 13-1h to 13-1j). Monolithic zirconia crowns were selected as the prosthetic solution. For stability and because of the bone augmentation in the site of the second premolar, the crowns were splinted.

Following removal of the healing abutments (Fig 13-1k) and after trying in the NobelPearl abutments, the screw channels were sealed with polytetrafluoroethylene (PTFE) and the abutments were prepared for cementation (Fig 13-1l). Figures 13-1m and 13-1n show the final restoration and abutments before insertion.

To achieve a tension- and bending-free connection between the restoration and the implants, the zirconia restorations were cemented to the abutments intraorally in a standard procedure with RelyX Unicem resin cement (3M ESPE). The PTFE was removed through the screw channel, and the entire restoration was removed as one piece. The cement could then be removed easily, and the final restorations were polished according to procedure. After this cleaning, the restoration was reinserted and the Vicarbo screw (Nobel Biocare) was torqued to 25 Ncm following manufacturer guidelines. The screw channel was closed again using a PTFE band (Fig 13-1o) and finally covered with composite resin. Figures 13-1p and 13-1q show the final restoration after screw channel closure and sealing with composite. The total treatment time was 4 months.

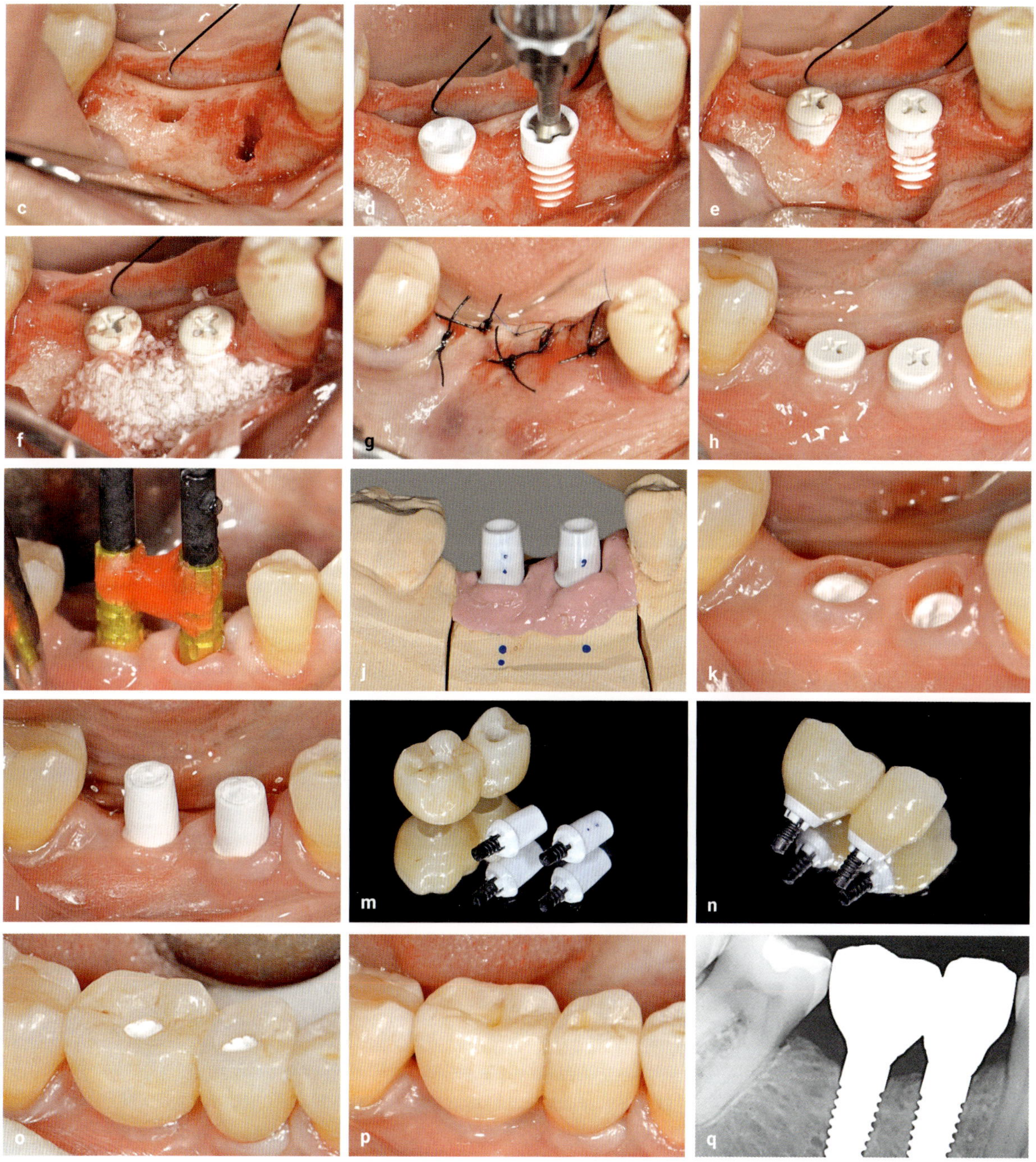

FIG 13-1 *(cont)* › *(c)* Sufficient bone for implant placement in the site of the first molar and a lateral defect in the site of the second premolar. *(d)* Freehand placement of a NobelPearl implant using a NobelPearl Inter-X implant driver following preparation of the implant sites. *(e)* NobelPearl Inter-X cover screws in place. *(f)* Horizontal bone augmentation using deproteinized bovine bone. *(g)* With a two-piece implant system, primary wound closure is possible. *(h)* Healthy soft tissue 2 weeks after reentry. *(i)* NobelPearl Open Tray Inter-X impression copings placed on the implants and fixed for precision. *(j)* Abutments placed on the master cast with a gingival mask. *(k)* Healthy and thick keratinized peri-implant mucosa following removal of the NobelPearl healing abutments. *(l)* The screw channels were sealed with PTFE, and NobelPearl abutments were prepared for cementation. *(m and n)* Final restoration and abutments before insertion. *(o)* For the final placement of the restoration, the screw is torqued at 25 Ncm and the screw channel is closed again with a PTFE band. *(p)* Final restoration in place after screw channel closure and sealing with composite resin. *(q)* Radiograph after delivery of the restoration. →

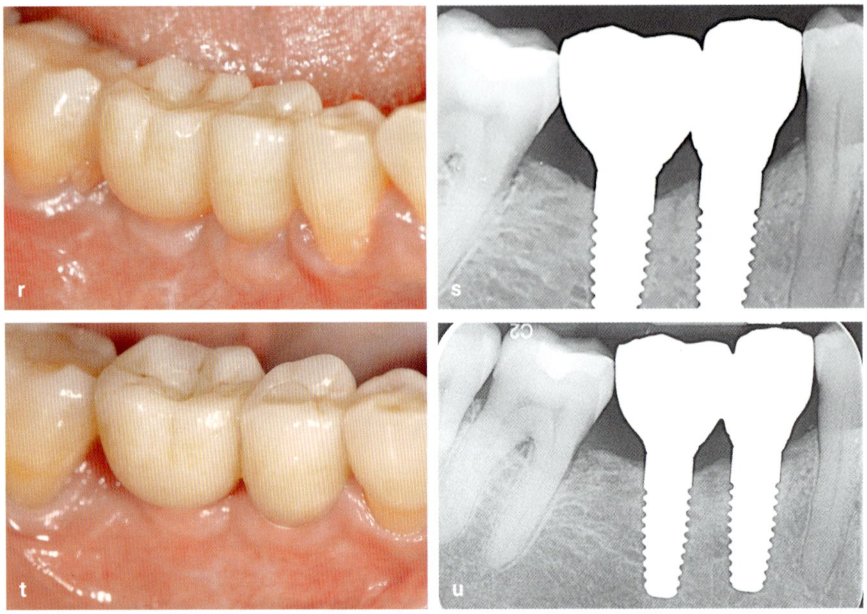

FIG 13-1 *(cont)* › *(r)* Excellent esthetics at the 1-year follow-up. Note the healthy soft tissue and natural-looking prosthesis. *(s)* The 1-year follow-up radiograph shows stable bone levels. *(t)* Excellent esthetics at the 5-year follow-up. Note the healthy soft tissue and natural-looking prosthesis. *(u)* The 5-year follow-up radiograph shows stable bone levels.

CLINICAL OUTCOMES

The results were beautiful and esthetic, and the patient was highly satisfied at the 1- and 5-year follow-ups (Figs 13-1r to 13-1u). No inflammation or prosthetic problems occurred during the follow-up periods. The results were favorable in this case of a metal- and cement-free, screw-retained and removable restoration. If problems such as chipping or subsequent color changes become evident in this type of restoration, they can be easily corrected, just as with titanium implants.

CONCLUSION

The NobelPearl Tapered dental implant system is designed for a broad range of indications, from single to multiple units. It performed very well in this case and supported splinted crowns after bone augmentation. The surgical and prosthetic protocols are comparable to those of titanium implants. These are important factors for the successful integration of a new dental implant system in daily dental practice.

The rationale for using the NobelPearl Tapered dental implant system in the present case is summarized here:

- The NobelPearl system is designed to support a natural appearance of the soft tissue, especially in patients with a thin mucosal phenotype.[1] Zirconia is generally associated with less plaque accumulation[2] and bacterial adhesion[2,3] than titanium.
- The surface of NobelPearl implants is microroughened and hydrophilic for successful osseointegration, while the implant collar is partially machined.

This design is optimal for achieving excellent soft tissue attachment and a minimal inflammatory response.[4]

- NobelPearl implants are made of alumina-toughened zirconia (ATZ) with improved hardness, bending strength, and toughness compared with tetragonal zirconia polycrystals (TZP).[5]
- NobelPearl offers great restorative flexibility thanks to its reversible and cement-free two-piece internal connection.
- The primary stability of the implant is good as a result of its non–self-cutting, tapered body, and the clinical protocol is comparable to that of titanium dental implants.
- NobelPearl is a completely metal-free solution, as even the screw is made of a carbon fiber–reinforced polymer designed for a strong ceramic-to-ceramic connection, which is highly biocompatible.

Restoration with a Custom Patent Implant

Company partner: Zircon Medical
Product: Patent
Clinician: Sebastian Horvath

Patent

THE PATENT DENTAL IMPLANT SYSTEM

In his landmark 2012 review examining the influence of various implant designs and materials on soft and hard tissue stability, Belgian researcher Professor Eric Rompen defined the specific characteristics that a dental implant system must possess to achieve long-term success and guarantee the preservation of stable marginal bone levels.[6] First, ceramic implant materials are preferable to materials such as titanium in the transgingival area. Second, tissue-level designs are more advantageous than bone-level designs with microgaps at the subgingival level. Third, implant systems that do not require the removal or replacement of prosthetic components are preferable.

The Patent Dental Implant System (Zircon Medical) successfully incorporates all the characteristics identified by Rompen as necessary for long-term implant treatment success. Patent is an entirely metal-free dental implant system, employing yttria-stabilized zirconia and an innovative prosthetic glass fiber abutment. Patent also has a true soft tissue–level design, with the crown margin and implant interfacing at the gingival level and its integrated abutment (the ferrule) incorporated inside the body of the crown at the supragingival level. In addition, using Patent implants does not involve any removal or replacement of prosthetic components, and cementation and preparation of the prosthetic components take place supragingivally.

Soft tissue seal

The peri-implant soft tissue serves as a defense barrier that shields the body against attacking pathogens from the outside world. The stronger the soft tissue

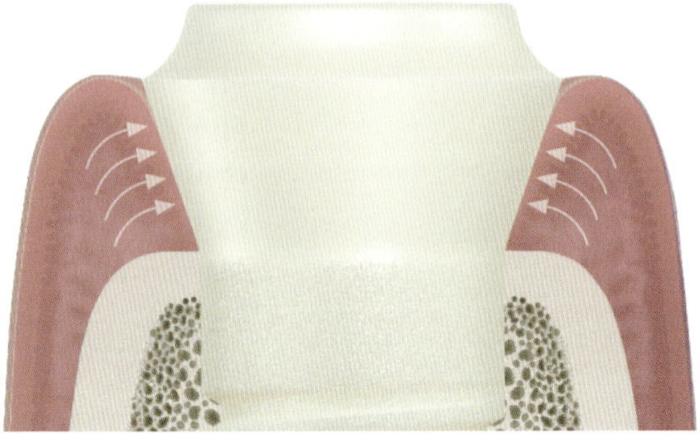

FIG 13-2 › The soft tissue seal that forms around Patent implants prevents pathogenic bacteria in the oral cavity from penetrating beyond the implant into the deeper tissue, where it would promote peri-implantitis and marginal bone loss, among other things.

adaptation to a dental implant is, the harder it is for pathogenic bacteria in the oral cavity to bypass the marginal epithelium and penetrate past the implant into deeper tissue, where they would promote peri-implant inflammation and marginal bone loss, among other things (Fig 13-2).

In histologic analyses, Glauser and Schüpbach[7] observed that the soft tissue seal around Patent implants remained supragingival after a healing period of 4 weeks and that this seal prevented the spread of plaque and calculus toward the underlying bone. In the titanium control implants, however, they observed a significant accumulation of plaque and calculus, which subsequently spread downward toward the marginal epithelium, the point at which the body begins to react. Furthermore, they found that the vertical histoarchitecture at the soft tissue—consisting of connective tissue, marginal epithelium, and sulcular epithelium (ie, the biologic width)—had a highly favorable structure around the Patent implants and was comparable in composition to that of the tissue around natural teeth.

Fast healing and rapid bone formation

A special patented manufacturing process is used to create an osteoconductive surface on the endosteal part of Patent implants. The surface roughness of 6 μm is significantly rougher than conventional ceramic implant surfaces. The surface is also hydrophilic, attracting autologous blood to a particularly high degree. As a result, a fibrin network begins to attach to the surface of the implants just a few minutes after placement, triggering rapid and successful bone formation via contact osteogenesis. The optimization of the early phase of bone healing by these special surface properties has been demonstrated in an animal model study by Glauser and Schüpbach.[7] The two researchers found bone-to-implant contact (BIC) of over 70% for Patent implants after a healing period of just 4 weeks.

Innovative prosthetic concept

In the two-piece Patent Dental Implant System, a glass fiber post is cemented into the 3C platform of the implant and prepared and restored like a natural tooth. The highly stable yet flexible glass fiber post has dentin-like properties and attenuates the masticatory forces transferred from the definitive restoration to the implant. In addition, Patent employs an intraoral impression-taking system that uses the 3C implant platform as the measuring reference rather than a scan body. This facilitates significantly faster and more accurate fabrication of the implant restoration. This system works with the most widely used laboratory software and saves significant time and costs.

Proven long-term success

The clinical success of Patent implants is supported by scientific studies. For example, Brüll et al[8] and Becker et al[9] observed in their 3- and 2-year studies, respectively, that the proportion of keratinized gingiva around Patent implants increased over time. They also reported significantly lower probing depths in gingival pockets around Patent implants and less bleeding on probing than around the natural teeth of the same patients. Long-term protection of the deeper tissue by the strong soft tissue seal around Patent implants has been proven by unique long-term studies. Karapataki et al[10] followed over 90 Patent implants over a functional period of up to 12 years and found that even after this long period of wear, none of the implants showed signs of peri-implantitis. In their long-term follow-up study, Becker et al[11] reported stable bone levels and healthy soft tissue conditions (mucosal recession < 1 mm) around Patent implants after a functional period of over 9 years. They also documented survival rates similar to those of titanium implants (95.8%).

CASE STUDY

A 54-year-old woman requested a general restoration of her teeth. As a part of this complex case, the mandibular right quadrant was restored. The patient reported that the old restoration had been placed about 20 years prior, after the right first molar was lost due to endodontic complications. A few years after placement of the restoration, the mandibular right second premolar was endodontically treated through the placed restoration. Now the patient reported increasing sensitivity in the second molar due to ill-fitting restoration margins (Figs 13-3a to 13-3c).

It was planned to restore the area with all-ceramic crowns in the sites of the second premolar and second molar, with an implant-retained restoration in the site of the first molar. The implant-retained restoration was planned to be a new fixed dental prosthesis to reduce the load on the endodontically treated second premolar and to reduce future risks by incorporating an endodontically treated tooth in a larger restoration. The surgical procedure is illustrated in Figs 13-3d to 13-3x.

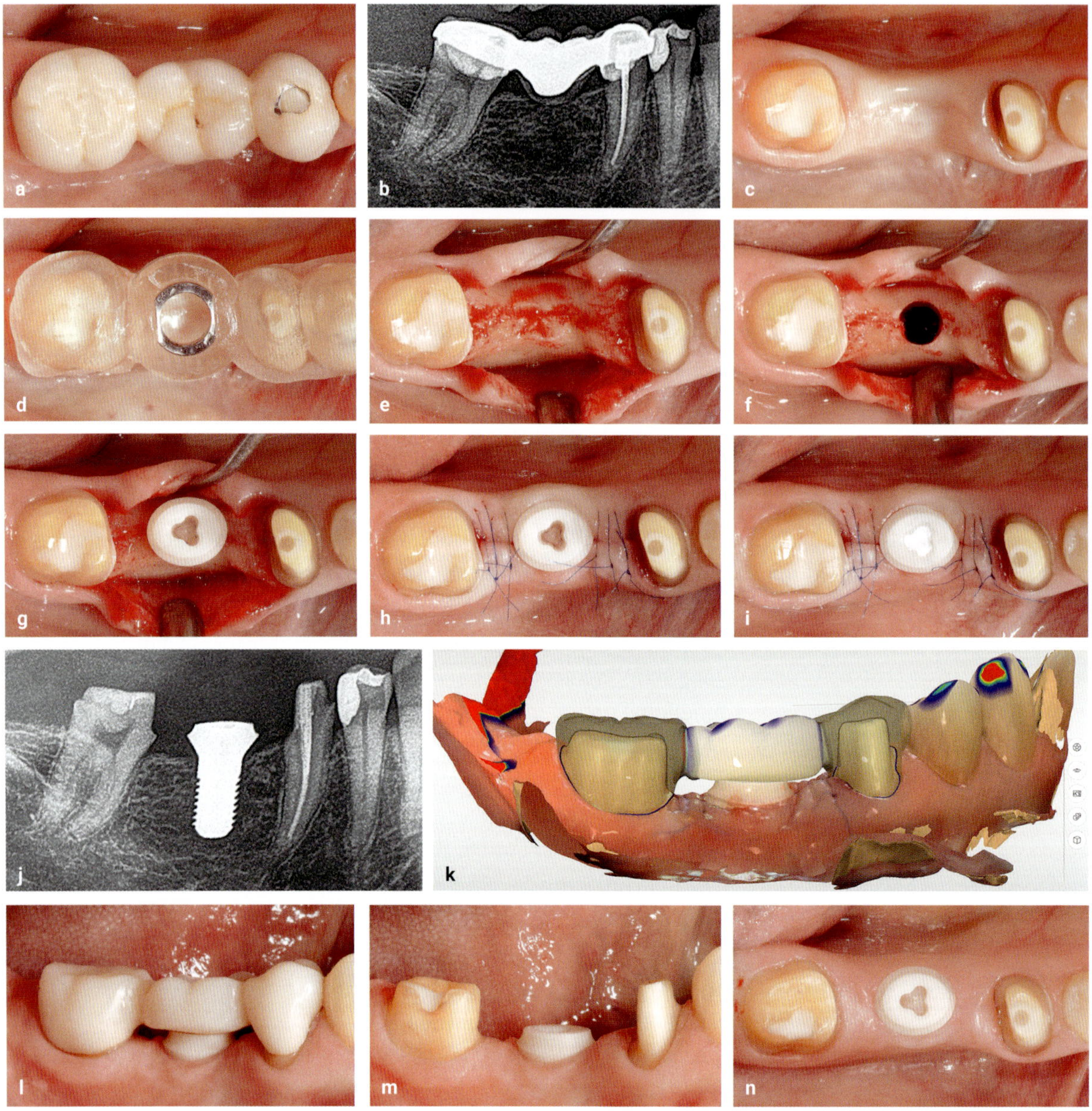

FIG 13-3 › *(a)* Initial situation in the mandibular right quadrant. The patient reported increasing sensitivity in the second molar. *(b)* Initial radiograph showing the mandibular right quadrant. Note the ill-fitting distal margin of the restoration in the site of the second molar. CBCT revealed sufficient bone volume in the site of the first molar to place an implant. *(c)* Clinical situation prior to surgery. *(d)* Surgical guide in place. *(e)* A full-thickness flap was elevated to gain access to the bone. *(f)* The osteotomy was performed using the drilling protocol for hard bone. *(g)* A custom Patent implant was placed, and sufficient primary stability (30 Ncm) was achieved. *(h)* Wound closure. *(i)* The 3C implant platform was sealed with PTFE tape. *(j)* Radiographic evaluation of the implant position. *(k)* In the area of the freshly placed implant, the provisional restoration was planned as a flat pontic with a distance of about 0.1 mm between the implant and the provisional restoration. *(l)* Clinical situation 3 months after implant placement. Healing was uneventful. *(m and n)* The implant was stable, and the surrounding soft tissue presented itself as healthy.

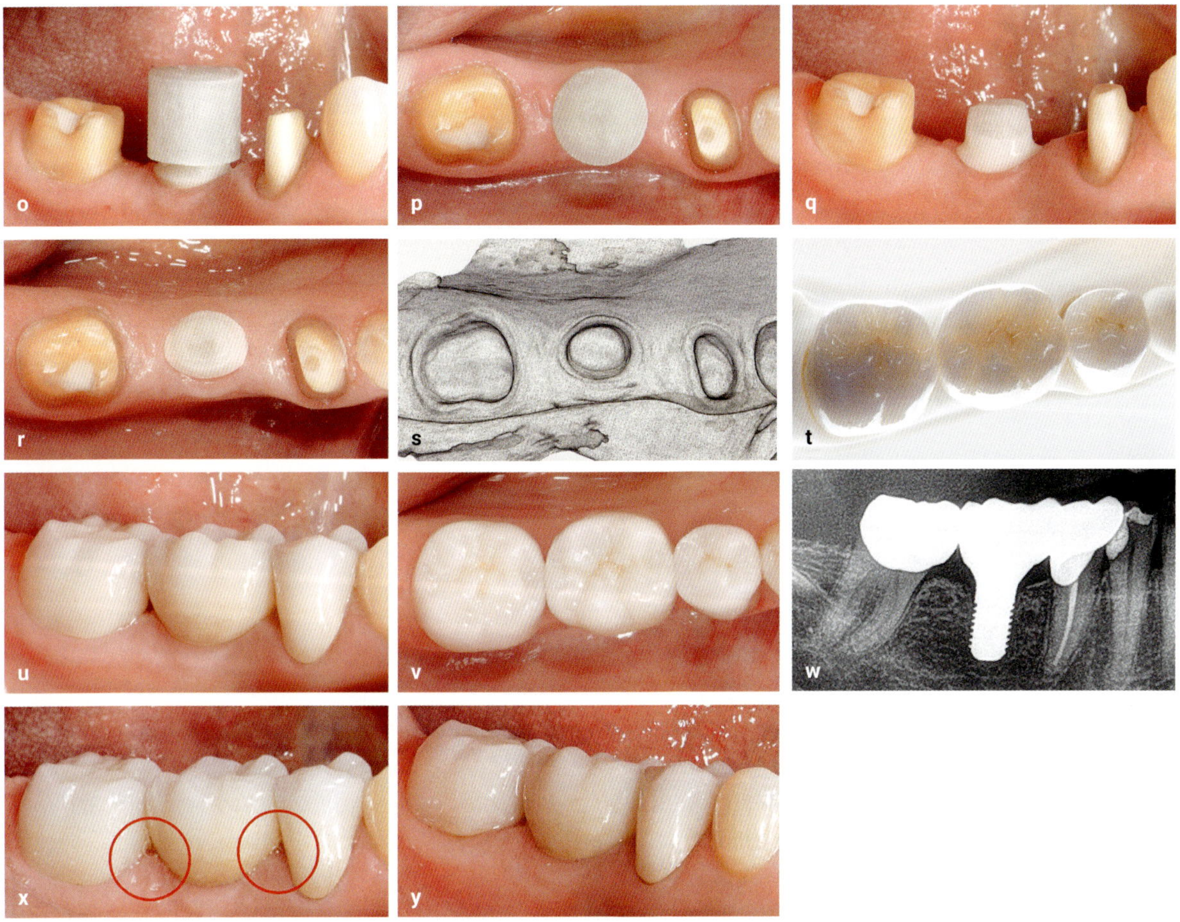

FIG 13-3 *(cont)* › *(o)* For the prosthetic reconstruction, a glass fiber post and core assembly was cemented on the implant. *(p)* The post and core assembly was prefabricated and tightly fitted into the implant connection. *(q and r)* Following this buildup, the implant was prepared for a full-crown restoration just like a natural tooth. *(s)* An intraoral scan was performed for the prosthetic workflow in the lab. *(t)* Three monolithic zirconia crowns were fabricated. (Ceramic work performed by Claus-Peter Schulz.) *(u and v)* Intraoral views of the treatment result. *(w)* Radiographic evaluation of the treatment result. *(x)* Results at the 1-year follow-up. *(y)* Results at the 3.5-year follow-up. The tissues are healthy and stable.

Metal-Free Implants in the Esthetic Zone with a 3.5-Year Follow-up

Company partner: Straumann
Product: Straumann PURE
Clinician: Juan Blanco Carrión

Healthy-looking oral soft tissues and pearly white teeth are deemed essential for a beautiful smile and good self-esteem, which directly contribute to better overall health-related quality of life.[12,13] Dental implants made of titanium and titanium alloys are considered the gold standard in implant dentistry due to their exceptional mechanical properties and long-term clinical success.[14] The main drawback of titanium implants is their dark gray color, which may occasionally be visible through the peri-implant mucosa, compromising esthetic outcomes, especially in the anterior region and areas with thin mucosa. Ceramic implants are designed to achieve a better esthetic outcome, and the published scientific evidence is vastly in support of their clinical application.[15–17] Clinical studies on ceramic implants have demonstrated exceptional outcomes, with survival rates from 97.6% to 100%.[15–19]

The Straumann PURE Ceramic Implant System results from more than 12 years of uncompromising research and development. This system combines quality, precision, strength, clinical success, and flexible treatment protocols to create an innovative solution to meet patient needs. Straumann PURE implants are made from yttria-stabilized tetragonal zirconia polycrystal (Y-TZP), which is an attractive metal-free alternative to titanium that exhibits better corrosion and wear resistance in addition to excellent flexural strength.[20–23] The compressive strength of zirconia implants has also been found to be adequate, and they can withstand occlusal loads for a longer period.[24] The ZLA surface of Straumann PURE implants is characterized by roughness values similar to the well-researched and proven Straumann SLA surface.[25] In preclinical studies, the ZLA surface demonstrated similar healing patterns, healing times, and osseointegration measured in terms of peri-implant bone density and BIC[26,27] (Fig 13-4).

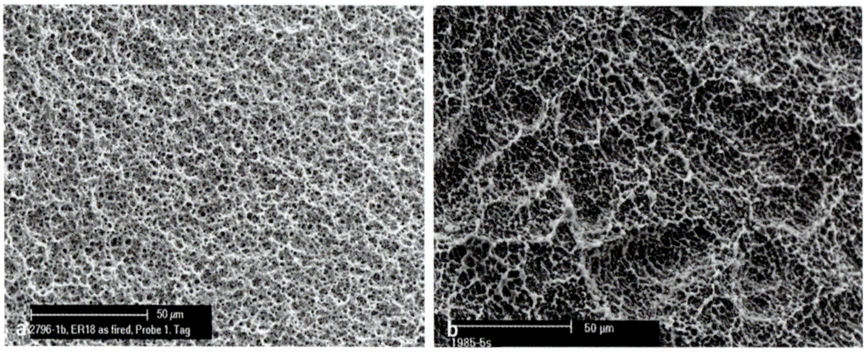

FIG 13-4 › Microrough intraosseous implant surfaces. *(a)* Zirconia ZLA surface. *(b)* Titanium SLA surface.

INITIAL PRESENTATION

A 55-year-old systemically healthy man presented to our clinic looking for a functional and esthetic metal-free solution for the edentulous areas exposed when he smiled. His dental history revealed the extraction of the maxillary right and left second premolars due to endodontic failure.

TREATMENT PLANNING

Clinical and radiographic assessments showed healed sites with optimal hard and soft tissue availability for placing two Straumann PURE ceramic implants with diameters of 4.1 × 12 mm (Figs 13-5a and 13-5b). The patient provided informed consent following an explanation of the procedure.

SURGICAL PROCEDURE

Supracrestal and intrasulcular incisions were made with the elevation of full-thickness mucoperiosteal flaps (Figs 13-5c and 13-5d). The implant sites were prepared following manufacturer guidelines (Fig 13-5e), and alignment pins were used as a reference for achieving the optimal prosthetically driven position of the implants. Healing abutments and simple sutures were placed to close the flaps (Figs 13-5f and 13-5g), and periapical radiographs were taken (Fig 13-5h).

The sutures were removed 1 week later, and ceramic healing abutments were placed.

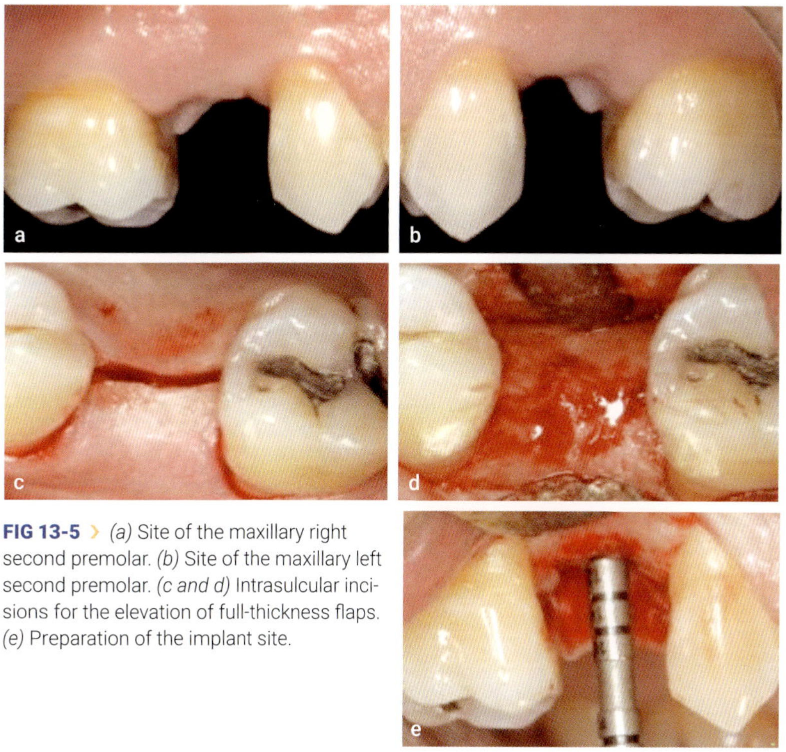

FIG 13-5 › *(a)* Site of the maxillary right second premolar. *(b)* Site of the maxillary left second premolar. *(c and d)* Intrasulcular incisions for the elevation of full-thickness flaps. *(e)* Preparation of the implant site.

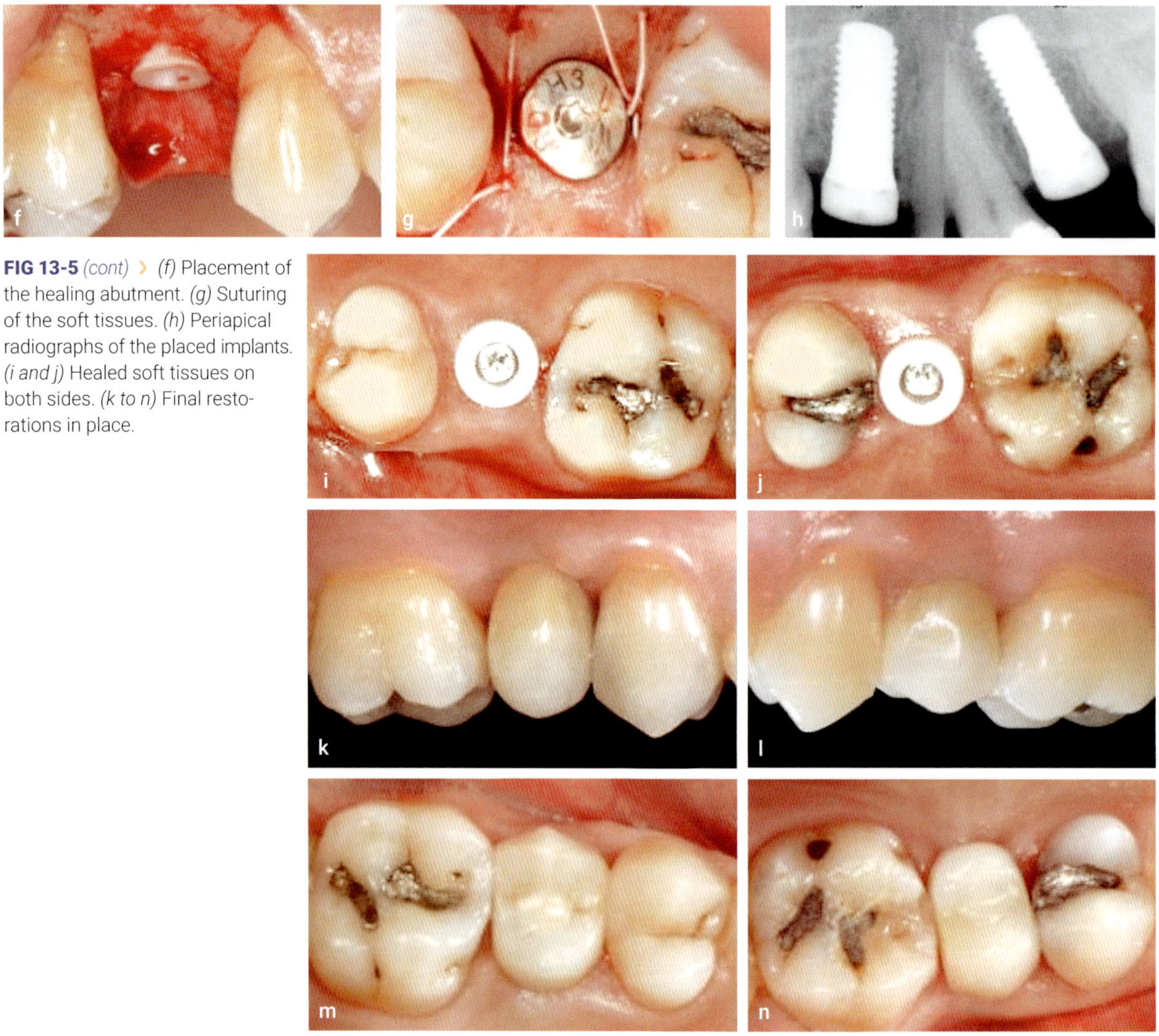

FIG 13-5 *(cont)* › *(f)* Placement of the healing abutment. *(g)* Suturing of the soft tissues. *(h)* Periapical radiographs of the placed implants. *(i and j)* Healed soft tissues on both sides. *(k to n)* Final restorations in place.

PROSTHETIC PROCEDURE

After soft tissue healing (Figs 13-5i and 13-5j), the patient attended a follow-up visit, and digital impressions were taken. This information was sent to the laboratory technician, who designed and milled the final restorations with Straumann PUREbase abutments.

The final restorations were screwed on the implants (Figs 13-5k to 13-5n), and a final radiograph was taken (Figs 13-5o and 13-5p). The patient was also given oral hygiene instructions and was enrolled in a yearly hygiene maintenance program.

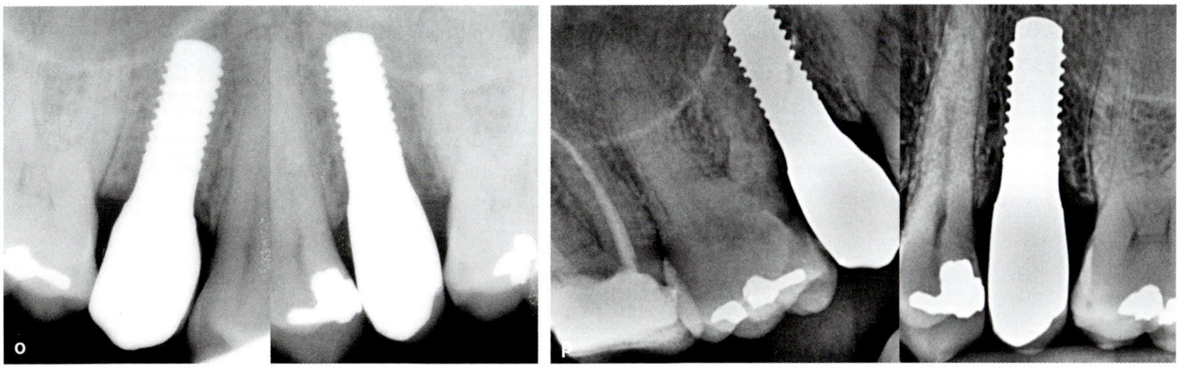

FIG 13-5 *(cont)* › *(o and p)* Radiographs with the implants and restorations in place.

TREATMENT OUTCOMES

The patient remained very satisfied with the functional and esthetic result of the procedure 3.5 years later. The periapical radiographs revealed excellent bone maintenance around the ceramic implants.

All-Ceramic Implant–Supported Dentures for Anterior Teeth with Severe Periodontal Damage

Company partner: CeramTec
Product: Zeramex XT
Clinician: Thomas Mehnert

Two-piece ceramic implants are receiving increasing attention due to their very good biologic and material properties. Thanks to their low plaque accumulation and excellent soft tissue biocompatibility, ceramic implants should be considered in preference to titanium implants for patients with periodontitis. This clinical case describes the successful use of two-piece ceramic implants.

CASE STUDY

A 59-year-old woman presented to our orthognathic surgery practice following a good experience with a previous ceramic implant in the site of the maxillary left first molar with sinus elevation. Despite having undergone a prior bone augmentation procedure performed by a high-profile expert in periodontology, the maxillary central incisors showed heavy periodontal damage (Stage III, 2020 S3 guidelines) and were not worth saving (Figs 13-6a and 13-6b).

A partial denture was considered too risky due to bone loss around the neighboring teeth. After a hygiene protocol was implemented and periodontal preparation of the teeth was performed, it was decided to restore the teeth using two-piece Zeramex XT ceramic implants.

SURGICAL PHASE

After extraction of the maxillary central incisors and curettage of the extraction sockets, the surgical sites were reopened 3 months later for placement of the two-piece XT ceramic implants with a diameter of 4.2 mm and a length of 12 mm, according to implant guidelines for the anterior maxilla and in compliance with the drilling protocol of the manufacturer. The vertical insertion depth was oriented around the mucous membrane thickness and the crestal bone of the neighboring teeth.

Due to the special thermal cauterization method used in their collar area, XT implants can be inserted between 1.6 and 0.6 mm supracrestal (Figs 13-6c and 13-6d). Simultaneous horizontal bone augmentation was performed with a mixture of autogenous bone chips harvested from the retromolar mandible, xenogeneic bone replacement material (Bio-Oss), and a collagen membrane (Jason, Straumann) (Fig 13-6e).

PROSTHETIC PHASE

The exposure was performed after 4 months using polyetheretherketone (PEEK) gingival formers (Fig 13-6f). After prolonged antiphlogistic therapy of the peri-implant gingiva with chlorhexidine due to recurrent bleeding, the individual gingival formers were molded based on the master cast featuring the gingival mask (Fig 13-6g).

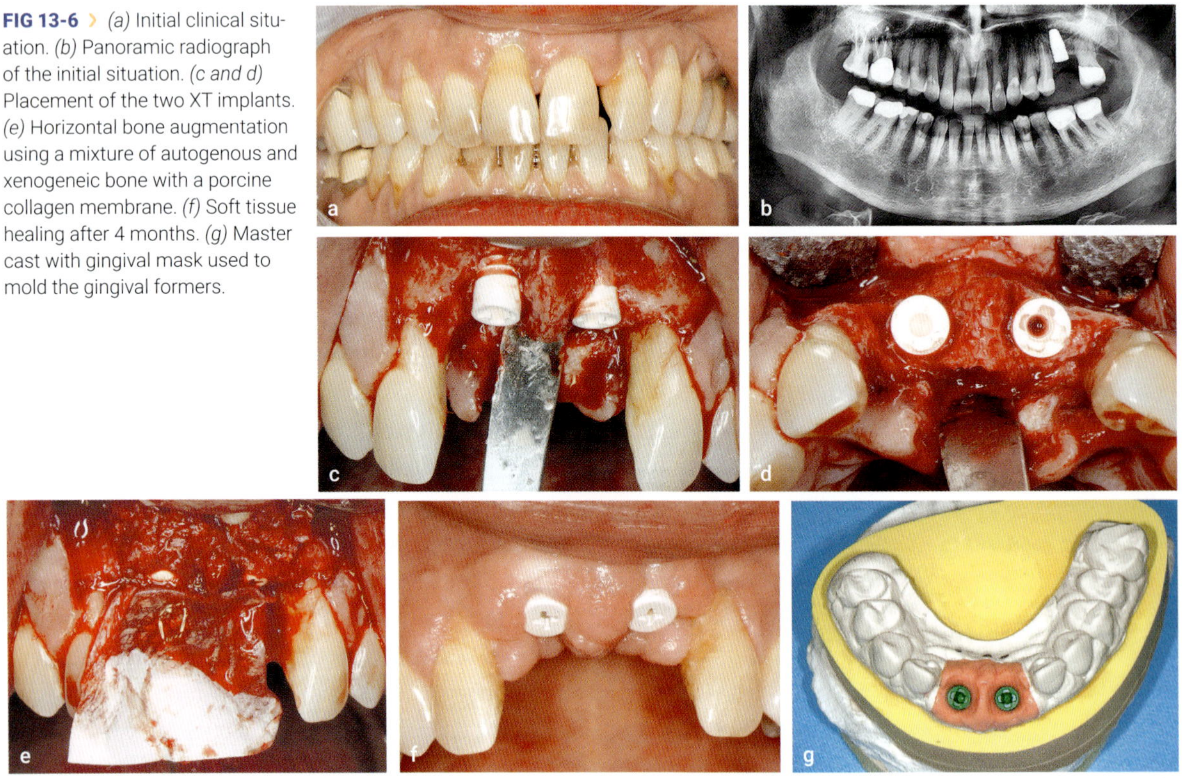

FIG 13-6 › *(a)* Initial clinical situation. *(b)* Panoramic radiograph of the initial situation. *(c and d)* Placement of the two XT implants. *(e)* Horizontal bone augmentation using a mixture of autogenous and xenogeneic bone with a porcine collagen membrane. *(f)* Soft tissue healing after 4 months. *(g)* Master cast with gingival mask used to mold the gingival formers.

In this case, the gingival formers were created with an injectable hybrid composite (Beautifil Flow Plus F03, Shofu Dental) based on PEEK abutments (Zeramex XT Provisional RB) with a maximum wearing time of 180 days and inserted into the mouth with the associated Vicarbo provisional screws (insertion torque maximum of 15 Ncm) (Figs 13-6h and 13-6i).

The individual zirconia abutments and the tooth crowns were created with CAD/CAM technology (3Shape software) according to the Labside method using the Zeramex XT Zerabase X RB (engaged) and RB scan bodies (Figs 13-6j and 13-6k).

The zirconia crowns were then pressed from Ivoclar Vivadent IPS e.max LT Press ingots and adjusted to match the neighboring crowns with Ivoclar Vivadent e.max enamel (Fig 13-6l). The individual definitive abutments were bonded to the matching Zeramex XT bonding platform with the Multilink Hybrid Abutment (Ivoclar Vivadent) and finally inserted into the mouth with the RB16550 Vicarbo screw at the specified torque (25 Ncm). The subsequent bonding of the ceramic crowns was performed with Panavia 21 (Kuraray) (Fig 13-6m).

FOLLOW-UP

Follow-up examinations after 6 and 12 months showed absolutely no inflammation (Fig 13-6n). Bleeding on probing was absent at both follow-ups. The patient was very satisfied with the two-piece ceramic crowns, which was reflected in her motivation to have them regularly inspected and professionally cleaned.

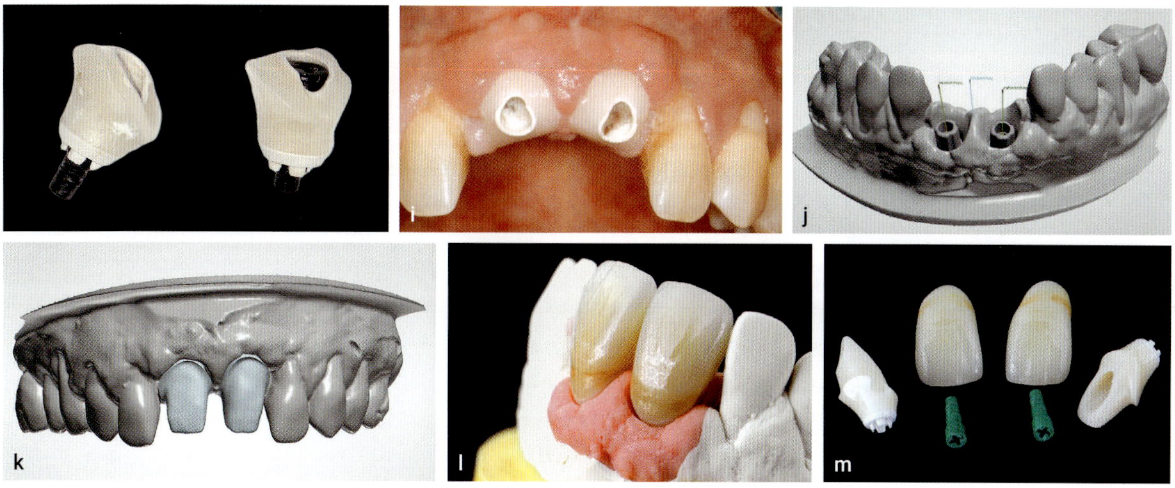

FIG 13-6 *(cont)* › *(h and i)* Extra- and intraoral views of the gingival formers. *(j and k)* Using CAD/CAM software to design the restoration. *(l)* Crowns created from the e.max ingots. *(m)* Crowns and abutments ready for placement.

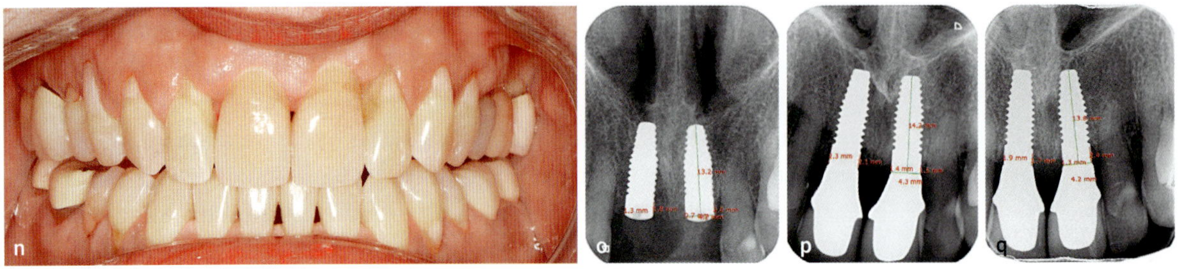

FIG 13-6 *(cont)* › *(n to q)* Intraoral view and radiographs after 12 months showing healthy tissues with no inflammation.

An assessment of the peri-implant bone structure with standardized radiographs (right-angle technique) and an evaluation using DBSWIN software (Dürr Dental) were also performed at 6 and 12 months after exposure (Figs 13-6o to 13-6q). After moderate bone loss in the first 6 months due to the restructuring process in the crestal area (which was expected based on the literature), bone levels stabilized after 12 months, with a very strong tendency toward remodeling.

SUMMARY

The advantages of two-piece ceramic implants over titanium implants are increasingly winning out in specific clinical scenarios. The very good biocompatibility of high-performance ceramic with the surrounding soft tissue means that ceramic implants can be used even in patients with prior periodontal damage as long as the appropriate protocols are followed. Periodontal rehabilitation of the teeth and regular professional cleaning are essential for success. A paradigm shift from titanium to ceramic implants is conceivable for this patient group in the future. My patients and I can look back on very positive clinical experiences involving over 400 Zeramex XT implants placed between 2017 and 2021.

Minimally Invasive Implant Placement in a Patient with High Expectations

Company partner: COHO Biomedical Technology
Product: ZiBone
Clinician: Franco Giancola

In recent years, patient demand for healthier and more attractive implants has led to the emergence of zirconia as the material of choice. Leading implant companies are increasingly offering zirconia systems with different surfaces, shapes, and sizes, in addition to traditional titanium implants to address various patient needs. Considerable progress has been made toward improving the osseointegration and reliability of zirconia implants, but it is up to clinicians to devise new operating strategies to achieve outstanding results.

The social and professional milieu of dental practices has undergone significant changes. Patients with the desire to regain their smiles and ability to chew with metal-free restorations present more often than ever with high health risks and/or very high expectations. Dentists are increasingly being called upon to treat patients with diabetes mellitus, heart disease, and allergies and patients suffering from severe osteoporosis and bone atrophy. In these situations, it is imperative to perform brief, minimally traumatic procedures without complications of any sort. In addition, work commitments and fast-paced lives lead many patients to demand high therapeutic standards. They want quick, effective procedures that don't force them to put their professional and social lives on hold. Finally, the high costs of running dental practices and rising incidences of litigation have caused many practitioners to minimize invasive treatments, reduce operating times, and strive to improve clinical results.

PATIENT EXPECTATIONS

Whenever patients set foot in a dental practice, they are making an overt plea for help to heal and restore impaired dental function or appearance. They share their health problems and express fears and desires. Implant surgery is a medical procedure that can be risky. Therefore, before operating, one must always remember Hippocrates' exhortation: "primum non nocere"—first do no harm. Dentists must rely on techniques and devices that promote healing and prevent damage to the tissues. Treatment plans must be shared with patients so they can provide informed consent. Patients must participate fully because clinical results depend on the materials used, the clinician's skill, the biology of the tissues, and also very much on patient collaboration.

SURGICAL TISSUE ENVIRONMENT

Aging, early tooth loss, and concomitant metabolic disorders often lead to inflamed gingival tissues, alveolar ridge atrophy, dental granulomas, and poor bone tissue quality. A winning therapeutic strategy requires an accurate evaluation of the local tissues. In case of infections (periodontitis, granulomas, or sinusitis), it is imperative to first heal the mouth with targeted periodontal treatments, extract affected teeth, and cleanse infected sockets. Ozone therapy sessions (local and systemic) and/or hyperbaric oxygen therapy are very beneficial for these patients. Nutraceuticals such as lithothamnion calcareum, vitamin D, ganoderma lucidum, and grapefruit seed extract improve tissue quality, promote wound healing, and improve implant osseointegration.

IMPLANT PLANNING

In patients with health problems, minimally invasive surgery is especially important. These patients are more fragile and tire quickly, so surgery must be minimally traumatic, fast, and free of complications. Only a careful case study, detailed surgical planning, and the best choice of materials will ensure clinical success.

In extensive implant rehabilitation cases, prosthetic surgical guides are indispensable. Anesthesia must be sufficient to prevent any pain during surgery without being excessive, which could cause undesirable side effects. Whenever possible, flapless techniques and magneto-dynamic surgery should be the first choices. To limit discomfort after surgery from pain, swelling, and bleeding, as well as to promote wound healing, systemic ozone therapy sessions and platelet growth factor infiltration (i-PRF) are recommended.

IMPLANT SITE PREPARATION

Because the body regards implants as a foreign body, acceptance by the host tissue must be encouraged to avoid excessive damage. Aggressive techniques and overheating of the bone can lead to bone necrosis, scarring, intense inflammatory processes with excessive pain, and even implant loss. Surgery should be carried out confidently and gently to facilitate normal wound healing with good outcomes. Clinicians must create the best conditions for good implant osseointegration to take place. Careful preparation is a fundamental step to ensure clinical success.

Gingival access

When bone conditions are optimal, a flapless technique should be used. The mucogingival incision is performed using circular zirconia mucotomes mounted on a micromotor contra-angle and rotated using tilting movements in contact with the cortical bone to sever all connective fibers. The incised tissue flap is then removed with a scalpel. In cases where a broader view of the surgical site is needed or if bone regeneration is required, the soft tissue incision is performed with zirconia scalpels angled at 15 degrees or with tissue trimmers mounted on a turbine and rotated quickly without irrigation.

Osteotomy

Zirconia burs are used in cases where the bone tissue is optimal or when it is necessary to harvest autogenous bone for guided bone regeneration. The cortical bone is penetrated with a rosette or lance drill positioned first obliquely to avoid slippage and then vertically to drill the bone to less than the needed depth. A depth gauge is inserted and a radiograph is taken to assess the angle and length of the preparation.

Next, a sequence of drills with increasing diameters is used until the right size for the chosen implant is achieved. The drills must be used without excessive pressure, in a back-and-forth motion, and without lateral angulation to avoid damaging the instrument. In cases of spongiosa and osteoporotic bone (maxilla), it is advisable to make an undersized preparation. Compact lamellar bone (mandible) requires an additional round of drilling with tappers to widen the implant osteotomy and avoid excessive tension.

CASE REPORT

The patient in this case was treated at different times, first in the maxilla and then in the mandible, and the treatment spanned several years. Implants (Zirkolith and ZiBone) were chosen based on patient needs and bone quality.

A 54-year-old woman requested replacement of her old crowns, which were no longer esthetically acceptable. She reported bad breath and gums that bled

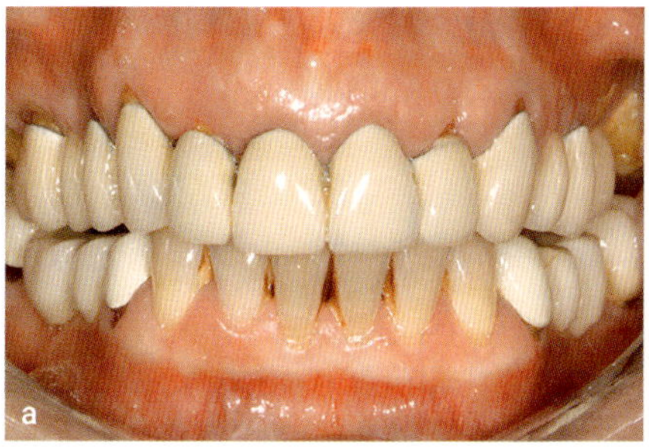

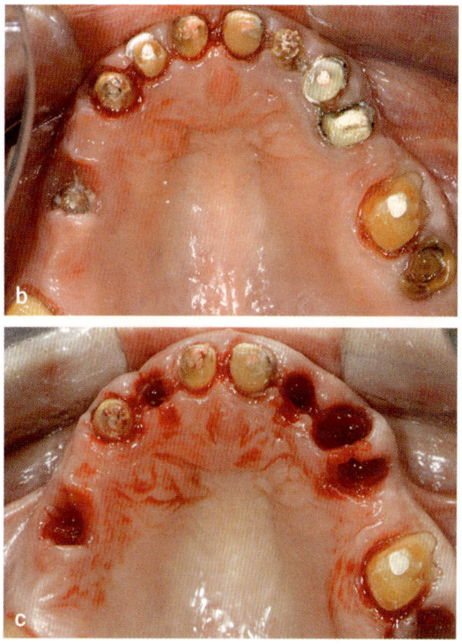

FIG 13-7 › *(a)* Clinical situation before surgery. *(b)* Occlusal view of the initial situation. *(c)* Well-preserved extraction sockets after tooth extraction.

easily. The patient also had high esthetic expectations and wanted only metal-free materials to be used in the treatment. Upon removal of the patient's original prostheses, numerous devitalized teeth with softened dentinal tissue, bleeding periodontal pockets, and generalized gingival recession were noted (Figs 13-7a and 13-7b). The radiologic study revealed horizontal bone atrophy of the alveolar ridges in the edentulous areas and periapical granulomas in correspondence with the devitalized teeth. The selected treatment plan was implant rehabilitation in progressive steps.

The affected teeth were extracted via an atraumatic piezosurgical technique, and the sockets were curetted with surgical spoons and disinfected according to a photodynamic method (HELBO Therapy, Bredent). Because the extraction sockets were well preserved (Fig 13-7c), it is was decided to immediately place the one-piece implants. Radiologic evaluation of the maxillary left arch showed reduced bone density (Type D3/D4), so the implant sites in that region were underprepared, and self-tapping Zirkolith Z5m(t) implants from Z-Systems (Fig 13-7d) were placed in the sites of the maxillary left canine and second premolar with insertion torques of 35 Ncm without irrigation. Subsequently, the flaps were sutured, the abutments were prepared, and a provisional previously prepared in the laboratory was adapted (Fig 13-7e). The sutures were removed at the first follow-up. The flaps were well closed, and the surrounding mucosa was healthy and well attached to the zirconia implants (Figs 13-7f and 13-7g).

Two months after the initial surgery, two additional two-piece Zirkolith Z5c implants were placed in the right side of the maxilla. The preparation was performed with zirconia burs after lifting the flaps (Figs 13-7h to 13-7i), and the implants were placed (Figs 13-7j to 13-7l). The implant abutments were shaped after complete osseointegration (Fig 13-7m).

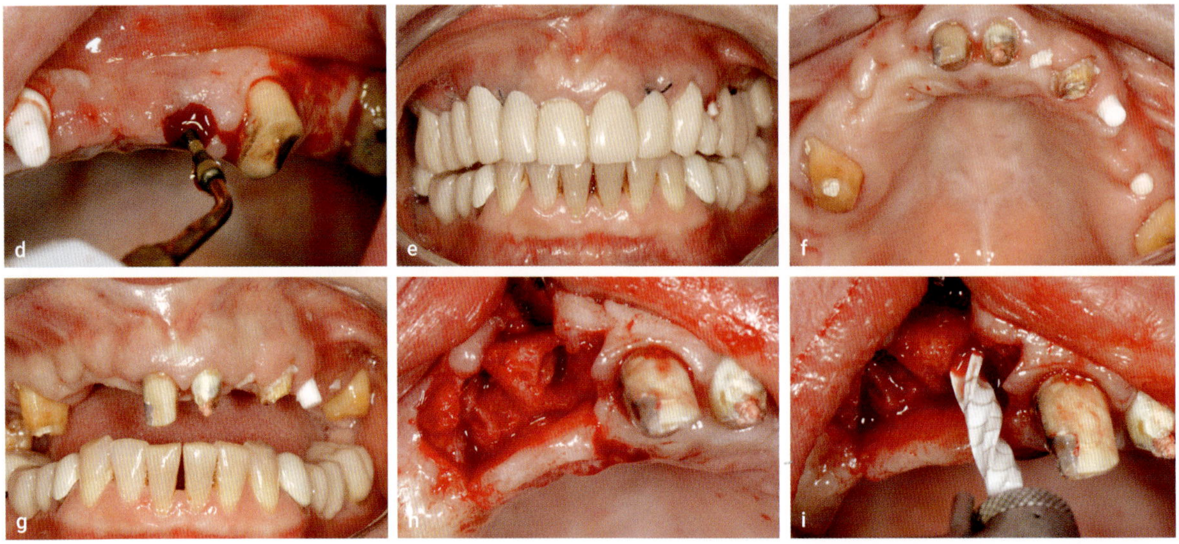

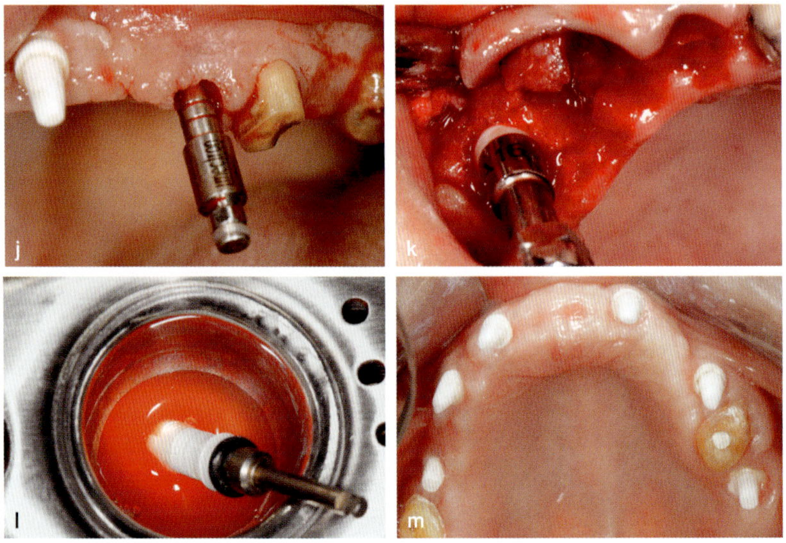

FIG 13-7 *(cont)* › *(d)* Initial osteotomy via Piezosurgery (insert 1MIS, Mectron). *(e)* Frontal view of the protective device after surgery. *(f)* Occlusal view after removal of the sutures. *(g)* Situation 15 days after surgery. *(h)* Lifting of the gingival flaps and cleaning of the extraction sockets. *(i)* Performance of the osteotomy with a zirconia drill at low speed without irrigation. *(j)* Condensing the jaw bone. *(k)* Slow insertion of the implants. *(l)* Bioactivation of the implant with injectable platelet-rich fibrin (i-PRF). *(m)* Implant abutments properly shaped using diamond burs under copious irrigation after complete osseointegration.

The patient, happy with the results of the implant placement in the maxilla 6 months later, decided to undergo rehabilitation of the edentulous areas of the mandible. The alveolar ridges were of greater density (Type D1/D2) and reduced thickness (Fig 13-7n), so it was decided to use smaller cylindrical one-piece ZiBone implants (Zr-I4011, COHO Biomedical Technology; Fig 13-7o) in the sites of the mandibular left and right second premolars and first molars.

Mucosal access was performed with a flapless technique using circular mucotomes mounted on a contra-angle (Fig 13-7p). The osteotomy was carried out with zirconia drills at low speed and without irrigation to the predefined dimensions (Figs 13-7q to 13-7s). The one-piece ZiBone implants were first screwed in mechanically with a micromotor and then with a manual ratchet (Figs 13-7t

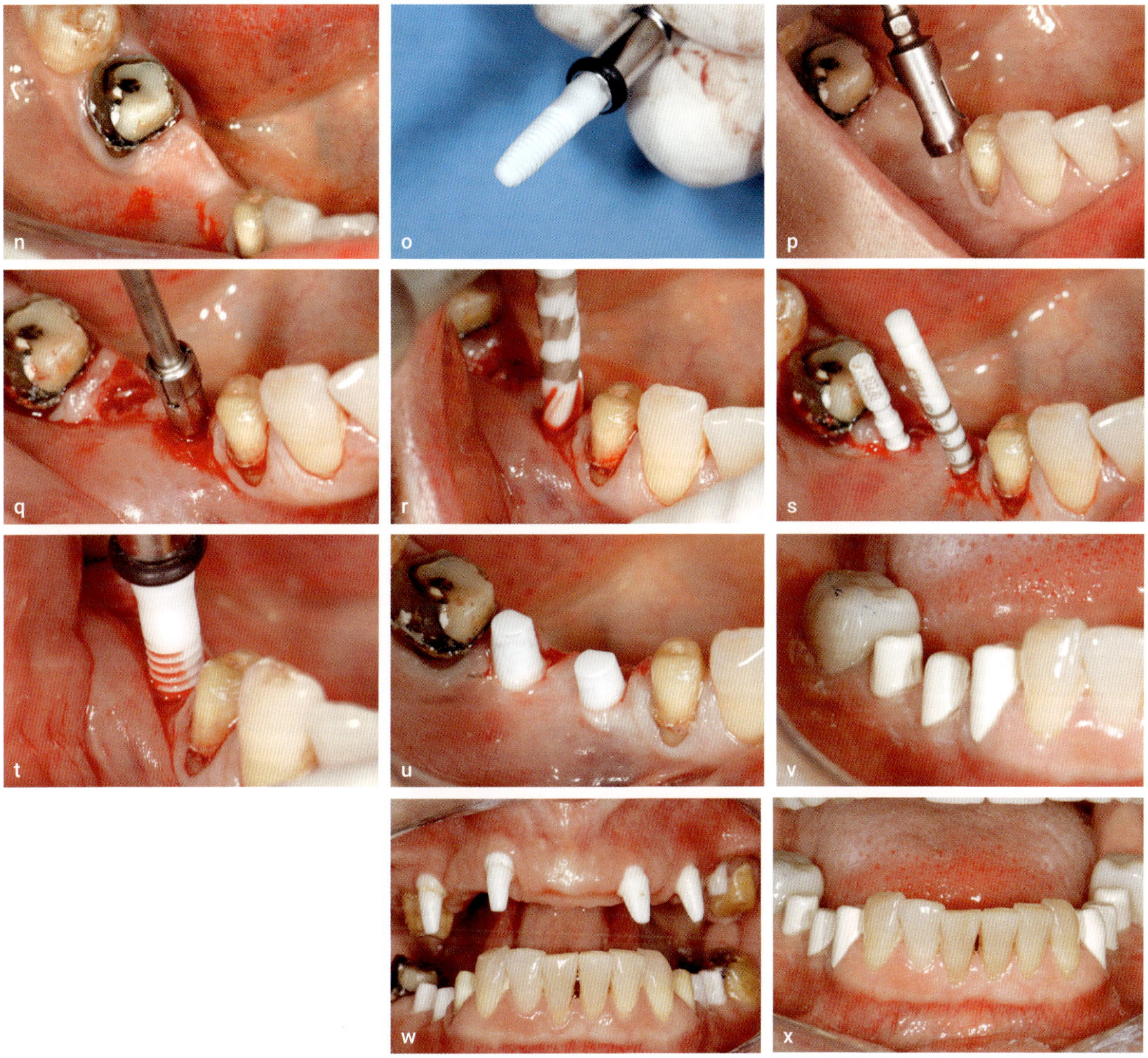

FIG 13-7 *(cont)* › *(n)* The edentulous area of the mandible before surgery. *(o)* One-piece ZiBone implant. *(p)* Gingival access using a circular metal mucotome for a flapless technique. *(q)* Initial osteotomy with a pilot drill. (r) Progressive enlargement of the implant site using a zirconia drill. *(s)* Depth gauges used to evaluate the correct length and positioning of the preparations. *(t)* Slowly screwing the implant in place. *(u)* Correct positioning of the ZiBone implants. *(v)* Zirconia implant abutments covered with PEEK caps to improve the structure and achieve excellent esthetics. *(w)* Frontal view of the implants in position. *(x)* View of the natural teeth and the PEEK caps on the zirconia abutments.

and 13-7u). The implants were subsequently protected with fixed resin devices until osseointegration was complete (Fig 13-7v).

The decision was made to complete prosthetic rehabilitation on the implants 2 years after starting treatment. Given the complexity of the work and the patient's desire for a metal-free prosthesis, all-zirconia crowns were fabricated. PEEK caps were positioned over the abutments (Figs 13-7w and 13-7x). PEEK is a high-density thermoplastic polymer with exceptional physical and chemical properties

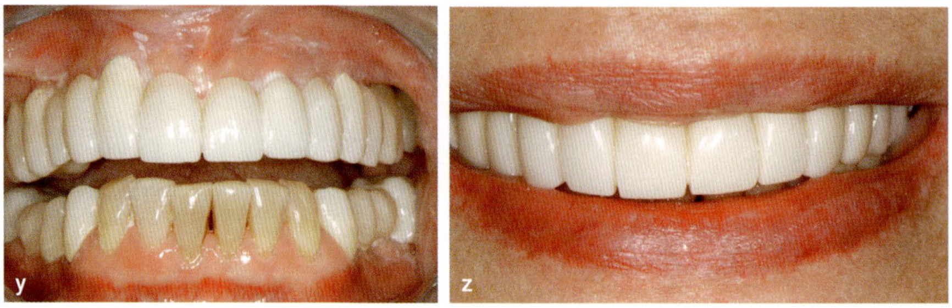

FIG 13-7 *(cont)* › *(y)* Frontal view after cementation of the zirconia crowns. *(z)* Patient's smile at the end of prosthetic implant rehabilitation.

with a linear aromatic semicrystalline structure. Its elasticity allows it to protect the implant from masticatory overload leading to peri-implantitis or fracture of the implant. PEEK's resistance to abrasion also makes it a suitable material for long-term rehabilitation.

At subsequent follow-ups, the gingiva appeared healthy and pink without any bleeding. The patient reported comfort when chewing and improved self-esteem thanks to a more esthetic smile. Clinical and radiologic evaluations after 1 year revealed excellent osseointegration of the implants, so we proceeded to take precision impressions and create a fixed prosthesis. Finally, two all-ceramic joined crowns were cemented onto the PEEK caps to provide elasticity to the structure and excellent esthetics (Figs 13-7y and 13-7z).

CONCLUSION

Zirconia implants on the market today have reached very high standards of reliability. Thanks to improvements in production processes and surface treatments, ceramic implants are very resistant to wear and integrate well with the surrounding bone. Placing two-piece zirconia implants in healthy patients with ideal bone conditions is quite simple. The challenge that will be confronted in the next few years is learning to use ceramic implants to successfully rehabilitate at-risk patients in a less traumatic way. Clinicians must have a thorough understanding of implant systems and acquire skills in minimally invasive surgical techniques for clinical success with minimal risk.

Considerations for Ceramic Implants

Company partner: Z-Systems
Product: Z-Lock, Z5 Implants
Clinician: Jochen Mellinghoff

Z-SYSTEMS swiss ceramic implants

Readers may wonder which ceramic implants and surgical instruments should be used to start working with ceramic implants. My path to ceramic implantology was triggered in 2000 by a patient who received all-ceramic crowns and partial crowns after a devitalized premolar was removed at another practice. The patient

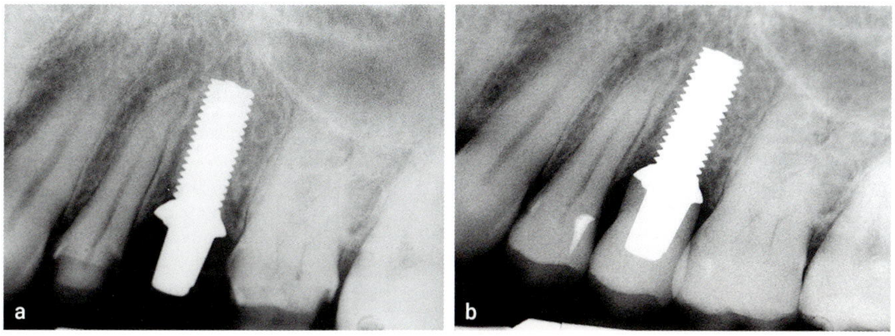

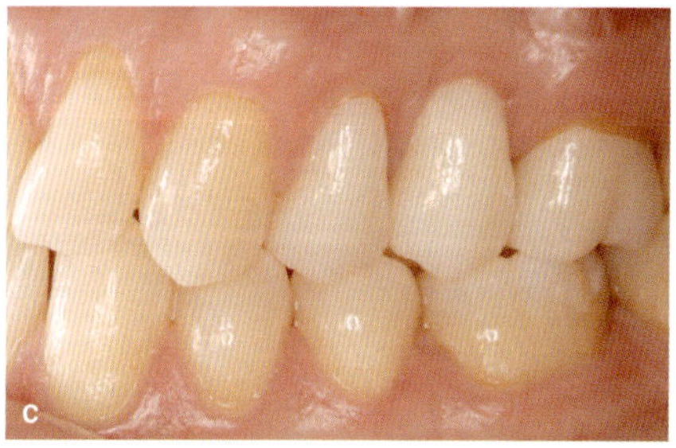

FIG 13-8 › *(a)* Implant in place. *(b)* Implant in place with crown. *(c)* Clinical and esthetic results.

requested that we replace the missing maxillary left second premolar with a ceramic implant. At the time, there were two ceramic implant systems to choose from: one from Professor Dr Sandhaus and one from the company Z-Systems. We decided to use the Z-Systems implants and never imagined that Professor Sandhaus, as a pioneer and trailblazer in the field of ceramic implants, would later become our mentor.

In accordance with the patient's request, he received a Z-Lock 3 implant in the site of the maxillary left second premolar in 2004, which was restored with a lithium disilicate crown, as illustrated in Fig 13-8.

As fate would have it, my own maxillary left first molar had to be removed in spring 2005 and was replaced with a Z-Systems ceramic implant at the end of the year, as illustrated in Fig 13-9.

Because the experience with ceramic implants in our practice was very positive, we started contributing to the team developing ceramic implantology over the years. This was dictated by the progress that had already been made in titanium implantology. All implants described in these cases are still in function today and represent 18 years of experience.

Implants with more aggressive threads (Z5m[t]) (Fig 13-10) were also introduced by Z-Systems. These implants offer improved primary stability and can be used minimally invasively in special indications.

The path from one- to two-piece ceramic implants was paved by dentists with clinical experience. Academic and industry research was concerned mainly with advancing developments in titanium implants. The use of angled abutments

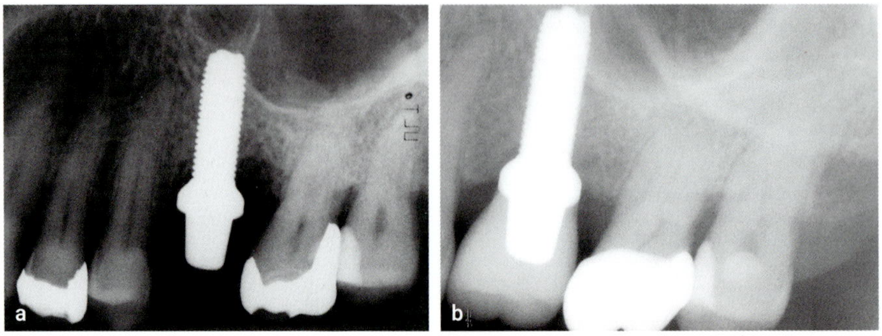

FIG 13-9 › *(a)* Implant in place. *(b)* Implant in place with crown. *(c)* Clinical and esthetic results.

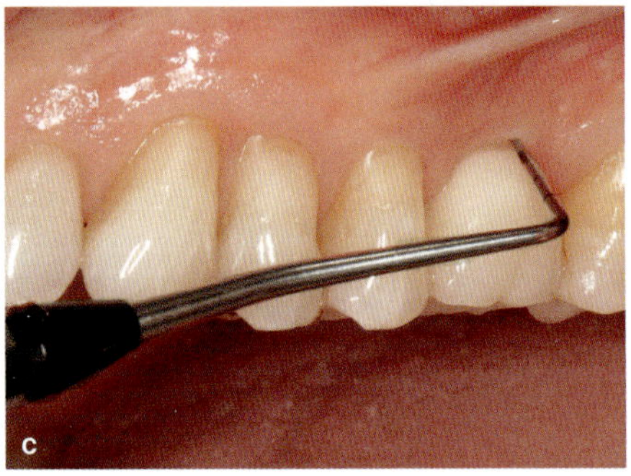

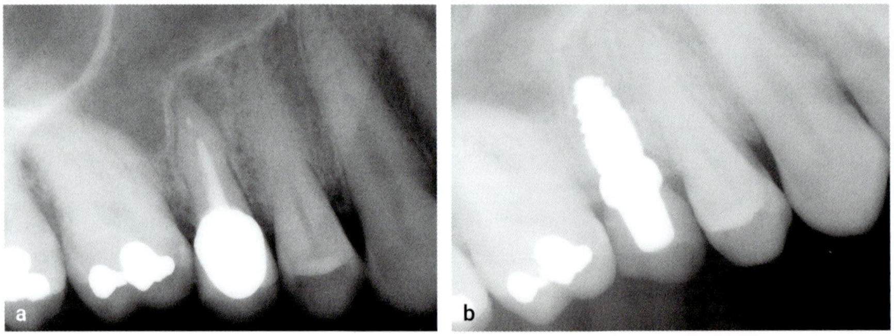

FIG 13-10 › *(a)* Preoperative radiograph. *(b)* Z5m(t) implant in place with crown. *(c)* Clinical and esthetic results.

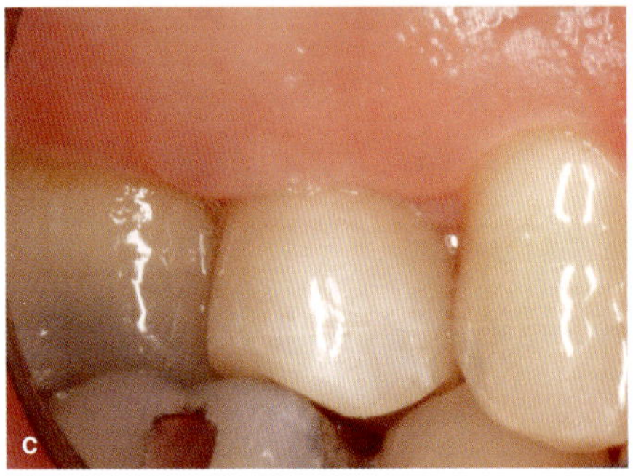

expanded the indications for ceramic implants. The increase in flexibility made it possible to use 15-degree abutments to compensate for insertion angles (Fig 13-11). The first screw-retained bone-level implants followed with the Z5s implants[32] (Fig 13-12).

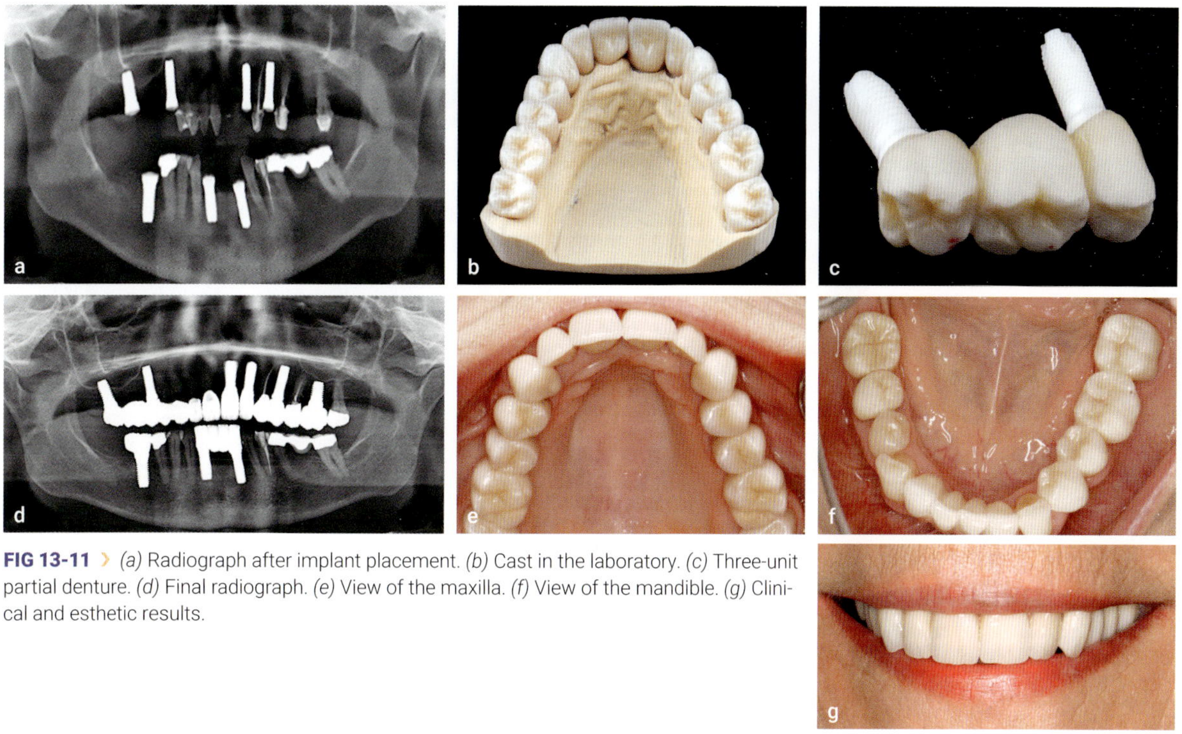

FIG 13-11 › *(a)* Radiograph after implant placement. *(b)* Cast in the laboratory. *(c)* Three-unit partial denture. *(d)* Final radiograph. *(e)* View of the maxilla. *(f)* View of the mandible. *(g)* Clinical and esthetic results.

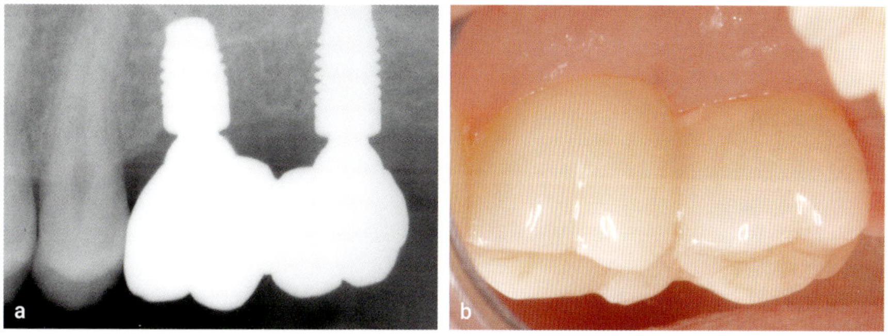

FIG 13-12 › *(a)* Radiograph of the Z5s implants in place. *(b)* Clinical and esthetic results.

In my experience, Z-Systems can meet the growing demands for user-friendly ceramic implants in implantology practices, even in demanding cases. Currently, four implant types are available, two one-piece options and two two-piece options, and each one is equipped with extensive accessories and the prosthetic components for analog and digital procedures (Fig 13-13). All systems presented in this chapter are highly advanced and can be used as an alternative to titanium implants.

FIG 13-13 › *(a)* Digital planning of Z-Systems implants. *(b)* Z5 BL implant in place. *(c)* Z5 BL implant with crown. *(d)* Clinical and esthetic results.

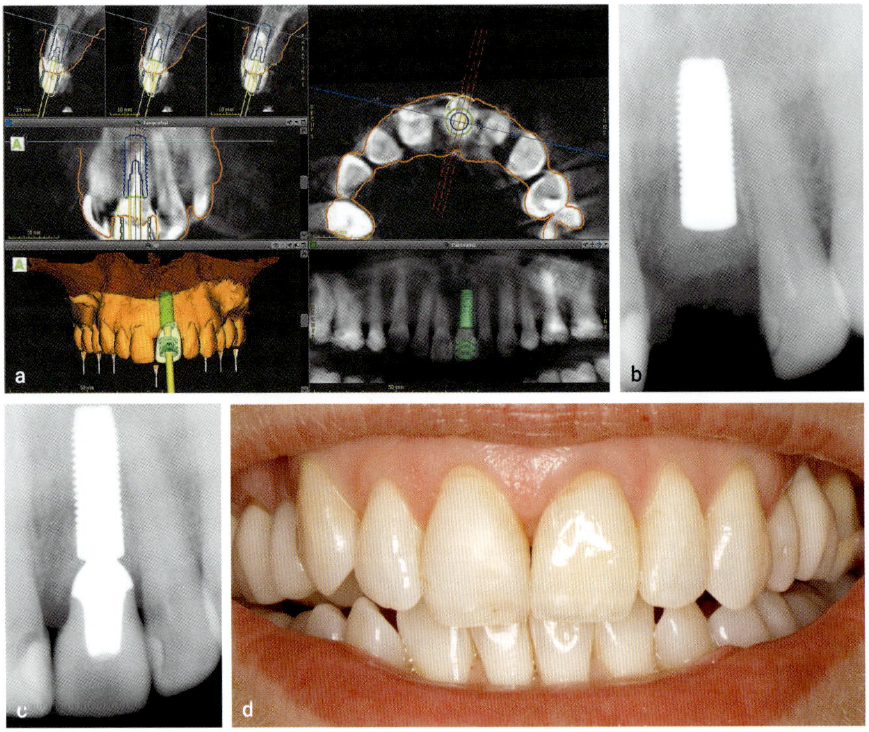

References

1. Cosgarea R, Gasparik C, Dudea D, Culic B, Dannewitz B, Sculean A. Peri-implant soft tissue colour around titanium and zirconia abutments: A prospective randomized controlled clinical study. Clin Oral Implants Res 2015;26:537–544.
2. Scarano A, Piattelli M, Caputi S, Favero GA, Piattelli A. Bacterial adhesion on commercially pure titanium and zirconium oxide disks: An in vivo human study. J Periodontol 2004;75:292–296.
3. Rimondini L, Cerroni L, Carrassi A, Torricelli P. Bacterial colonization of zirconia ceramic surfaces: An in vitro and in vivo study. Int J Oral Maxillofac Implants 2002;17:793–798.
4. Cionca N, Hashim D, Mombelli A. Zirconia dental implants: Where are we now, and where are we heading? Periodontol 2000 2017;73:241–258.
5. Spies BC, Sauter C, Wolkewitz M, Kohal RJ. Alumina reinforced zirconia implants: Effects of cyclic loading and abutment modification on fracture resistance. Dent Mater 2015;31:262–272.
6. Rompen E. The impact of the type and configuration of abutments and their (repeated) removal on the attachment level and marginal bone. Eur J Oral Implantol 2012;5(suppl):S83–S90.
7. Glauser R, Schüpbach P. Early bone formation around immediately placed two-piece tissue-level zirconia implants with a modified surface: An experimental study in the miniature pig mandible. Presented at Implant Dentistry for All: Honoring the Past—Treasuring the Present—Shaping the Future Academy of Osseointegration 2022 Annual Meeting, San Diego, 24–26 February 2022.
8. Brüll F, van Winkelhoff AJ, Cune MS. Zirconia dental implants: A clinical, radiographic, and microbiologic evaluation up to 3 years. Int J Oral Maxillofac Implants 2014;29:914–920.

9. Becker J, John G, Becker K, Mainusch S, Diedrichs G, Schwarz F. Clinical performance of two-piece zirconia implants in the posterior mandible and maxilla: A prospective cohort study over 2 years. Clin Oral Implants Res 2017;28:29–35.
10. Karapataki S, Vegh D, Payer M, Fahrenholz H, Antonoglou GN. Clinical performance of two-piece zirconia dental implants after 5 and up to 12 years. Int J Oral Maxillofac Implants 2023;38:1105–1114.
11. Becker J, John G, Becker K, Mainusch S, Diedrichs G, Schwarz F. Clinical performance of two-piece zirconium implants in the posterior mandible and maxilla: A prospective cohort study over nine years. Clin Oral Implants Res (in press).
12. Eli L, Bar-Tal Y, Kostovetzki I. At first glance: Social meanings of dental appearance. J Public Health Dent 2001;61:150–154.
13. Klages U, Bruckner A, Zentner A. Dental aesthetics, self-awareness, and oral health-related quality of life in young adults. Eur J Orthod 2004;26:507–514.
14. Steinemann SG. Titanium—The material of choice? Periodontol 2000 1998;17:7–21.
15. Bormann KH, Gellrich NC, Kniha H, Schild S, Weingart D, Gahlert M. A prospective clinical study to evaluate the performance of zirconium dioxide dental implants in single-tooth edentulous area: 3-year follow-up. BMC Oral Health 2018;18:181.
16. Roehling S, Ghazal G, Borer T, Thieringer F, Gahlert M. Implant supported fixed dental prostheses using a new monotype zirconia implant—A case report. Dent J (Basel) 2015;3:79–92.
17. Gahlert M, Kniha H, Weingart D, Schild S, Gellrich NC, Bormann KH. A prospective clinical study to evaluate the performance of zirconium dioxide dental implants in single-tooth gaps. Clin Oral Implants Res 2016;27:e176–e184.
18. Kniha K, Kniha H, Möhlhenrich SC, Milz S, Hölzle F, Modabber A. Papilla and alveolar crest levels in immediate versus delayed single-tooth zirconia implants. Int J Oral Maxillofac Surg 2017;46:1039–1044.
19. Kniha K, Modabber A, Kniha H, Möhlhenrich SC, Hölzle F, Milz S. Dimensions of hard and soft tissue around adjacent, compared with single-tooth, zirconia implants. Br J Oral Maxillofac Surg 2018;56:43–47.
20. Christel P, Meunier A, Heller M, Torre JP, Peille CN. Mechanical properties and short-term in-vivo evaluation of yttrium-oxide-partially-stabilized zirconia. J Biomed Mater Res 1989;23:45–61.
21. Cionca N, Hashim D, Mombelli A. Zirconia dental implants: Where are we now, and where are we heading? Periodontol 2000 2017;73:241–258.
22. Apratim A, Eachempati P, Krishnappa Salian KK, Singh V, Chhabra S, Shah S. Zirconia in dental implantology: A review. J Int Soc Prev Community Dent 2015;5:147–156.
23. Kohal RJ, Klaus G, Strub JR. Zirconia-implant-supported all-ceramic crowns withstand long-term load: A pilot investigation. Clin Oral Implants Res 2006;17:565–571.
24. Kohal RJ, Papavasiliou G, Kamposiora P, Tripodakis A, Strub JR. Three-dimensional computerized stress analysis of commercially pure titanium and yttrium-partially stabilized zirconia implants. Int J Prosthodont 2002;15:189–194.
25. Beger B, Goetz H, Morlock M, Schiegnitz E, Al-Nawas B. In vitro surface characteristics and impurity analysis of five different commercially available dental zirconia implants. Int J Implant Dent 2018;4:13.
26. Gahlert M, Roehling S, Sprecher CM, Kniha H, Milz S, Bormann K. In vivo performance of zirconia and titanium implants: A histomorphometric study in mini pig maxillae. Clin Oral Implants Res 2012;23:281–286.
27. Gahlert M, Röhling S, Wieland M, Sprecher CM, Kniha H, Milz S. Osseointegration of zirconia and titanium dental implants: A histological and histomorphometrical study in the maxilla of pigs. Clin Oral Implants Res 2009;20:1247–1253.

INDEX

Page references followed by "f" denote figures; those followed by "t" denote tables.